Current Clinical Psychiatry

MW00830730

Series editor: Jerrold F. Rosenbaum

For other titles published in this series, go to
www.springer.com/series/7634

John F. Kelly • William L. White
Editors

Addiction Recovery Management

Theory, Research and Practice

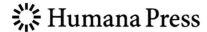 Humana Press

Editors
John F. Kelly
Harvard Medical School
MGH-Harvard Center for Addiction
Medicine
Boston, MA
USA
jkelly11@partners.org

William L. White
Lighthouse Institute
Chestnut Health Systems
Bloomington, IL
USA ·
billlwhite@aol.com

ISBN 978-1-60327-959-8   e-ISBN 978-1-60327-960-4
DOI 10.1007/978-1-60327-960-4
Springer New York Dordrecht Heidelberg London

Printed on acid-free paper

Humana Press is part of Springer Science+Business Media (www.springer.com)

Foreword

As a Senator, Barack Obama ruffled some feathers when he opined that eigth grade graduation ceremonies were overblown because the kids "weren't done yet." Years later, when we had the privilege to work for President Obama in the White House Office of National Drug Control Policy, his comments came back to us as we contemplated "addiction treatment and drug court graduation ceremonies" during which patients who had completed a residential stay or a drug court term were hugged and cheered in front of weeping relatives. Despite the pomp and circumstance, they too "weren't done yet." Recovery, like education, should not be the subject of closing ceremonies when years of toil, learning, and reward still lay ahead. At some point, it becomes not just unwise but also unethical to promise suffering people and their families otherwise. This volume makes this point in a compelling fashion and provides an exciting alternative path forward in the care of addiction.

As the chapters in this book establish, neuroscientific and epidemiologic evidence, clinical knowledge, and the lived experience of addicted people have long suggested that the course of serious substance use disorders tends to be chronic rather than short-term. Yet over the decades that this evidence about the nature of the illness has accumulated, the fundamental nature of the treatment offered, the insurance provided and the evaluations conducted on the US addiction treatment system remained largely the same. The system is well suited for managing the short-term crises of addiction, stabilizing addicted patients, and providing a small amount of aftercare. Indeed, given the nature of most funding streams, it might be simpler to say that it does precisely what it is paid to do.

Despite those flaws, that system has helped many people, especially when the initial treatment has been the doorway to the grandfather of all "recovery-oriented systems of care," Alcoholics Anonymous. But the more common outcome has been short-term intervention leading to repeated relapses and readmissions. To paraphrase the title of a chapter in this volume, if we had really believed at the outset that addiction were a chronic disorder, we would have designed a much different treatment and recovery support system with meaningful connection to partners in the health care and social welfare systems who provided long-term monitoring and management.

Simply hanging this entire problem on the US addiction treatment system would be both simplistic and unfair. The lack of financially and clinically attractive models for delivering effective continuing medical care is not peculiar to the addiction field – this is a general problem throughout the US health care system. Many diabetic patients cycle in and out of the hospital, many myocardial infarct patients do not receive adequate cardiac rehabilitation, and many asthmatic children are taken regularly by frightened parents to the emergency room. Further, although many people have diagnosed the problems of the acute care oriented addiction treatment system, far fewer have come up with concrete solutions. This book is the first serious effort within our field to answer that call, and the lessons here are potentially valuable for the rest of general health care.

In the pages that follow, national leaders in the recovery field assemble the growing evidence base, put forward specific models of care and, perhaps most importantly, take on directly the enormous system-level challenges of trying to re-engineer sclerotic infrastructure (both physical and philosophical), using inspiring real-world examples from the State of Connecticut and the City of Philadelphia. Though much remains to be done, there is great reason for optimism. First, the passing of the Affordable Care Act (aka "Health-care reform") signals the end of financial and clinical segregation of treatments for mental and substance use disorders from the rest of health care. Second, the rigorous insurance parity regulations contained in the Affordable Care Act and the Paul Wellstone Pete Domenici Mental Health Parity and Addiction Equity Act will help move behavioral health care up from its second-class status within health insurance benefits and reimbursement. The present moment is thus an unprecedented opportunity to expand the quantity and quality of addiction treatment and recovery support services. Yet in the midst of these victories we must simultaneously be humble because the hard truth is that virtually everything we know about long-term recovery management currently fits in a single book, albeit a truly excellent one.

Keith Humphreys
A. Thomas McLellan

Contents

1 Introduction: The Theory, Science, and Practice of Recovery
  Management 1
  William L. White and John F. Kelly

Part I Theoretical Foundations of Recovery Management

2 Addiction Treatment and Recovery Careers 9
  Yih-Ing Hser and M. Douglas Anglin

3 Integrating Addiction Treatment and Mutual Aid Recovery
  Resources 31
  Lee Ann Kaskutas and Meenakshi Subbaraman

4 Processes that Promote Recovery from Addictive Disorders 45
  Rudolf H. Moos

5 Recovery Management: What If We *Really* Believed
  That Addiction Was a Chronic Disorder? 67
  William L. White and John F. Kelly

Part II Research Approaches and Findings

6 Recovery Management Checkups with Adult Chronic
  Substance Users 87
  Christy K. Scott and Michael L. Dennis

7 Assertive Continuing Care for Adolescents 103
  Mark D. Godley and Susan H. Godley

8   Long-Term Trajectories of Adolescent Recovery...................... 127
    Sandra A. Brown, Danielle E. Ramo, and Kristen G. Anderson

9   Residential Recovery Homes/Oxford Houses 143
    Leonard A. Jason, Bradley D. Olson, David G. Mueller,
    Lisa Walt, and Darrin M. Aase

10 Continuing Care and Recovery 163
    James R. McKay

Part III   Recovery Management in Practice

11 Recovery-Focused Behavioral Health System Transformation:
    A Framework for Change and Lessons Learned
    from Philadelphia 187
    Ijeoma Achara-Abrahams, Arthur C. Evans,
    and Joan Kenerson King

12 Connecticut's Journey to a Statewide Recovery-Oriented
    Health-care System: Strategies, Successes, and Challenges........... 209
    Thomas A. Kirk

13 Implementing Recovery Management in a Treatment
    Organization 235
    Michael Boyle, David Loveland, and Susan George

14 Peer-Based Recovery Support Services Within a Recovery
    Community Organization: The CCAR Experience.................... 259
    Phil Valentine

15 The Physician Health Program: A Replicable Model
    of Sustained Recovery Management 281
    Gregory E. Skipper and Robert L. DuPont

Part IV   Future Directions in Recovery Management

16 Recovery Management and the Future of Addiction
    Treatment and Recovery in the USA 303
    John F. Kelly and William L. White

Appendix 317

Index.. 319

Contributors

Darrin M. Aase, PhD
Center for Community Research, DePaul University and Professor,
Psychology Department, DePaul University, Chicago, IL

Ijeoma Achara-Abrahams, PsyD
Department of Behavioral Health and Mental Retardation Services,
1101 Market St., 7th Floor, Philadelphia, PA 19107, USA

Kristen G. Anderson, PhD
Assistant Professor, Department of Psychology, Reed College, Portland, OR

M. Douglas Anglin, PhD
Professor and Associate Director, Department of Psychiatry and Behavioral,
UCLA Integrated Substance Abuse Programs, Los Angeles, CA

Michael Boyle, MA
Fayette Companies, 600 Fayette Street, Peoria, IL 61603, USA

Sandra A. Brown, PhD
Department of Psychiatry and Psychology, University of California,
San Diego, and Psychology Service VA San Diego Healthcare System,
San Diego, CA, USA

Michael L. Dennis, PhD
Senior Research Psychologist and Director of the Global Appraisal
of Individual Needs (GAIN) Coordinating Center, Chestnut Health Systems,
Bloomington, IL

Robert L. Dupont, MD
Medical Director and President, Institute for Behavior and Health,
Rockville, MD

Arthur C. Evans, PhD
Director, Department of Behavioral Health and Mental Retardations
Services, Philadelphia, PA

Susan George, PhD
Vice President of Clinical Services, Fayette Companies, Peoria, IL

Mark D. Godley, PhD
Lighthouse Institute, Chestnut Health Systems, 448 Wylie Drive,
Normal, IL 61761, USA

Susan H. Godley, RhD
Senior Research Scientist, Chestnut Health Systems, Bloomington, IL

Yih-Ing Hser, PhD
Department of Psychiatry and Behavioral Sciences,
UCLA Integrated Substance Abuse Programs,
1640 S. Sepulveda Blvd., Suite 200, Los Angeles, CA 90025, USA

Keith Humphreys, PhD
VA Palo Alto Health Care System and Stanford University
School of Medicine, Stanford, CA

Leonard A. Jason, PhD
Psychology Department, Center for Community Research, DePaul University,
990 W. Fullerton Ave., Chicago, IL 60614, USA

Lee Ann Kaskutas, DrPH
Alcohol Research Group, Public Health Institute, 6475 Christie Avenue,
Suite 400, Emeryville, CA 94608, USA

John F. Kelly, PhD
Massachusetts General Hospital, Center for Addiction Medicine,
60 Staniford Street Suite 120, Boston, MA 02114, USA

Joan Kenerson King, APRN-BC
Owner, Joan Kenerson King Consulting and Counseling,
Consultant Department of Behavioral Health/Mental Retardation Services,
Philadelphia, PA

Thomas A. Kirk, PhD
Department of Mental Health and Addiction Services,
100 Sorghum Hill Drive, Cheshire, CT 06410, USA

David Loveland, PhD
Director of Research, Fayette Companies, Peoria, IL

James R. Mckay, PhD
Center on the Continuum of Care in the Addictions,
University of Pennsylvania, 3440 Market Street,
Suite 370, Philadelphia, PA 19104, USA

Tom Mclellan, PhD
Director Treatment Research Institute, and Professor of Psychiatry,
University of Pennsylvania School of Medicine, Philadelphia, PA

Rudolf H. Moos, PhD
Stanford University and Department of Veterans Affairs,
Center for Health Care Evaluation, 795 Willow Rd. (152-MPD),
Menlo Park, CA 94025, USA

David G. Mueller, PhD
Center for Community Research, DePaul University and Professor,
Psychology Department, DePaul University, Chicago, IL

Bradley D. Olson, PhD
National Louis University, Chicago, IL

Danielle E. Ramo, PhD
Postdoctoral Scholar, University of California, San Francisco, CA

Christy K. Scott, PhD
Lighthouse Institute, Chestnut Health Systems, 720 W. Chestnut Street,
Bloomington, IL 61701, USA

Gregory E. Skipper, MD
Alabama Physician Health Program (Medical Director),
Medical Association of the State of Alabama, 19 S. Jackson St,
Montgomery, AL 36104, USA

Meenakshi Subbaraman, MS
Pre-Doctoral Fellow, Alcohol Research Group and PhD Candidate,
Division of Epidemiology, School of Public Health, University
of California Berkeley, CA

Phil Valentine
Connecticut Community for Addiction Recovery, Hartford, CT, USA

Lisa Walt, PhD
Center for Community Research, DePaul University; Professor,
Psychology Department, DePaul University, Chicago, IL

William L. White, MA
Lighthouse Institute, Chestnut Health Systems, Bloomington, IL, USA

Chapter 1
Introduction: The Theory, Science, and Practice of Recovery Management

William L. White and John F. Kelly

Abstract Today, almost 14,000 specialized addiction programs treat approximately two million individuals a year in the United States. This treatment spans a wide diversity of settings, levels of care, service philosophies, and techniques. However, most share an acute-care model of intervention, characterized by a single episode of self-contained and unlinked intervention focused on symptom reduction and delivered within a short timeframe. Impressions are given that long-term recovery should be achievable following such acute intervention. This model is now being challenged, and calls are increasing to extend the design of addiction treatment to a model of sustained recovery management that is comparable to how other chronic primary health disorders are effectively managed. *Recovery management* is a philosophy of organizing treatment and recovery supports to enhance early engagement, recovery initiation and maintenance, and the quality of personal/ family life in the long-term. This chapter provides an overview of this book highlighting the theory, science, and practice of recovery management and exploring how it is being incorporated into larger "systems transformation" processes. This is the first academic text designed specifically to focus on recovery management as a philosophy of professional treatment and a framework for recovery management.

Keywords Addiction treatment models · Acute-care · Recovery management · Systems of care · Chronic illness

Introduction

An elaborate system of inebriate homes and asylums, private addiction cure institutes, religiously sponsored missions and inebriate colonies, and bottled and boxed "home cures" for alcohol and drug addiction flourished in the United Sates during the

W.L. White (✉)
Lighthouse Institute, Chestnut Health Systems, Bloomington, IL, USA
e-mail: bwhite@chestnut.org

J.F. Kelly and W.L. White (eds.), *Addiction Recovery Management: Theory, Research and Practice*, Current Clinical Psychiatry, DOI 10.1007/978-1-60327-960-4_1,
© Springer Science+Business Media, LLC 2011

mid-nineteenth century only to collapse in the opening decades of the twentieth century [1]. A new generation of addiction treatment and recovery advocates coalesced in the mid-twentieth century to lay the foundation for the resurrection of modern addiction treatment. What began as two social movements (one focused on alcoholism and the other focused on narcotic addiction and rising youthful "polydrug abuse") were subsequently integrated, professionalized, commercialized, and supported by federal, state, and local governments, as well as private systems of healthcare reimbursement. Today, almost 14,000 specialized addiction programs treat approximately two million individuals a year at an annual cost in the range of 11 billion dollars [2, 3]. This treatment spans a wide diversity of institutional settings, levels of care, service philosophies, and service techniques which are collectively supported by administrative, management, regulatory, education, training, and research infrastructures that have become industries in their own right.

References to these thousands of direct service and support institutions as a specialized "system of care", however, grossly misrepresent their level of integration or even coordination. Yet, most of these programs do have something in common; they share an acute-care (AC) model of intervention that has dominated specialized addiction treatment. White and McLellan [4] define this model in terms of seven core characteristics:

- Services are delivered "programmatically" in a uniform series of encapsulated activities (screening, admission, a single-point-in-time assessment, a short course of minimally individualized treatment, discharge, and brief "aftercare" followed by termination of the service relationship).
- The intervention is focused on symptom elimination for a single primary problem.
- Professional experts direct and dominate the assessment, treatment planning, and service delivery decision making.
- Services transpire over a short (and historically ever-shorter) period of time – usually as a function of a prearranged, time-limited insurance payment designed specifically for addiction disorders and "carved out" from general medical insurance.
- The individual/family/community is given the impression at discharge ("graduation") that "cure has occurred": long-term recovery is viewed as personally self-sustainable without ongoing professional assistance.
- The intervention is evaluated at a short-term, single-point-in-time follow-up that compares pretreatment status with discharge status and posttreatment status, months – or at best a few years – following professional intervention.
- Posttreatment relapse and readmission are viewed as the failure (noncompliance) of the individual rather than possible flaws in the design or execution of the treatment protocol.

That acute-care model is now being challenged. There is a revolution underway in the design and delivery of addiction treatment in the United States. That revolution promises to change how severe alcohol and other drug (AOD) problems and the people experiencing such problems are viewed and treated.

The impetus for such change comes from multiple sources. A new recovery advocacy movement is calling for addiction treatment to become reconnected to the larger and more enduring process of personal and family recovery [5]. Frontline practitioners lament working in addiction treatment institutions that seem to care more about margin (financial profit and regulatory compliance) than mission (recovery outcomes) – more about a progress note signed by the right color of ink than whether those being served are actually making progress [6]. Research critiques of addiction treatment from within the field are calling for a "fundamental shift in thinking" [7], a "paradigm shift" [8], a "seismic shift rather than a mere tinkering" [9], and a "sea change in the culture of addiction service delivery" [10]. Administrative, regulatory, and funding authorities are calling for a redesign of addiction treatment in response to a growing population of individuals repeatedly recycling through addiction treatment at great cost with no measurable long-term recovery outcomes. After two decades of hearing the treatment industry's central mantra, "Treatment Works," most know someone for whom addiction treatment did not work and the public at large has grown weary of the rich and famous regularly cycling into "rehab." Addiction treatment's probationary status as a social institution is set to be severely tested.

Within this cultural and professional context, calls are increasing to extend the design of addiction treatment from a model of acute biopsychosocial stabilization to a model of sustained recovery management that is comparable to how other chronic primary health disorders are effectively managed.

> *Recovery management* is a philosophy of organizing addiction treatment and recovery support services to enhance early prerecovery engagement, recovery initiation, *long-term* recovery maintenance, and the quality of personal/family life in long-term recovery [11].

There are simultaneous calls to embrace these recovery management philosophies within larger recovery-oriented systems of care.

> *Recovery-oriented systems of care* are networks of indigenous and professional support designed to initiate, sustain, and enhance the quality of *long-term* addiction recovery for individuals and families and to create values and policies in the larger cultural and policy environment that are supportive of these recovery processes. The "system" in this phrase is not a federal, state, or local agency, but a macro-level organization of the larger cultural and community environment in which long-term recovery is nested [11].

The purpose of this book is to provide a primer on the theory, science, and practice of recovery management and to explore how recovery management is being incorporated into larger behavioral health "systems transformation" processes. This movement has until now been chronicled only on the pages of scientific journals and government monographs, through papers posted on recovery advocacy web sites (e.g., Faces and Voices of Recovery) and through presentations at professional conferences. This is the first academic text designed specifically to explore recovery management as a philosophy of professional treatment and a framework for recovery self-management.

Part I includes several chapters that cover seven foundational premises of recovery management:

1. AOD problems present in transient and chronic forms; sustained recovery management is not appropriately applied to the former, but is particularly well suited for the latter. Not everyone with an AOD problem needs sustained recovery management support, or needs to the same degree, but persons with high personal vulnerability, high problem severity/complexity, and low recovery capital[1] will benefit greatly from sustained and assertive forms of monitoring and support.

2. The course of severe substance-use disorders and their successful resolution can span decades. This is highlighted in detail in Chap. 2 by Hser and Anglin who provide a theoretical and data-based presentation of addiction and recovery trajectories spanning decades.

3. Severe AOD problems have been long depicted as a "chronic, progressive disease" but have been treated primarily as an acute condition resembling the treatment of traumatic injury or a bacterial infection [13, 14].

4. Recovery from severe substance-use disorders is enhanced through assertive linkages from formal addiction treatment services to indigenous recovery supports in the community. In Chap. 3, Lee Ann Kaskutas and Meenakshi Subbaraman describe such linkages and the long-term resulting benefits. (In Part II, Godley provides research findings on assertive approaches with young people).

5. The course of addiction and the process of long-term recovery can be explained in large part by a variety of social processes that have commonalities across multiple theories. In Chap. 4, Rudolf Moos discusses how the social processes associated with several prominent theories are reflected in the active ingredients that underlie how community contexts, especially family members, friends, and mutual-help groups promote relapse, remission, and recovery.

6. Most people discharged from addiction treatment are precariously balanced between recovery and readdiction in the weeks, months, and year following their discharge ([15], See [11] for a review).

7. Strategies used in the treatment of other chronic health conditions can be adapted to enhance long-term recovery outcomes for severe substance-use disorders. In Chap. 5, White and Kelly describe how such strategies constitute significant changes in the current core services practices of addiction treatment.

Part II summarizes scientific studies that support the movement toward sustained recovery management. Christy Scott and Michael Dennis highlight the results of a series of experiments utilizing posttreatment recovery checkups with adults as a strategy of long-term recovery support. The chapters by Sandra Brown and colleagues, and Mark Godley, review the research that has been conducted on long-term recovery trajectories of adolescents followed up across the high-risk substance use period of emerging adulthood and that provides evidence for assertive linkage approaches to posttreatment continuing care for adolescents. In the concluding chapters in Part II, Leonard Jason and colleagues note the emergence

----

[1]Recovery capital encompasses the quantity and quality of internal and external resources that can be mobilized to initiate and sustain recovery from addiction [12].

of new recovery support institutions and review the studies his research group has conducted on the growing network of Oxford Houses in the United States, and James McKay summarizes the outcomes of the scientific studies that have been conducted to evaluate the effects of continuing care interventions for adults.

Part III moves from the theoretical conceptualization and research studies related to recovery management to the real-world efforts to implement recovery management and recovery-oriented systems of care. In Chaps. 11 and 12, Kirk and Achara-Abrahams and colleagues describe the recovery-focused systems transformation effort each has led, respectively, in the State of Connecticut and the City of Philadelphia. In Chap. 13, Boyle describes the rationale, methods, and outcomes linked to the implementation of a recovery management philosophy within a local behavioral health-care organization in Peoria, Illinois. In Chap. 14, Valentine describes the peer-based recovery support services piloted within the Connecticut Community of Addiction Recovery – a grassroots recovery advocacy and support organization. In the final chapter in Part II, DuPont and Skipper describe the Physician Health Program (PHP) as a model of extended recovery management that has generated the highest recovery rates in the scientific literature. They suggest that major elements of the PHP could be adapted for mass application to addiction treatment programs throughout the United States.

Part IV contains a final chapter in which Kelly and White discuss recovery management and the future of addiction treatment. They draw six key conclusions:

1. RM and ROSC are part of a larger shift toward a recovery paradigm reflected in growth and diversification of recovery mutual aid groups, new recovery support institutions, and a new recovery advocacy movement that reflects the cultural and political awakening of individuals and families in recovery.
2. The addiction treatment industry has oversold the long-term recovery outcomes that can be achieved for people with severe AOD problems from a brief episode of professionally directed biopsychosocial stabilization.
3. The acute-care model is culturally, economically, and politically unsustainable.
4. Approaches of sustained recovery management hold great promise in enhancing long-term recovery outcomes for persons with severe substance-use disorders and low natural recovery capital.
5. The process of transforming addiction treatment from an acute-care model to a model of sustained recovery management is already underway as evidenced by federal, state, and local "systems transformation" efforts and growing calls for a recovery-focused research agenda to guide and support these transformation efforts.
6. That transformation effort will take years to achieve and, as work in the State of Connecticut and the City of Philadelphia illustrate, will involve sustained processes of conceptual alignment, practice alignment, and contextual alignment (policy, regulations, funding mechanisms, and stakeholder relationships).

The future of addiction treatment as a social institution may rest with its ability or inability to move toward treatment of addiction via a model of sustained recovery management.

In closing this introduction, we would like to acknowledge and thank all of the authors who contributed to this volume. Their collective efforts have exerted an enormous influence on the evolution of modern addiction treatment and recovery. We would also like to thank Julie Yeterian, Sarah Dow, and Julie Sloane for their help in the preparation of this volume.

References

1. White W. Slaying the dragon: the history of addiction treatment and recovery in America. Bloomington, IL: Chestnut Health Systems; 1998.
2. Mark TL, Levit KR, Coffey RM, et al. National expenditures for mental health services and substance abuse treatment, 1993–2003 SAMHSA Publication No. SMA 07-4227. Rockville, MD: Substance Abuse and Mental Health Services Administration; 2007.
3. Substance Abuse and Mental Health Services Administration, Office of Applied Studies. The ADSS cost study: costs of substance abuse treatment in the specialty sector, analytic series A-20, DHHS Publication No. (SMA) 03-3762. Rockville, MD; 2003.
4. White W, McLellan AT. Addiction as a chronic disease: key messages for clients, families and referral sources. Counselor. 2008;9(3):24–33.
5. White W. Let's go make some history: chronicles of the new addiction recovery advocacy movement. Washington, DC: Johnson Institute and Faces and Voices of Recovery; 2006.
6. White W. The treatment renewal movement. Counselor. 2002;3(1):59–61.
7. Moos RH. Addictive disorders in context: principles and puzzles of effective treatment and recovery. Psychol Addict Behav. 2003;17:3–12.
8. Dennis ML, Scott CK, Funk R, Foss MA. The duration and correlates of addiction and treatment careers. J Subst Abuse Treat. 2005;28 Suppl 1:S51–62.
9. Humphreys K. Closing remarks: swimming to the horizon – reflections on a special series. Addiction. 2006;101:1238–40.
10. Miller WR. Bring addiction treatment out of the closet. Addiction. 2007;102:863–9.
11. White W. Recovery management and recovery-oriented systems of care: scientific rationale and promising practices. Pittsburgh, PA: Northeast Addiction Technology Transfer Center, Great Lakes Addiction Technology Transfer Center, Philadelphia Department of Behavioral Health & Mental Retardation Services; 2008.
12. Granfield R, Cloud W. Coming clean: overcoming addiction without treatment. New York: New York University Press; 1999.
13. Dennis ML, Scott CK. Managing addiction as a chronic condition. Addict Sci Clin Pract. 2007;4(1):45–55.
14. McLellan AT, Lewis DC, O'Brien CP, Kleber HD. Drug dependence, a chronic medical illness: implications for treatment, insurance, and outcomes evaluation. J Am Med Assoc. 2000;284(13):1689–95.
15. Scott CK, Foss MA, Dennis ML. Pathways in the relapse – treatment – recovery cycle over 3 years. J Subst Abuse Treat. 2005;28 Suppl 1:S63–72.

Part I
Theoretical Foundations of
Recovery Management

Chapter 2
Addiction Treatment and Recovery Careers

Yih-Ing Hser and M. Douglas Anglin

Abstract Recovery from addiction is a complex and dynamic process, with considerable variations across individuals. Despite historical and recent surge of interest in recovery among many stakeholders in the addiction field, empirical research on recovery has been limited. The varying definitions of recovery across different stakeholder groups best illustrate the wide-ranging thinking on recovery, yet how recovery is conceptualized, promoted, and achieved has important implications for how treatment systems should be structured, delivered, and evaluated. The concept of addiction as a chronic illness is redefining the fundamental way we view drug abuse and its treatment. Currently, many efforts are directed toward determining how to provide a continuity of treatment and how to measure if treatment systems are successfully addressing addiction as a chronic disease. In this chapter, we describe empirical patterns of drug use trajectories over the life course, discuss the diverse ways of conceptualizing recovery, and identify key aspects of addiction that require attention as we investigate and treat addiction to promote long-term, stable recovery.

Keywords Addiction recovery management · Addiction recovery · Addiction as a chronic illness · Continuity of care

Introduction

Illicit drug use continues to be a top public concern, directly or indirectly affecting individuals, families, and communities, with detrimental effects that may persist across generations. Patterns of substance abuse are extremely heterogeneous, with

Y.-I. Hser (✉)
Department of Psychiatry and Behavioral Sciences, UCLA Integrated Substance Abuse Programs, 1640 S. Sepulveda Blvd., Suite 200, Los Angeles, CA 90025, USA
e-mail: yhser@ucla.edu

J.F. Kelly and W.L. White (eds.), *Addiction Recovery Management: Theory, Research and Practice*, Current Clinical Psychiatry, DOI 10.1007/978-1-60327-960-4_2, © Springer Science+Business Media, LLC 2011 many individuals having used drugs and stopped the use, but for others, addiction becomes a chronic and recurring condition [1–6], oftentimes spanning decades of an individual's lifetime [3–5, 7]. While various treatment options are now available and have been shown to be effective, most treatment effects are short-lived. Many dependent users cycle through several treatments before they achieve more stable recovery, resulting in prolonged adverse consequences associated with addiction. The traditional acute care model of drug abuse treatment appears ill suited to address the chronic condition. As such, focus has increasingly turned toward embracing long-term and continuity-of-care models for understanding and treating drug addiction [3, 8, 9]. Meanwhile, the field is increasingly interested in recovery, shifting from the focus on pathology to more positive outcomes such as well-being or quality of life [10, 11]. Recovery-oriented systems of care have been emerging, promoted, and in several states, implemented [12].

Recovery from addiction is a complex and dynamic process, with considerable variations across individuals. Despite historical and recent surge of interest in recovery among many stakeholders in the addiction field, empirical research on recovery has been limited. The varying definitions of recovery across different stakeholder groups best illustrate the wide-ranging thinking on recovery, yet how recovery is conceptualized, promoted, and achieved has important implications for how treatment systems should be structured, delivered, and evaluated. Consequently, while the vision to broadening the systems of care to support long-term recovery is admirable, strategies for implementation remain to be developed and effectiveness empirically investigated. In this chapter, we describe empirical patterns of drug use trajectories over the life course, discuss the diverse ways of conceptualizing recovery, and identify key aspects of addiction and recovery that require attention as we investigate and treat addiction as a chronic disease and move toward a recovery-oriented system of care that supports long-term, stable recovery.

We describe and discuss relevant issues from a life course perspective, which uses a more integrated systems approach to studying substance abuse and recovery. This perspective takes into account varied and multiple factors that might contribute to abstinence, relapse, or stable recovery, which will be helpful given the complex nature of substance use and its dynamic interplay with various social systems [9]. The approach complements the shift in the treatment and research paradigms from short-term "snapshots" of substance use and treatment episodes to long-term developmental patterns of behavior and outcomes over time, and it takes into consideration factors that may shape or be shaped by these pathways.

A Life Course Conceptual Framework

The life course perspective has roots in the social sciences, and its application to addiction most closely resembles the approach applied in the developmental criminology research studying criminal careers. Key life course concepts include developmental trajectories, transitions and turning points, and their relationships to one another. The life course approach applied in the study of drug use emphasizes long-term patterns of continuity and change that can be both gradual and radical in relation to transitions in terms of social roles (e.g., parent, offender) over the life span [9, 13]. This approach is particularly appropriate given the now widely accepted perspective that drug addiction is a chronic and recurring condition for many, which necessitates a chronic disease management view [6].

Elder [14] defines life course as interconnected trajectories as people age. Trajectories are interdependent sequences of events in different life domains. In the developmental criminology literature, Sampson and Laub [15] refer to trajectories as "long-term patterns and sequences of behavioral transition" (p. 351), which are affected by the degree of *social capital* (individuals' interpersonal relations and institutional ties, i.e., to family, work) available to an individual [16]. Social capital is important because personal change does not happen in a vacuum, but it is influenced by the social context that can facilitate or impede recovery from addiction; the resources developed through the structure and functions of social relationships are part of an individual's "recovery capital" [17, 18]. Transitions are changes in stages or roles (e.g., getting a new job; becoming abstinent) that are short term. Some transitions can lead to turning points that engender long-term behavioral change. The essential characteristic of a turning point is that it redirects a trajectory; it is not simply a temporary detour [19].

Recovery involves a lifestyle change, which implies a long-term commitment that is consistent with the life course perspective. From the life course perspective, questions about the process of transition into recovery concern whether the initiation of recovery is a drawn-out process versus a dramatic transformation, and whether those changes are triggered by critical events as turning points. Questions about maintaining recovery include whether there are variations in the recovery trajectory and what are the underlying factors or mechanisms. Identifying what constitutes a turning point toward recovery is of great interest. The life course perspective also has the advantage of recognizing developmental stage as protective and risk factors may differ across the life span. Thus, the life course perspective offers a rich source of theoretical concepts, terminologies, and measures for the study of addiction and recovery careers.

Drug Use Trajectories

Guided by the life course perspective, we have conducted several studies to empirically investigate developmental trajectories of drug use [5, 20]. It is important to note that whereas drug use persists over the lifespan for some, for others it may decelerate gradually or dramatically and then may cease entirely, or it may exhibit a recurring pattern of repeated acceleration and deceleration with periods of abstinence. Longitudinal studies that allow the depiction of long-term patterns of drug use, however, are limited. Below, we use data from our own studies and those in the public domain to illustrate empirical findings of the overall drug use trajectories for both the general population and drug-dependent samples, followed with distinctive trajectories among drug users.

Drug Use Trajectories Among the General Population

Based on the National Survey of Drug Use and Health (NSDUH), marijuana is the most prevalently used drug in the general population. While substance use generally peaks in the late teens to young adulthood (Fig. 2.1), most drug use begins before age 15 [21]. To further illustrate the longitudinal patterns of alcohol and drug use among the general population, we analyzed the National Longitudinal Survey of Youth (NLSY79). NLSY79 is a nationally representative sample of 12,686 young men and women who were 14–22 years old when they were first surveyed in 1979 [22]. Individuals were surveyed annually from 1979 to 1994 and biennially from 1996 to the present. The survey has collected extensive information about youths' labor market behaviors, and in certain years, about alcohol and drug use. Heavy alcohol use (more than six drinks in one occasion) is the most prevalent problem among the general population, followed by marijuana, cocaine, and heroin use, which is consistently at a very low level. As shown in Fig. 2.2, alcohol and marijuana use peeked during the teens, and cocaine use occurred mostly during young adulthood; use of all substances gradually declines as the cohort aged, although declines covered different age periods and occurred at different rates over time.

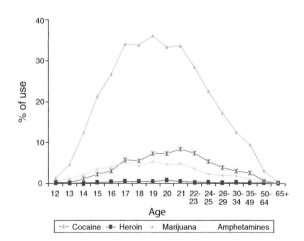

Fig. 2.1 Past-year drug use by age (National Survey of Drug Use & Health, 2002, $N = 54,079$)

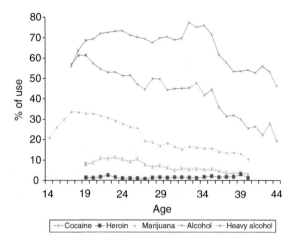

Fig. 2.2 Past-year alcohol and drug use over time (National Longitudinal Survey of Youth, NLSY79, $N = 12,686$)

Drug Use Trajectories Among Drug-Dependent Users

In contrast to the use patterns among the general population, research findings have generally shown that severe or dependent users tend to persist in their drug use, often for substantial periods of their lifespan. The UCLA Center for Advancing Longitudinal Drug Abuse Research (CALDAR) has accumulated data from several long-term follow-up studies. Using CALDAR data combined from five longitudinal studies ($N = 1,797$), we were able to compare the trajectories of primary heroin, cocaine, and methamphetamine (meth) use over the first 10 years after initiation [20, 23]. The study findings showed that heroin addiction is characterized by long periods of regular use (13–18 days per month over 10 years), while stimulants such as cocaine (8–11 days) and meth (around 12 days) are generally used at a lower frequency and are reflective of an episodic pattern (e.g., weekend users) (see Fig. 2.3). The use of alcohol and marijuana also persisted, although generally at a lower level than the primary drug. Despite the varying levels of use, the group means of use for all three types of primary drugs appear to suggest a persistent pattern of use over a long period of time (e.g., at least for the first 10 years of the addiction careers observed in the study), which supports the chronic nature of addiction to heroin, cocaine, and meth. These findings also suggest that the treatment activities and approaches for individuals with a diagnosis of opiate addiction (almost daily use) should be different from that for those dependent on stimulants (episodic use).

Distinctive Trajectories Among Drug Users

Although our work and other studies often show convergent findings on the persistence of drug use typically over a long period, some addicts may cease their

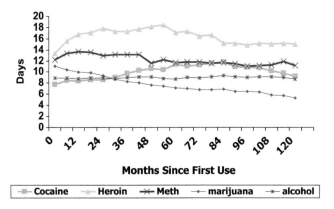

Fig. 2.3 Days using per month over 10 years since first use ($N = 1{,}797$)

drug use careers earlier than others [5]. Recent advances in analytic methods, particularly the application of growth mixture modeling in the analysis of longitudinal data, have allowed researchers to identify distinct trajectories of behavior over extended time [24–27]. Examples of this methodology include applications to the study of developmental trajectories of cigarette smoking [28, 29], alcohol use [30], and marijuana use [31, 32] from adolescence to young adulthood. These studies generally demonstrate the importance of examining subgroups, particularly their associated risk factors and subsequent outcomes.

Applying growth mixture modeling to the CALDAR longitudinal dataset ($N = 1{,}797$), we were able to reveal heterogeneous trajectory groups (Fig. 2.4): those who prolonged their drug use at a relatively low level (on average, less than once per month; 5% of the sample) or at a moderate level (about 5 days per month; 35%); those who decreased (14%) or increased (14%) drug use over long periods of time; and yet others who persisted in high levels of use (about 15 days per month; 30%) even over decades [20]. Heroin users were most likely to be in the high-use group (52%), and cocaine (50%) and meth (35%) users are most likely to be in the moderate-use group. Drug users in the high-use group had the earliest onset of arrest and primary drug use, spent the longest time incarcerated and the shortest time employed, and many of them (44%) had their first drug treatment in prison. In contrast, users in the low-use group were the smallest group and were oldest when first arrested, spent the least time in prison, and had the longest duration of employment.

Other studies on the onset of drug use have shown that adolescents who begin drug use at early ages typically use drugs more frequently, escalate to higher levels of use more quickly, and are more likely to persist in using [33, 34]. Similarly, we have also found that users who persistently used a high level of heroin, cocaine, or meth had earlier onsets of use of these drugs [35]. Most importantly, while quitting drug use can be facilitated by formal treatment and/or self-help participation, few people (about 25%) had these experiences in the 10 years following first use [20]. We turn back to this point later when we discuss the treatment and cumulative treatment effects.

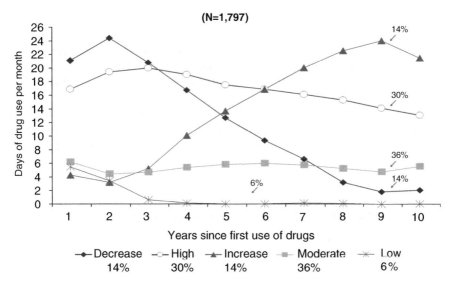

Fig. 2.4 Five distinctive drug use trajectories ($N = 1,797$)

Recovery Careers

Until recently, stable cessation and recovery has received little attention in drug abuse research. Thus, it is not surprising that despite the theoretical and policy importance of understanding why people initiate recovery and are able to maintain recovery, we do not have robust conceptual models or rich empirical investigations of recovery.

Conceptualization and Definitions of Recovery

Although the topic of recovery has been around for decades, a recent surge in interest has inspired the first serious attempts to define recovery from addiction. In defining recovery, some stakeholders consider abstinence from illicit drug use to be the only factor in determining recovery, while others believe recovery requires abstinence from alcohol and tobacco as well as any other drugs. Yet others suggest that recovery should be more broadly defined and that improved health and quality of life (e.g., employment) should be the primary criteria [10–12, 36, 37]. In 2005, the Substance Abuse and Mental Health Services Administration's Center for Substance Abuse Treatment (SAMHSA/CSAT) held a National Summit on Recovery, which convened over 100 individuals representing a variety of stakeholders in the addiction treatment and recovery field. While it was acknowledged that individuals may choose to define recovery differently, as a starting point for further discussion, the consensus definition embraced the concept of recovery as *a process of change through which an individual achieves abstinence and improved health, wellness, and quality of life* [12].

Apparently, the meaning and measures of these concepts need to be developed or operationalized for research purposes. For example, when does recovery begin and how long must abstinence be maintained for a person to be considered fully "recovered?" Some maintain that individuals who intend to make changes be considered "in recovery," while most others take into consideration a certain period of time (e.g., 1–2 years) of abstinence and/or improvement in other life domains. Some studies have suggested that 5 years of abstinence may be critical to indicate the likelihood of a "complete" recovery [35, 38]. These different ways of viewing or defining recovery have implications not only for research but for how treatment systems should be structured, delivered, and evaluated to optimize recovery.

Long-Term Follow-Up Studies Informing Recovery

Long-term follow-up studies on substance use and addiction have been limited, and most of those that exist are based on treatment cohorts. Although natural recovery or spontaneous recovery (i.e., recovery without treatment) is possible and likely widespread particularly among less severe users [39], most literature reviewed in this chapter is based on treatment samples where most empirical data are available. Results of these long-term follow-up studies generally show that relapse is problematic even after decades and that the risk of death is high [4]. Abstinence rates vary by the duration criteria used in studies. In a 10-year follow-up study of 200 alcoholics who received inpatient treatment, 51% were abstinent at the time of the follow-up but only 10% reported being abstinent for 3 or more years [40]. Based on an 8-year follow-up study, Dennis et al. [38] reported on the outcomes among a cohort of 1,326 substance users receiving treatment. At the follow-up, 501 (or 37.8%) were abstinent from alcohol and illicit drugs, of them 142 individuals (10.7% of the sample) had been abstinent for at least 3 years, and only 77 (or 5.8%) had been abstinent for 5 years or more. In a 12-year follow-up of cocaine-dependent sample [41], 22.3% tested positive for cocaine, and slightly more than one half (51.9%) had achieved stable recovery by maintaining abstinence from cocaine for more than 5 years. In a 33-year follow-up study [4], we examined life course cessation among heroin addicts and showed that eventual cessation of heroin use is a slow process and may not occur for some older addicts. Opiate use patterns of the cohort were remarkably stable; by 50–60 years of age, only about half of the sample interviewed tested negative for heroin.

Predictors of Recovery

Besides treatment and self-help group participation, few studies have examined the predictors of recovery. It seems obvious that the longer the period of nonuse, the less likely it is that an individual will relapse [4, 42, 43]. Several studies have found that social and personal resources that persons possess can be instrumental in overcoming substance dependence.

Studies by Scott et al. [45] support that cumulative time of abstinence is a strong predictor of future recovery. They found that the duration of abstinence at a given interview was among the best predictors of maintaining abstinence over the subsequent year, with the likelihood of sustaining abstinence for another 12 months increasing from 36% among those with less than a year of abstinence to 86% among those with 3 or more years of abstinence. Yet even after 3–7 years of abstinence, 14% per year continued to relapse. As the length of abstinence increased, days in employment increased, with commensurate reduction in the number of days of incarceration, the amount of crime, high-cost service utilization (e.g., emergency department, hospital, jail), and their consequent costs to society [44, 45]. Similarly, based on our 33-year follow-up data, we examined the likelihood of eventual cessation of heroin use (during the period between 1985/86 and 1996/97) associated with the lengths of abstinence before the 1985/86 interview [4]. The rate of abstinence in 1996/97 was 15.3% among the 85 subjects who reported active use at the 1985/86 follow-up, was 16.7% among the 66 who reported abstinence for up to 5 years, 75% among the 36 men who reported abstinence for 6–15 years, and 72.2% among the 34 men abstinent for more than 15 years. Thus, increased durations of abstinence predict future abstinence, yet even among those abstinent for as long as 15 years, one-quarter had eventually relapsed at the subsequent observation point.

Using a cross-sectional design, Laudet et al. [46] conducted a survey with 51 individuals between the ages of 23 and 74 in various stages of recovery and found that those with long-term (vs. short-term) abstinence were more likely to have experienced hitting bottom (e.g., more consequences and poor quality of life). Engagement in 12-step was also important after the initiation of abstinence. Another qualitative study [17] included 46 individuals who overcame their addiction to alcohol and drugs without treatment. The study found that these individuals' recovery process appeared to be typically triggered by assorted personal problems, experienced as turning points for the desire to change, which was then sustained with ongoing strategies such as alternative activities, changing social networks, and increased reliance on family and nonusing friends.

Scott et al. [45] also reported that treatment predicted recovery initiation but not maintenance. Conversely, 12-step participation predicts maintenance of abstinence but not initiation. On the other hand, Moos and Moos [47] compared the long-term remission among treated and untreated drinkers and reported a 62% remission rate in helped drinkers compared with 43% in the drinkers who did not seek help from treatment services. In the untreated group, those who improved had more personal resources and fewer alcohol-related deficits, leading the authors to conclude that the likelihood of relapse rises in the absence of personal and social resources that reflect maintenance factors for stable remission.

Hser [35] compared and contrasted the recovery group (defined as abstinent for at least 5 years prior to the interview at the 33-year follow-up) and the nonrecovery groups. The two groups did not differ in deviant behaviors and family/school problems in their earlier lives. Both groups tried formal treatment and self-directed recovery ("self-treatment"), often many times. While the nonrecovered addicts were significantly more likely to use substances in coping with stressful conditions, to have spouses who also abused drugs, and to lack non-drug-using social support, stable recovery 10 years later was predicted only by ethnicity, self-efficacy, and psychological well-being. These findings suggest that in addition to early intervention efforts to curtail heroin addiction, increasing self-efficacy and addressing psychological problems are likely to enhance the odds of maintaining long-term stable recovery.

Theory-Based Processes Promoting Recovery

As noted in the above literature, there are many predictors of recovery from substance use disorders, although most predictor identification research has not been guided by theory [48]. Focusing on protective resources that may facilitate recovery, Moos [48] examined four relevant theories and identified their common elements. These theories are the social control theory, behavioral economics and behavioral choice theory, social learning theory, and stress and coping theory. The common social processes indicated by these theories include the provision of support, goal direction, and monitoring, engagement in rewarding activities other than substance use, exposure to abstinence-oriented norms and models, and attempts to build self-efficacy and coping skills. These social processes enhance the development of personal and social resources that protect individuals against the reemergence of substance use and abuse. Dr. Moos noted that these findings are similar to factors shown to aid recovery in long-term follow-up of men with alcohol use disorder identified by Vaillant [49, 50]. These considerations have implications for tailoring treatment and continuing care to strengthen the protective resources that promote recovery.

Studies in the criminal careers research, on the other hand, have suggested that developmental transitions (e.g., into adolescence or adulthood) and critical life events (e.g., employment, marriage, military service) are turning points that modify life trajectories and redirect behavior paths. In examining trajectories of offending over the life course of delinquent males followed from ages 7 to 70, Sampson and Laub [51] found that while crime declined with age for all offender groups, childhood prognoses account poorly for long-term trajectories of offending. Instead, the dynamics of life course transitions and turning points were better determinants of long-term outcomes.

Similarly, in the 33-year follow-up study of heroin addicts, we tested several hypotheses regarding stable recovery from heroin use [36]. Problems with family and school in earlier life did not predict recovery in later life periods, even though they are often demonstrated to be key risks for later problems in life in other studies. Our findings of the high prevalence of continued heroin use in this aging sample and the lack of association of older age with recovery are consistent with others that have suggested that the concept of maturing out does not apply to many heroin addicts [52–54]. The substitution hypothesis also received little support from our data, as most recovered individuals in our sample demonstrated lower levels of use of alcohol or other drugs [4], in contrast to those of the nonrecovered individuals. Our findings are consistent with prior studies on relapse documenting that negative emotional states (depression, anxiety) and lack of constructive coping skills are risk factors, while self-efficacy and adequate social support are protective factors in maintaining stable recovery.

Individuals cope with stressors through their identified and preferred coping strategies, and what seems to separate the two groups is that the recovery group was more likely to have a non-drug-using supportive network, to use substance-free strategies to cope with stressful conditions, and to have greater self-confidence and determination to stay away from heroin, while the nonrecovery group relied on drugs to deal with stress. Thus, developing stress-coping strategies, identifying personal and social resources, and engaging in prosocial activities should all be considered as parts of effective strategies for achieving and maintaining stable recovery. Such findings also provide empirical support for relapse prevention interventions and clinical practice that incorporate these components.

The life course perspective suggests further theoretical consideration that takes into account the issue of life stages. For example, both the developmental criminology and our long-term follow-up study of heroin addicts found that childhood prognoses do not account for long-term trajectories. The CALDAR longitudinal dataset also demonstrates few earlier experiences in deviant behaviors and family or school problems predicted distinctive patterns of trajectories [9], suggesting that predictors of recovery status for different groups may vary depending on the stage of the life course. These phenomena could be due to dynamics of turning points over individuals' life course or due to risk and protective factors changing across life stages. These theoretical alternatives need to be further examined in future research to more precisely ascertain determinants of recovery or their relative importance.

Addiction Treatment

While there are many pathways to recovery and formal treatment is only one discrete aspect to recovery, effective treatment can facilitate recovery. Evaluation studies consistently support the effectiveness of drug abuse treatment [1, 3, 55–57]. At the same time, high relapse rates and readmission to treatment raise the question: Is drug abuse treatment based on an acute care model suited to address the chronic condition? Noting the similarities between chronic addiction and other chronic illness, the field has increasingly called for shifting to the chronic care or management approach akin to the model used in the treatment of other chronic conditions [6, 9, 58]. In this section, we describe the state of addiction treatment, its effectiveness, and current movement toward a recovery-supported system of care.

Current Treatment Services for Drug Addiction

The past three decades of efforts to curtail drug use and related problems in the USA have given rise to a wide range of treatment options. Individuals with drug problems may choose from a host of treatment programs including hospital-based inpatient stays, residential care, outpatient drug-free (nonmethadone) treatment, day treatment, narcotics substitution therapy (mostly methadone maintenance, also including buprenorphine), and self-help group meetings. Services available at such programs may include drug education; individual, group, and family counseling and cognitive-behavioral therapy; specialized medical care; educational and vocational training; relapse prevention training; social and community support; and pharmacotherapy. Formal treatment programs usually provide a combination of such service components, although the quality and quantity of these services vary greatly from program to program.

The increasing recognition that drug addiction is a chronic relapsing disorder has also resulted in increased availability of aftercare programs. Although some individuals with drug disorders are able to achieve sustained recoveries after receiving treatment, for many others, drug addiction is characterized by periods of abstinence followed by relapse and reentry into the treatment system. Thus, individuals are generally encouraged to participate in some form of aftercare extending beyond the formal treatment episode. The primary goal of this phase is to maintain the gains that have been achieved in treatment and to prevent relapse. Most aftercare programs, regardless of the treatment setting of the primary care, have usually consisted of outpatient aftercare group therapy sessions and participation in self-help programs such as Alcoholics Anonymous (AA), Cocaine Anonymous (CA), or Narcotics Anonymous (NA). These programs support the individual's efforts to become and remain drug-free.

Despite the existence of various services and options, programs often operate in isolation, and cross-referral among programs has been limited [59, 60]. Patients may not be admitted to the program most appropriate for them, and dropout rates have been high. Even for patients who have completed treatment, once discharged, they may not receive continued care until they relapse and are then readmitted to yet another treatment.

Treatment Outcomes and Cumulative Treatment Effects

Many treatment evaluation studies have provided evidence of the overall effectiveness of drug treatment [1, 55–58, 61]. No single treatment type works best for all patients, however, and the most consistent finding in treatment evaluation research is that the length of stay in treatment is positively associated with more favorable treatment outcomes. For some addicts, treatment may be a turning point toward stable recovery. For others, treatment effects tend to be short-lived [3, 6] as many relapse after treatment.

Given the high relapse rates following treatment, it is not surprising that many drug users experience several episodes of treatment [9, 62]. In fact, research on drug addiction reveals that drug treatment is rarely a one-time event. Instead, many drug-dependent individuals are involved in treatment multiple times over their addiction careers, with each treatment episode of varying lengths of stay [3]. For these individuals, multiple treatment episodes may be necessary to achieve incremental improvement and eventual cessation.

A treatment career approach to understanding how best to intervene with drug use is broadly intended to encompass the complexity of diverse addiction patterns, especially those dynamic phenomena pertaining to recovery from the chronic, relapsing nature of addiction. Examining the incremental and cumulative effects of multiple treatment episodes over an extended time (i.e., the treatment career) complements the usual focus on single episodes of treatment used in conventional outcome evaluations [3, 9].

The challenge in assessing cumulative treatment effects in the observational studies is that those multiple treatment episodes generally do not stand alone over the life course. Multiple treatments are often the results of drug use and related problems; even though a given treatment may reduce drug use, subsequent drug use may result in additional treatment. As a result, different treatment profiles of subjects may reflect some different dynamic processes. This dynamic process poses challenges in statistical methodology when the cumulative effect is investigated assessing past treatments according to drug use outcome (e.g., abstinence) at a later time. One standard approach to this problem is to apply regression analysis predicting the mean of drug use outcome at a later stage as a function of those past treatments. We developed and applied a marginal structural model [63–65] to the CALDAR longitudinal data to unbiasedly estimate the causal effect of cumulative treatments on a later drug use outcome in the presence of time-dependent confounders that are themselves affected by past treatments [63, 65]. Our study [66] demonstrated that the cumulative treatment occurring over the previous 10 years significantly increased the likelihood of drug use abstinence in the subsequent 5-year period.

The cumulative treatment effects are indicative of the need for multiple treatment episodes, at least for many addicts. As mentioned earlier, however, most treatment programs in the current service delivery system lack interconnection, so the multiple treatments that patients receive likely occur as a result of relapse as opposed to planned continuing care. Previous studies have shown that multiple treatments in a continuing care arrangement produced more favorable outcomes than non-coordinated discrete treatments [67]. Efforts to integrate treatment components to develop coordinated long-term care should take these findings into consideration.

Emerging Long-Term Care Models

Long-term care models responding to the need for treating addiction as a chronic disorder are still being developed. The long-term care concept has a range of definitions including continuing care, aftercare, step-down care, stepped care, extended intervention, disease management model, or chronic care model. Narcotics replacement treatment (e.g., methadone maintenance, buprenorphine) is medically assisted care intended for long-term maintenance, but is only for opioid dependence. Self-help has long been available and has received wide support not only in the recovery community but also in the treatment field. In this section, we briefly discuss several other long-term care interventions that recently underwent empirical investigations, as well as the recent emerging recovery-oriented systems of care.

Long-Term Care Interventions

Studies have shown improved treatment outcomes associated with successive treatments that provide an orderly progression of services (i.e., inpatient, followed by residential treatment, outpatient treatment, and self-help group participation) [68]. Research efforts are increasingly documenting how continuing care (or aftercare) maintains progress achieved in the formal phase of treatment [69]. The Recovery Management Checkups (RMC) developed by Dennis and Scott [8] consisted of quarterly assessments after intake and referring those with problems to linkage managers with the aim for ongoing monitoring and linking them back to treatment. The intervention has shown that patients receiving RMC are more likely to return to treatment, stayed in treatment longer, and demonstrated improved outcomes. Another line of research involves telephone interventions delivered following the formal treatment. These phone interventions provide counseling over the phone, are cheap, and are appealing to the patients. There is evidence of association with improved outcomes, although it might be more appropriate for less severe patients [70]. While the empirical literature in this area is still limited, overall findings appear to be promising. Innovative methods should be further explored. The fast-growing internet technologies and other electronic devices provide great opportunities to engage and network with patients because of the wide access and more appealing interaction mechanism, particularly among young people.

Recovery-Oriented Systems of Care

Consistent with the current discussions on reconceptualizing and restructuring treatment delivery systems to better address addiction as a chronic condition, major efforts are being led by SAMHSA to foster the redesign and development of recovery-oriented systems of care (ROSC; CSAT, p. 8) [12] in order to support sustained recovery. Several states are transitioning to recovery oriented services with the vision of changing from intense episodes of acute specialty care to multisystem, person-centered, continuum of care, and from addressing pathology to promoting global health/wellness. Continuing the current and past recommendations, ROSC promotes evidence-based interventions, comprehensive services (e.g., employment, mental health), and accountability. Conceptually, there is a shift from deficits to strength-based emphasis, and with greater consumer involvements. Other major areas unique to ROSC that differ from the current system include, for example, the following:

- Involvement of consumers in the management of their own health care; individuals, in collaboration with their caregivers, assume responsibility for wellness management for a variety of conditions.
- Mutual aid or peer support groups (recovery coaches, recovery support specialist, community recovery support centers) are explicitly promoted.
- Recovery support services delivered within recovery-oriented systems of care are nonclinical services that may be provided to individuals not requiring or seeking treatment. They may also be provided during and after treatment.

While the vision and goals for sustained support for recovery are admirable, these concepts and procedures need to be operationalized and strategically developed. For example, quality of care is a promising outcome bringing addiction research and treatment further into the realm of public health. However, if addiction treatment providers are being held accountable for improved quality of life of their patients, what are the mechanisms and resources for service providers to achieve such performance goals? Additional issues include allocation of resources for long-term and comprehensive services and defining measureable outcomes. Perhaps the most important question is whether this system would produce better outcomes. ROSC as an evidence-based practice requires a system-level outcome evaluation.

Implications and Future Research

The typical person seeking addiction treatment evolves from a drug user, to an abuser, to an addicted person over a period of years. During this course, it is common for them to develop social, health, mental health, and legal problems. Those psychosocial complications affect how responsive the patient will be to treatment and the likelihood of relapse after treatment. A comprehensive treatment delivery system should have a variety of treatment programs and services available to meet patients' diverse needs at various phases of recovery. Additionally, because drug addiction is typically a chronic disorder characterized by occasional relapses, a short-term, one-time treatment often is not sufficient. Many addicted individuals require prolonged treatment and multiple treatment episodes to achieve long-term abstinence and fully restored functioning. An effective treatment delivery system needs to incorporate strategies to sustain long-term treatment effectiveness.

In this chapter, we have reviewed empirical research findings regarding drug use and recovery trajectories and related factors. We also describe the current and emerging treatment service systems. The findings on efficacy of cumulative treatment versus single episode assessment support a comprehensive service system including a long-term care approach that supports and maintains stable recovery for different drug use disorders and patient populations. Still, many aspects of recovery or the care system in support of recovery require further development and empirical support. Below we provide some research questions to be addressed in future research.

Improving Understanding of Recovery

The literature on life course theory and addiction has identified many key concepts and domains that provide a preliminary basis for a conceptual framework for understanding the drug use and recovery trajectories and turning points. Much of the empirical evidence supporting the various components and relationships is still lacking. As mentioned earlier, considerable research has been conducted in understanding onset and relapse, and research is only recently starting to accumulate regarding distinct long-term patterns of substance use and recovery trajectories. However, we do not understand the relationship between internal and external processes that contribute to recovery careers, turning points, or the lack of them. We have limited knowledge and virtually no empirical evidence about the nature and timing of recovery, related factors (e.g., social capital, stage in life, human agency, self-awareness), and the underlying mechanisms that sustain or lead to changes in drug use behavior toward recovery over the life course.

Future research should address the following research questions: What constitutes the empirical support for different ways of conceptualizing recovery, in what contexts, and their implications for research, policy, and practice? Specifically, should abstinence be considered only from a particular drug or from all substances? How long an abstinence period is necessary to predict long-term stable recovery? What factors impact patterns of abstinence and relapse in the context of other indicators such as quality of life? Are there patterns of recovery that include improvements in quality of life, employment, social support, and family relationships, as well as reductions in substance use over time (apart from abstinence)?

Developing Empirically Based Long-Term Care Strategies

The recovery-oriented systems of care (ROSC) movement has incorporated many well-accepted concepts such as integrated and comprehensive services, accountability, and evidence-based practices, and it has been broadened by including the larger communities, particularly the recovery communities. The evidence base supporting practices to promote long-term recovery is still rather limited. Additionally, current treatment programs are often isolated entities, and cross-referring is an exception rather than the rule. Furthermore, patients' willingness to accept and comply with ROSC-type long-term care is largely unknown. Strategies are needed to shape the systems to make the "continuity of care" and "disease management" acceptable, accessible, and efficient.

Longitudinal intervention studies are needed to more effectively adapt treatment strategies suited to specific stages of drug use over the life course in order to facilitate long-lasting recovery. Longitudinal studies are needed that experimentally test a series of interventions with random assignment contingent upon response to the prior intervention and patient's preference. As with medical model treatment dealing with other brain diseases, the treatment for drug dependence faces the challenge of recommending a sequence of treatments for those who do not satisfactorily respond to initial treatment attempt. Unproductive and unsubstantiated variation in treatment practices can be reduced and outcomes improved if such treatment sequence recommendations can be empirically based on better efficacy, acceptability, or cost. Further, clinical trials protocol development should consider patient preferences to more closely represent decision-making processes that occur in actual clinical practice by preserving the central role that patients play in negotiating treatment decisions. Clinicians, particularly in mental health, have increasingly recognized the value of patient-directed care as a means to empower patients as well as improve the therapeutic alliance, treatment adherence, and outcomes [71]. This integrative approach, demonstrated by a series of articles testing interventions for depressed patients [72], appears promising and serves as an excellent example for addiction research.

Finally, individual or group differences always need to be considered in clinical practice to optimize the likelihood of recovery. Research needs to address how patterns and mechanisms of recovery differ by individuals' characteristics (e.g.,gender, ethnicity/race, psychiatric comorbidity, and HIV risk profiles) and with regard to their service system interactions.

Summary

- The life-course drug use perspective offers a rich framework guiding the study of recovery in terms of transitions (to incorporate developmental and social context), turning points (to characterize changes), and social capital (to characterize the potential role of social ties).
- For many addicted drug users, drug addiction persists over a long period of time. Thus, studying long-term dynamic changes over the life course allows for characterizing distinctive patterns of drug use trajectories and identifying critical factors contributing to persistence or change over the life span.
- There are distinctive trajectory patterns of drug use and recovery over the life course.
- Developing stress-coping strategies, identifying personal and social resources, and engaging in prosocial activities should all be considered as parts of effective strategies for achieving and maintaining stable recovery.
- Risk and protective factors related to initiating and sustaining recovery may vary depending on the life stage.

- Periods of no use are aided by treatment and self-help participation for heroin, cocaine, and meth users, but few of these users receive treatment (about 25%) during the 10 years after first use.
- Cumulative treatment (or total duration of treatment summed across episodes) is associated with favorable outcomes in subsequent periods.
- Post-treatment continuity of care (e.g., phone monitoring, self-help groups) is effective in reducing drug use and forestalling relapse.
- Innovative longitudinal intervention strategies need to be developed.

Acknowledgment This work was supported in part by the UCLA Center for Advancing Longitudinal Drug Abuse Research (CALDAR) under grant P30DA016383 (PI: Hser) from the National Institute on Drug Abuse (NIDA). Dr. Hser is also supported by a NIDA Senior Scientist Award (K05DA017648).

References

1. Anglin MD, Hser Y. Treatment of drug abuse. In: Tonry M, Wilson JQ, editors. Drugs and crime, vol. 13. Chicago, IL: University of Chicago Press; 1990. p. 393–460.
2. Compton WM, Glantz M, Delany P. Addiction as a chronic illness: putting the concept into action. Eval Program Plan. 2003;26:353–4.
3. Hser Y, Anglin MD, Grella CE, Longshore D, Prendergast ML. Drug treatment careers: a conceptual framework and existing research findings. J Subst Abuse Treat. 1997;14:543–58.
4. Hser Y, Hoffman V, Grella CE, Anglin MD. A 33-year follow-up of narcotics addicts. Arch Gen Psychiatry. 2001;58:503–8.
5. Hser Y, Huang D, Chou C, Anglin MD. Trajectories of heroin addiction: growth mixture modeling results based on a 33-year follow-up study. Eval Rev. 2007;31:548–63.
6. McLellan AT, Lewis DC, O'Brien CP, Kleber HD. Drug dependence, a chronic medical illness: implications for treatment, insurance, and outcomes evaluation. JAMA. 2000;284:1689–95.
7. Dennis M, Scott C. Managing addiction as a chronic condition. Addict Sci Clin Pract. 2007;4(1):45–55.
8. Scott CK, Dennis ML. Recovery Management Checkup (RMC) protocol for people with chronic substance use disorders. Bloomington, IL: Chestnut Health Systems; 2002.
9. Hser Y, Longshore D, Anglin MD. The life course perspective on drug use: a conceptual framework for understanding drug use trajectories. Eval Rev. 2007;31:515–47.
10. Laudet AB. What does recovery mean to you? lessons from the recovery experience for research and practice. J Subst Abuse Treat. 2007;33:243–56.
11. White WL. Addiction recovery: its definition and conceptual boundaries. J Subst Abuse Treat. 2007;33:229–41.
12. Center for Substance Abuse Treatment. National Summit on Recovery: 2005 Conference Report. DHHS Publication No. (SMA) 07-4276. Rockville, MD: Substance Abuse and Mental Health Services Administration; 2007.
13. Teruya C, Hser YI. Turning points in the life course: current findings and future directions in drug use research. Curr Drug Abuse Rev. 2010; [Epub ahead of print]
14. Elder Jr GH. Perspectives in the life course. In: Elder GH, editor. Life course dynamics. Ithaca, NY: Cornell University Press; 1985. p. 23–49.
15. Sampson RJ, Laub JH. Socioeconomic achievements in the life course of disadvantaged men: military service as a turning point, 1940–1965. Am Sociol Rev. 1996;61:347–67.

16. Laub JH, Sampson RJ. Turning points in the life course: why change matters to the study of crime. Criminology. 1993;31:301–25.
17. Cloud W, Granfield R. The social process of exiting addiction: a life course perspective. In: Blomqvist J, Koski-Jannes A, Ojesjo L, editors. Addiction and life course. Helsinki, Finland: Nordic Council on Alcohol and Drug Research; 2004. p. 185–202.
18. Granfield R, Cloud W. Social context and "natural recovery": the role of social capital in the resolution of drug-associated problems. Subst Use Misuse. 2001;36:1543–70.
19. Wheaton B, Gotlib IH. Trajectories and turning points over the life course: concepts and themes. In: Gotlib IH, Wheaton B, editors. Stress and adversity over the life course: trajectories and turning points. New York, NY: Cambridge University Press; 1997. p. 1–25.
20. Hser Y, Huang D, Brecht M, Li L, Evans E. Contrasting trajectories of heroin, cocaine, and methamphetamine use. J Addict Dis. 2008;27:13–21.
21. Substance Abuse and Mental Health Services Administration. Overview of findings from the 2002 National Survey on Drug Use and Health (Office of Applied Studies, NHSDA Series H-21, DHHS Publication No. SMA 03-3774). Rockville, MD: SAMHSA; 2003.
22. Center for Human Resource Research. NLSY97 Codebook Supplement Main File Round 8, Prepared for the U.S. Department of Labor, by Center for Human Resource Research. Columbus, OH: The Ohio State University; 2006.
23. Hser Y, Evans E, Huang D, Brecht M, Li L. Comparing the dynamic course of heroin, cocaine, and methamphetamine use over 10 years. Addict Behav. 2008;33:1581–9.
24. Nagin DS. Analyzing developmental trajectories: semi-parametric group-based approach. Psychol Methods. 1999;4:39–177.
25. Nagin DS. Group-based modeling of development. Cambridge, MA: Harvard University Press; 2005.
26. Muthen B. Latent variable analysis: growth mixture modeling and related techniques for longitudinal data. In: Kaplan D, editor. Handbook of quantitative methodology for the social sciences. Newbury Park, CA: Sage Publications; 2004. p. 345–68.
27. Muthen B, Asparouhov T. Growth mixture analysis: models with non-Gaussian random effects. In: Fitzmaurice G, Davidian M, Verbeke G, Molenberghs G, editors. Advances in longitudinal data analysis. Boca Raton, FL: Chapman & Hall/CRC Press; 2006.
28. Chassin L, Presson CC, Pitts SC, Sherman SJ. The natural history of cigarette smoking from adolescence to adulthood in a midwestern community sample: multiple trajectories and their psychosocial correlates. Health Psychol. 2000;19:223–31.
29. Orlando M, Tucker JS, Ellickson PL, Klein DJ. Developmental trajectories of cigarette smoking and their correlates from early adolescence to young adulthood. J Consult Clin Psychol. 2004;72(3):400–10.
30. Chassin L, Pitts SC, Prost J. Binge drinking trajectories from adolescence to emerging adulthood in a high-risk sample: predictors and substance abuse outcomes. J Consult Clin Psychol. 2002;70:67–78.
31. Hix-Small H, Duncan TE, Duncan SC, Okut H. A multivariate associative finite growth mixture modeling approach examining adolescent alcohol and marijuana use. J Psychopathol Behav Assess. 2004;26:255–70.
32. Ellickson PL, Martino SC, Collins RL. Marijuana use from adolescence to young adulthood: multiple developmental trajectories and their associated outcomes. Health Psychol. 2004;23:299–307.
33. Anthony JC, Petronis KR. Early-onset drug use and risk of later drug problems. Drug Alcohol Depend. 1995;40:9–15.
34. Yu J, Williford WR. The age of alcohol onset and alcohol, cigarette, and marijuana use patterns: an analysis of drug use progression of young adults in New York State. Int J Addict. 1992;27:1313–23.
35. Hser Y. Predicting long-term stable recovery from heroin addiction: findings from a 33-year follow-up study. J Addict Dis. 2007;26:51–60.

36. The Betty Ford Institute Consensus Panel. What is recovery? A working definition from the Betty Ford Institute. J Subst Abuse Treat. 2007;33:221–8.
37. World Health Organization (WHO). Basic documents. 35th ed. Geneva, Switzerland: WHO; 1985.
38. Dennis ML, Foss MA, Scott CK. An eight-year perspective on the relationship between the duration of abstinence and other aspects of recovery. Eval Rev. 2007;31:585–612.
39. Sobell L, Cunningham JA, Sobell MB. Recovery from alcohol problems with and without treatment: prevalence in two population surveys. Am J Public Health. 1996;7:966–72.
40. Cross G, Morgan C, Moonye A, Martin C, Rafter J. Alcoholism treatment: a ten-year follow-up study. Alcohol Clin Exp Res. 1990;14:169–73.
41. Hser Y, Stark ME, Paredes A, Huang D, Anglin MD, Rawson R. A 12-year follow-up of a treated cocaine-dependent sample. J Subst Abuse Treat. 2006;30:219–26.
42. Scott CK, Foss MA, Dennis ML. Pathways in the relapse–treatment–recovery cycle over 3 years. J Subst Abuse Treat. 2005;28:S63–72.
43. Weisner C, Ray GT, Mertens JR, Satre DD, Moore C. Short-term alcohol and drug treatment outcomes predict long-term outcome. Drug Alcohol Depend. 2003;1071(3):281–94.
44. Salome HJ, French MT, Scott C, et al. Investigating the economic costs and benefits of addiction treatment: econometric analysis of the Chicago Target Cities project. Eval Program Plann. 2003;26(3):325–38.
45. Scott CK, Foss MA, Dennis ML. Factors influencing initial and longer-term responses to substance abuse treatment: a path analysis. Eval Program Plann. 2003;26:287–96.
46. Laudet A, Savage R, Mahmood D. Pathways to long-term recovery: a preliminary investigation. J Psychoactive Drugs. 2002;34:305–11.
47. Moos RH, Moos BS. Rates and predictors of relapse after natural and treated remission from alcohol use disorders. Addiction. 2006;101:212–22.
48. Moos RH. Theory-based processes that promote the remission of substance use disorders. Clin Psychol Rev. 2007;27:537–51.
49. Vaillant GE. A long-term follow-up of male alcohol abuse. Arch Gen Psychiatry. 1996;53:243–9.
50. Vaillant G. A 60-year follow-up of alcoholic men. Addiction. 2003;98:1043–51.
51. Sampson RJ, Laub JH. Life-course desisters? Trajectories of crime among delinquent boys followed to age 70. Criminology. 2003;41:555.
52. Simpson DD, Sells SB. Opioid addiction and treatment: a 12-year follow-up. Malabar, FL: Krieger; 1990.
53. Termorshuizen F, Krol A, Prins M, van Ameijden EJ. Long-term outcome of chronic drug use: The Amsterdam Cohort Study among Drug Users. Am J Epidemiol. 2005;161:271–9.
54. Winick C. Maturing out of narcotic addiction. Bull Narc. 1962;14:1–8.
55. Anglin MD, Hser Y. Legal coercion and drug abuse treatment: research findings and social policy implications. In: Inciardi J, editor. Handbook of drug control in the United States. Westport, CT: Greenwood Press; 1990. p. 151–76.
56. Simpson DD, Joe GW, Fletcher BW, Hubbard RL, Anglin MD. A national evaluation of treatment outcomes for cocaine dependence. Arch Gen Psychiatry. 1999;56:507–14.
57. Simpson DD, Joe GW, Broome KM. A national 5-year follow-up of treatment outcomes for cocaine dependence. Arch Gen Psychiatry. 2002;59:538–44.
58. Institute of Medicine (IOM). Improving the quality of health care for mental and substance-use conditions. Washington, DC: National Academy Press; 2006.
59. Rawson, R. Building a treatment system: elements and challenges. Presentation at the Hawaii Addiction Conference/AAPI Workgroup Scientific Conference; May 2009; Honolulu, Hawaii.
60. McLellan AT, Carise D, Kleber HD. Can the national addiction treatment infrastructure support the public's demand for quality care? J Subst Abuse Treat. 2003;25:117–21.
61. Gerstein DR, Harwood HJ. National Academy of Sciences, Institute of Medicine, Division of Health Care Services, Committee for the Substance Abuse Coverage Study, Washington, DC.

Treating drug problems, vol. 1: a study of the evolution, effectiveness, and financing of public and private drug treatment systems. Washington, DC: National Academy Press; 1990.

62. Anglin MD, Hser Y, Grella CE. Drug addiction and treatment careers among clients in the Drug Abuse Treatment Outcome Study (DATOS). Psychol Addict Behav. 1997;11:30823.

63. Robins JM. Causal inference from complex longitudinal data. In: Berkane M, editor. Latent variable modeling and applications to causality. Lecture notes in statistics, vol. 120. New York, NY: Springer; 1997. p. 69–117.

64. Robins JM. Marginal structural models versus structural nested models as tools for causal inference. In: Halloran E, editor. Statistical models in epidemiology. New York, NY: Springer; 1999. p. 95–134.

65. Robins JM, Hernán MA, Brumback B. Marginal structural models and causal inference in epidemiology. Epidemiology. 2000;11:550–60.

66. Li L, Evans E, Hser Y. A marginal structural modeling approach to assess the cumulative effect of drug treatment on later drug use abstinence. J Drug Issues. 2010;40(1):221–40.

67. Hser Y, Huang D, Teruya C, Anglin MD. Diversity of drug abuse treatment utilization patterns and outcomes. Eval Program Plann. 2004;27:309–19.

68. Khalsa ME, Paredes A, Anglin MD, Potepan P, Potter C. Combinations of treatment modalities and therapeutic outcome for cocaine dependence. In: Tims FM, Leukefeld CG, editors. Cocaine treatment: research and clinical perspectives. Rockville, MD: National Institute on Drug Abuse; 1993. p. 237–59. NIDA Research Monograph 135.

69. McKay JR. Is there a case for extended interventions for alcohol and drug use disorders? Addiction. 2005;100:1594–610.

70. McKay JR, Merikle E, Mulvaney FD, Weiss RV, Koppenhaver JM. Factors accounting for cocaine use two years following initiation of continuing care. Addiction. 2001;96:213–25.

71. Wagner EH, Austin BT, Von Korff M. Organizing care for patients with chronic illness. Milbank Q. 1996;74:511–44.

72. Rush AJ, Koran LM, Keller MB, et al. The treatment of chronic depression, part I. Study design and rationale for evaluating the comparative efficacy of sertraline and imipramine as acute, crossover, continuation and maintenance phase therapies. J Clin Psychiatry. 1993;59:589–97.

Chapter 3
Integrating Addiction Treatment and Mutual Aid Recovery Resources

Lee Ann Kaskutas and Meenakshi Subbaraman

Abstract The most widely used source of help for alcohol problems is Alcoholics Anonymous (AA), and much formal treatment has adapted AA's methods and concepts. Usually many people seek help from AA at the recommendation of a treatment professional. Even treatment programs that historically have not been 12-step-oriented, such as Therapeutic Communities, may recommend AA or mutual help alternatives post-treatment. Because evidence shows that individuals are more likely to attend these groups after treatment if they are introduced to them during treatment interventions to facilitate 12-step involvement are needed. Twelve-step facilitation can vary, focusing on introducing clients to the 12-step philosophy, helping them work the intial steps of the program, or helping them connect with the fellowship of individuals they encounter in AA. Randomized trials of 12-step facilitation consistently demonstrate abstinence rates 10% higher (or more) than the usual care conditions at 1-year follow-up, with even stronger results in particular subgroups such as those with prior treatment episodes. Manuals are available that guide counselors through these 12-step facilitation interventions, increasing the likelihood that treatment programs will incorporate evidence-based practices which increase clients' AA involvement during and post-treatment, and reduce relapse. This chapter describes these interventions and summarizes the trial results. Unfortunately, there has been less progress in developing ways to facilitate the utilization of non-12-step alternatives such as Women For Sobriety, Life Ring, or SMART Recovery, which are less widely available yet offer another supportive environment. This is an important area of future research.

Keywords Addiction recovery management · Alcoholics Anonymous · Twelve-step facilitation

L.A. Kaskutas (✉)
Alcohol Research Group, Public Health Institute, 6475 Christie Avenue,
Suite 400, Emeryville, CA 94608, USA
e-mail: lkaskutas@arg.org

J.F. Kelly and W.L. White (eds.), *Addiction Recovery Management: Theory, Research and Practice*, Current Clinical Psychiatry, DOI 10.1007/978-1-60327-960-4_3,
© Springer Science+Business Media, LLC 2011

Introduction

Treatment for alcohol and drug dependence has evolved over time, driven first by unmet need, then by professionalization and market forces, and more recently by research findings. One constant throughout this history is reliance on non-professional mutual aid groups, such as the 12-step programs of Alcoholics Anonymous (AA) and Narcotics Anonymous (NA), both for a theoretical framework of long-term recovery management for treating addiction and also as a free source of post-treatment aftercare. This chapter provides a brief social construction of this history and then reports on the effectiveness of interventions to facilitate clients' entry into 12-step programs.

Brief History of 12-Step Treatment

Pre-AA mutual aid groups for recovery flourished in the nineteenth century alongside a large network of inebriate asylums, inebriate homes, and private addiction cure institutes; however, both the voluntary and the professional recovery support resources collapsed in the USA in the early decades of the twentieth century. The advent of AA in 1935 led to a population of alcoholics who were no longer drinking and who believed that the best way to stay that way was to help other alcoholics [1]. This is AA's 12th step: *Having had a spiritual awakening as the result of these steps, we tried to carry this message to alcoholics, and to practice these principles in all our affairs* [2].

The rise of alcohol problems following the repeal of Prohibition led to new alcoholism treatment models in the 1940s and early 1950s. These models included outpatient clinics and a new approach to inpatient treatment that emerged from three institutions in the state of Minnesota (Pioneer House, Hazelden, and Willmar State Hospital). "Minnesota Model" programs were led by a multidisciplinary team of medical and mental health professionals as well as recovering counselors [3, 4]. A competing approach, the California Social Model, deliberately avoids professional staff and relies exclusively on recovering staff [5]. With either model, clients attend AA meetings and begin to work the steps during treatment, and are advised to continue their connection with AA after leaving treatment [6]. A third approach, the Therapeutic Community, initially eschewed the 12 steps [7], but was staffed by recovering addicts as well as professionals similar to the Minnesota Model [8]. Importantly, the methods for introducing clients to AA vary even within these models of treatment, in which counselors were generally left to their own best judgment to accomplish this important hand-off.

The biggest change in treatment over the years has been in the intensity of treatment allowed by public payors and private insurers. This has been driven by research that has been unable to document clear benefits for 28-day residential programs over less costly outpatient options [9, 10], and by managed care organizations that restrict even the number of outpatient visits a patient can expect. Because of this, even the Therapeutic Community approach now recommends attendance at 12-step groups following discharge, and even during treatment [11]. Recognizing that it is unrealistic to expect patients to remain abstinent following such relatively constrained treatment episodes, the most recent move in the specialty treatment field has been to argue for a continuing care model akin to how other medical conditions such as diabetes are conceptualized [12]. However, in the absence of funding for long-term aftercare, 12-step groups and the fellowship of AA and NA members become an attractive alternative that offers ongoing support post-treatment.

Involvement in AA and NA has been associated with alcohol and drug abstinence in numerous observational studies (e.g., [13–17]). Because of reductions in treatment intensity and length, as well as limited funding for aftercare treatment associated with managed care and today's climate of fiscal constraint [18, 19], 12-step groups are especially crucial in supplementing specialty treatment. Importantly, participation in peer-led 12-step organizations has been shown to mobilize some of the same kinds of intrinsic mechanisms of behavior change that are mobilized by professionally-led interventions (e.g., coping, self-efficacy, motivation for abstinence) [20]. Additionally, such resources are typically more easily accessible, especially at times of high relapse risk when professional help is often not available (e.g., evenings, weekends, and holidays).

However, most treatment graduates severely underutilize 12-step groups, dropping out of AA/NA after having been exposed during their stays in formal treatment [21–24]. This has incited interest in manual-guided twelve step facilitation (TSF) interventions that uniformly introduce clients to AA and NA in a way that not only sustains meeting attendance but also promotes involvement in the prescribed AA activities (such as having AA friends) that are associated with better drinking outcomes [25].

Though not completely consistent, results from trials of TSF approaches are optimistic. A brief review of these findings is presented here. Our review is organized by delivery format: individual (one-on-one) and group delivery.

Individual Format

Project MATCH

First, let us consider Project MATCH, a large multi-site trial of alcohol dependent individuals, which included a TSF condition that focused on the first three steps of AA/NA during 12 individual (1-on-1) sessions [22]. The project consisted of two groups of subjects: aftercare patients who had recently completed inpatient treatment (the "aftercare arm"; $n = 774$); and outpatients who were recruited directly (the "outpatient arm"; $n = 952$). Superior results were evident for TSF only among the outpatient group: At both the 1- and 3-year follow-up interviews, outpatients who had been randomized to TSF had significantly higher alcohol abstinence rates than those randomized to Motivational Enhancement Therapy (MET), which is designed to increase motivation to stop drinking, or Cognitive Behavior Therapy (CBT), a behavioral approach (e.g., 36, 27, and 24%, respectively, were abstinent at 3 years; $p < 0.007$[1]). No differences in abstinence emerged among aftercare patients, who had attended 12-step-oriented inpatient treatment prior to joining Project MATCH [22] and were followed up for only 1 year.

One explanation for the null finding in the aftercare arm is that TSF's mechanism of action, meeting attendance, was high in all three conditions ([22], p. 192), and thus, differential abstinence rates could not emerge. This may suggest that the Project MATCH TSF content may not sufficiently exceed what is conveyed during usual inpatient treatment, in terms of accepting or being comfortable with the 12-step approach (specifically, the first three steps).

In addition to these overall effects, TSF results were superior for two subgroups of the outpatient arm: among those without psychiatric problems, abstinence rates were higher for TSF subjects at 1 year [26], but not at 3 years [27]; at higher levels of psychiatric severity, the TSF effect faded. Among those whose social networks were supportive of drinking, TSF subjects had higher abstinence at 3 years [27], but not at 1 year [26]; the higher rates of AA attendance for these TSF subjects seems to have inoculated them from potentially negative influences of their social network [28]. These results suggest a need to consider the effects of TSF interventions among subgroups based on their psychiatric severity and social network characteristics.

Intensive Referral

Another study, conducted in Department of Veterans Affairs outpatient clinics, randomized 345 incoming patients with substance use disorders to standard AA referral (which involved giving patients the AA/NA meeting schedules and encouraging attendance) or to an intensive referral condition in which patients were arranged to attend a meeting with a self-help group volunteer [29]. Both conditions were delivered in five individual-format sessions.

Significantly more patients in the intensive referral condition were abstinent from drugs at 6 months (78 vs. 70%, $p < 0.05$; [29]) and from both alcohol and drugs at both the 6- and 12-month follow-up interviews (51 and 41%, respectively; [30]). Higher abstinence rates were not obtained in the intensive referral condition for alcohol at 6 months [29], and comparisons of 12-month abstinence from alcohol were not reported [30]. However, intensive referral patients showed more

---

[1]$p < 0.05$ is recognized as statistically significant. Statistical significance refers to the probability of obtaining results at least as extreme as the observed results assuming there is truly no relationship between treatment and outcomes. A low p-value implies a low probability of the relationship arising purely by chance and suggests that treatment significantly affects outcomes.

improvement on another alcohol- and drug-related outcome, addiction severity [31], with decreases in alcohol and in drug problem severity from baseline to either follow-up interview, which was higher for the intensive referral condition [29, 30].

Intensive referral was especially effective in reducing problem severity by 6 months among those with less prior AA meeting attendance [29]. This finding coincides with the pattern of effects for TSF in Project MATCH, where TSF was superior only for outpatients who (unlike the aftercare arm) had not been exposed to AA during a recent stay in inpatient treatment.

Motivational Interviewing

A third, smaller study of alcohol dependent patients in a detoxification unit ($n = 48$) compared standard motivational interviewing techniques for promoting AA/NA participation in a single, individual-format, 6-min TSF session to a brief (5 min) advice condition to attend AA/NA [32]. Those with less prior 12-step involvement benefited more (i.e., had less drinking at 6-month follow-up) from TSF, whereas those with more prior exposure to AA and NA benefited more from the brief advice condition [32].

Findings from Timko and Kahler's studies suggest a need for considering 12-step facilitation effects disaggregated based on prior AA exposure levels. It may be that the TSF content in Kahler's study was enough of an introduction to AA/NA to help 12-step newcomers get involved in AA/NA; but, as with Project MATCH TSF in the aftercare arm, its content did not add significantly to what those with more prior AA/NA experience already knew and understood about AA, nor did it serve to counter negative lingering first impressions.

Individual TSF for Cocaine Dependence

Another study in the Department of Veterans Affairs focused on cocaine dependence, and delivered Project MATCH-based TSF and CBT in a combined group and individual format [33]. The treatment lasted 12 weeks with three groups and one individual session each week. African American patients with strong religious beliefs and individuals with low abstract reasoning abilities did better in TSF, while outcomes favored CBT in the overall sample ($n = 128$), and among both depressed clients and those with high abstract reasoning.

Given the spiritual content of 12-step groups such as AA, and the high levels of religiosity among the treated African Americans [34–36], the superior findings for African Americans in TSF makes sense. Similarly, CBT's foci on mood management and coping strategies should be especially helpful for those who are depressed and for individuals who are able to apply general (abstract) coping techniques to their own situations [33]. There were only 26 non-African American subjects in the sample, so they did not analyze that group alone. Nonetheless, Maude-Griffin's results point out a need to consider the effectiveness of 12-step facilitation interventions separately by ethnicity and by religious beliefs.

Twelve-Step Directive

Within a skills-focused individual treatment program, Walitzer and colleagues randomized 169 alcohol-dependent participants to receive one of three treatments: a 12-step based directive condition based on Project MATCH TSF, a 12-step-oriented MET where participants received about half of the AA-related material than those in the 12-step directive condition, or usual care which did not focus on AA especially [37]. All conditions were manual-guided and involved 12 weekly sessions. Participants in the 12-step directive (but not in MET) had higher rates of AA attendance, more involvement in AA activities during the 12-month follow-up, and more days abstinent than the usual care group (80% abstinent days vs. 65%).

Group Format

All five of the above TSF studies required individual sessions with substance abuse counselors, ranging in intensity from a single 6-min session [32], to three 50-min sessions [29] and twelve 90-min sessions [33, 38, 39]. Since most treatment today is delivered in group format [40–43], it is likely that treatment programs would not be able to sustain all but the briefest of these interventions without the support of a research study, as they would require funding for counselor's time that is not otherwise available.

Group Project MATCH

In recognition of this concern, Brown and colleagues [44] have implemented a 10-week, group-format version of the individual-format TSF intervention used in Project MATCH. The intervention was delivered as a form of aftercare treatment following inpatient or outpatient treatments, and was compared to a relapse prevention (RP) condition ($n = 133$). There were no main effects for condition at their 6-month follow-up, but several subgroups did better in the TSF condition than in RP: women (less severe alcohol problems at follow-up); those with high levels of psychiatric problem severity (higher levels of total abstinence from alcohol and drugs at 6 months); and those with multiple substance use profiles (less severe alcohol and drug problems at the 6-month follow-up). Brown and colleagues also found that patient preference mattered: patients who said they preferred TSF and were randomized to the TSF condition had better outcomes than those who said they preferred RP but were randomized to TSF; the same was true for preferring RP. This highlights a need to consider client preference in determining referral practices to 12-step groups.

Group TSF for Cocaine Dependence

An earlier study similarly focused on the first three steps of AA/NA/CA (Cocaine Anonymous) and compared it to RP, delivering seventeen 2-h group sessions to 110 outpatients whose drug of choice was cocaine [45]. Alcohol, marijuana, and cocaine use were studied at 12 weeks and 6 months. No differences in drug use emerged between conditions, but less alcohol use was reported over time among those who had been randomized to TSF than to RP (e.g., at 12 weeks, 47% were abstinent in the TSF condition vs. 25% in RP). No subgroup analyses were conducted.

Note that the majority of the above TSF interventions focus on introducing clients to the first three steps of AA. It is possible that the mixed results illustrated in the TSF trials reported above may arise, at least in part, from this emphasis. These key first steps recommend that individuals admit they are powerless over alcohol and surrender to a higher power for relief from the obsession to drink. These are concepts that frequently arise in AA meetings, and about which many new members receive counsel from AA sponsors and other experienced AA members.

Making AA Easier/MAAEZ

MAAEZ was developed by the first author (LAK) of this chapter. MAAEZ questions the wisdom of developing a 12-step facilitation intervention that focuses on the steps and thus replicates what AA and NA members already do so well. MAAEZ instead concentrates on tangibly helping clients to interact with people they will meet in AA/NA. MAAEZ must be delivered by individuals who are themselves active in AA or NA. MAAEZ is manual-guided, with an *Introduction* session and four "core" sessions (*Spirituality, Principles Not Personalities, Sponsorship*, and *Living Sober*). Clients return to the *Introductory* session week 6 as program graduates to share their MAAEZ and AA experiences with the MAAEZ newcomers [46].

MAAEZ was studied in existing residential, day treatment, and outpatient programs ($n = 508$) [46]. At the 12-month follow-up, bivariate analyses showed that more clients in MAAEZ than in usual care reported past-30-day abstinence from alcohol ($p = 0.012$), drugs ($p = 0.009$), and both ($p = 0.045$). In multivariate analyses, odds of abstinence from alcohol (OR = 1.85) and from drugs

(OR = 2.21) were significantly higher for MAAEZ participants; abstinence odds also increased significantly for each additional MAAEZ session received. The MAAEZ effect size was similar to those reported in Project MATCH [22] and the Veterans Affairs intensive referral study [29, 30], that is, about an 8–10% higher abstinence rate than the comparison group(s). Furthermore, subgroup analyses showed that those with more prior AA exposure, severe psychiatric problems, and atheists/agnostics benefited particularly from MAAEZ [46].

Differences in Sub-group Effects

A number of 12-step enhancement studies reviewed above also considered whether particular groups respond better to treatment than others. In some cases, findings are similar across studies. For example, the MAAEZ findings were consistent with the results of Brown et al. who found more alcohol and drug abstinence among those with high psychological distress who had been randomized to their 10-week TSF intervention [44]. However, other TSF studies have had quite different results with respect to psychiatric comorbidity. Project MATCH found that TSF was only helpful for those without psychopathology [26, 47], and Maude-Griffin's psychiatric analysis reported that depressed clients had done better in CBT than in TSF [33]. Many have voiced concern that AA may be inappropriate for those with psychiatric problems [48, 49], but empirical evidence of AA's effectiveness has begun to illustrate the opposite [50–52].

Results also are inconsistent in terms of prior AA and treatment involvement. For example, TSF results in Project MATCH and in the Veterans Affairs Intensive Referral study favored those with less prior AA meeting exposure, rather than more, while the opposite was the case with MAAEZ. Similarly, MAAEZ was more effective among those with prior (vs. no) treatment episodes. Perhaps MAAEZ's focus on connecting with the AA fellowship and culture gave these retracted clients a new perspective of AA and its members; this new way of viewing AA may not have been open or familiar in their past experiences with AA (and treatment). Given that almost half of the AA newcomers drop out in less than a month; [53] and that treatment clients often require more than one treatment episode (72% among those recruited in long-term residential programs in the MAAEZ study alone), interventions that tangibly encourage clients to try AA again, with an open mind and with new behaviors, are needed. Based on anecdotal evidence and our own observations at AA meetings and among treatment clients, quite a few people who have attended AA (some for years) always sit around the edges of meetings, arrive late and leave early, and never actually connect with other program members. MAAEZ may meet the needs of these people particularly.

Carrie Randall and colleagues have reported that many alcoholics suffer from social anxiety [54], so it makes sense that such individuals may not know how to go about introducing themselves at AA meetings. Timko's intensive referral intervention linked clients to AA members who would meet them at meetings; this may be exactly what a 12-step neophyte needs to kick-start a relationship with AA. MAAEZ results suggest that those with more prior AA exposure may need more than that.

Similarly, in Project MATCH clients were taught about acceptance and surrender, concepts helpful to a relative AA newcomer but somewhat well-worn to those with more AA attendance and experience. Kahler's finding of a positive effect for a TSF intervention only among those with minimal prior AA/NA experience [32] supports this interpretation. Since different types of 12-step facilitation appear appropriate in relation to past AA experience, providers may want to consider matching different TSF approaches based on prior AA exposure.

Another area of different subgroup effects pertains to religiosity. Those who were atheist, agnostic, or unsure of their religious beliefs benefited more from MAAEZ, whereas Maude-Griffin found that those with strong religious beliefs did better in TSF. However, Maude-Griffin studied African American clients for whom church and religiosity are prevalent sources of social and emotional support. Nonetheless, the MAAEZ *Spirituality* session may have presented clients with a new, more neutral, and open-minded way of experiencing the discussions of god and spirituality that inevitably occur in AA (indeed, this was a focus of the session) and hence was more effective among secularists. While AA may attract more of those predisposed to religion, religiosity may not necessarily moderate or influence AA's effect [55, 56].

Finally, there was a significantly higher MAAEZ effect for those without heavy alcohol and drug users in their social network. This is unlike Project MATCH, which found a greater TSF effect among those high in network support for drinking. MAAEZ was based on the Theory of Planned Behavior [57], and addresses resistance to 12-step groups by changing participants' attitudes, subjective norms, and perceived control regarding 12-step involvement. Perhaps changes in social network characteristics and in how study clients viewed consequences of their AA/NA involvement (including what their friends would think) may explain MAAEZ effects in part.

As the other chapters in this book have documented, people professionally treated for substance use disorders remain precariously balanced between recovery and relapse following the discharge from treatment. As currently designed, the utility of addiction treatment is limited by high post-treatment relapse and re-admission rates, and what are all too often prolonged addiction and treatment careers. Assertive linkage to AA and other recovery mutual aid groups can help individuals transition from brief experiments in sobriety (recovery initiation) to stable and sustainable recovery maintenance, and an enhanced quality of life in long-term recovery. To achieve that goal will require closer connections between the worlds of professional treatment and indigenous recovery support institutions, and the establishment of assertive linkage procedures to enhanced engagement and retention with these indigenous community resources. Their wide availability makes them a useful recovery management tool and provides a long-term recovery ally.

Summary of Key Points

- There are several proven techniques for enhancing 12-step participation. Some 12-step facilitation (TSF) interventions are delivered in group-format by recovering counselors, but most are one-on-one with professional therapists.
- The content of 12-step facilitation also varies. Most focus on introducing clients to the 12-step philosophy and helping them to follow the initial steps of the program, but several help them to connect with the fellowship of individuals they encounter in AA.
- Despite different approaches in delivery format and focus, all 12-step enhancement protocols seem to have the same magnitude of effect in relation to drinking outcomes.
- Certain subgroups of people, such as those with more prior AA attendance and those with higher psychological severity, appear to benefit more from certain types of 12-step enhancement interventions but not others.
- Many of these interventions are free, are manual-guided, and readily available for use.

References

1. McElrath D. The Minnesota model. J Psychoactive Drugs. 1997;29(2):141–4.
2. Alcoholics Anonymous World Services. Twelve steps and twelve traditions. New York: Alcoholics Anonymous Publishing; 1991.
3. Anderson DJ, McGovern JP, DuPont RL. The origins of the Minnesota Model of addiction treatment – a first person account. J Addict Dis. 1999;18:107–14.
4. Spicer J. The Minnesota model: the evolution of the multidisciplinary approach to addiction recovery. Center City, MN: Hazelden Foundation; 1993.
5. Borkman TJ, Kaskutas LA, Room J, Barrows D. An historical and developmental analysis of social model programs. J Subst Abuse Treat. 1998;15(1):7–17.
6. Borkman TJ, Kaskutas LA, Owen P. Contrasting and converging philosophies of three models of alcohol/other drugs treatment: Minnesota Model, Social Model, and addiction Therapeutic Communities. Alcohol Treat Q. 2007;25(3):21–38.
7. Janzen R. The rise and fall of Synanon: a California utopia. Baltimore, MD: The Johns Hopkins Press; 2001.
8. De Leon G. Therapeutic communities for addiction: a theoretical framework. Int J Addict. 1995;30(12):1603–45.
9. McKay JR, Alterman AI, McLellan AT, Snider EC, O'Brien CP. The effect of random versus nonrandom assignment in a comparison of inpatient and day hospital rehabilitation for male alcoholics. J Consult Clin Psychol. 1995;63(1):70–8.
10. Putt CA. Outcome research in substance abuse treatment. In: Dowd ET, Rugle L, editors. Comparative treatments of substance abuse. New York: Springer Publishing Company; 1999. p. 8–49.
11. Troyer TN, Acampora AP, O'Connor LE, Berry JW. The changing relationship between therapeutic communities and 12-step programs: a survey. J Psychoactive Drugs. 1995;27 (2):177–80.

12. McLellan AT, Lewis DC, O'Brien CP, Kleber HD. Drug dependence, a chronic medical illness: implications for treatment, insurance, and outcomes evaluation. J Am Med Assoc. 2000;284(13):1689–95.
13. Thurstin AH, Alfano AM, Nerviano VJ. The efficacy of AA attendance for aftercare of inpatient alcoholics: some follow-up data. Int J Addict. 1987;22(11):1083–90.
14. Ouimette PC, Moos RH, Finney JW. Influence of outpatient treatment and 12-step group involvement on one-year substance abuse treatment outcomes. J Stud Alcohol. 1998;59(5):513–22.
15. Timko C, Moos RH, Finney JW, Lesar MD. Long-term outcomes of alcohol use disorders: comparing untreated individuals with those in Alcoholics Anonymous and formal treatment. J Stud Alcohol. 2000;61(4):529–40.
16. Kaskutas LA, Ammon LN, Weisner C. A naturalistic analysis comparing outcomes at substance abuse treatment programs with differing philosophies: social and clinical model perspectives. Int J Self Help Self Care. 2004;2(2):111–33.
17. Moos RH, Moos BS. Participation in treatment and Alcoholics Anonymous: a 16-year follow-up of initially untreated individuals. J Clin Psychol. 2006;62(6):735–50.
18. Schmidt L, Weisner C. Developments in alcoholism treatment: a ten year review. In: Galanter M, editor. Recent developments in alcoholism. New York: Plenum; 1993. p. 369–96.
19. Weisner C, McCarty D, Schmidt L. New directions in alcohol and drug treatment under managed care. Am J Manag Care. 1999;5(Special issue):SP57–69.
20. Kelly JF, Magill M, Stout RL. How do people recover from alcohol dependence? A systematic review of the research on mechanisms of behavior change in Alcoholics Anonymous. Addiction Research and Theory 2009;17(3):236–259.
21. Moos R, Schaefer J, Andrassy J, Moos B. Outpatient mental health care, self-help groups, and patients' one-year treatment outcomes. J Clin Psychol. 2001;57(3):273–87.
22 Tonigan JS, Connors GJ, Miller WR. Participation and involvement in Alcoholics Anonymous. In: Babor TF, del Boca FK, editors. Treatment matching in alcoholism. New York: Cambridge University Press; 2003. p. 184–204.
23. Kelly JF, Moos RH. Dropout from 12-step self-help groups: prevalence, predictors, and counteracting treatment influences. J Subst Abuse Treat. 2003;24:241–50.
24. Kaskutas LA, Ammon LN, Delucchi K, Room R, Bond J, Weisner C. Alcoholics Anonymous careers: patterns of AA involvement five years after treatment entry. Alcohol Clin Exp Res. 2005;29(11):1983–90.
25. Kaskutas LA, Bond J, Humphreys K. Social networks as mediators of the effect of Alcoholics Anonymous. Addiction. 2002;97(7):891–900.
26. Project MATCH Research Group. Matching alcoholism treatment to client heterogeneity: project MATCH posttreatment drinking outcomes. J Stud Alcohol. 1997;58(1):7–29.
27. Project MATCH Research Group. Matching alcoholism treatments to client heterogeneity: project MATCH three-year drinking outcomes. Alcohol Clin Exp Res. 1998;22(6):1300–11.
28. Longabaugh R, Wirtz PW, Zweben A, Stout RL. Network support for drinking, Alcoholics Anonymous and long-term matching effects. Addiction. 1998;93(9):1313–33.
29. Timko C, DeBenedetti A, Billow R. Intensive referral to 12-step self-help groups and 6-month substance use disorder outcomes. Addiction. 2006;101:678–88.
30. Timko C, Debenedetti A. A randomized controlled trial of intensive referral to12-step self-help groups: one-year outcomes. Drug Alcohol Depend. 2007;90(2–3):270–9.
31. McLellan AT, Luborsky L, Woody GE, O'Brien CP. An improved diagnostic instrument for substance abuse patients: the Addiction Severity Index. J Nerv Ment Dis. 1980;168:26–33.
32. Kahler CW, Read JP, Ramsey SE, Stuart GL, McCrady BS. Motivational enhancement for 12-step involvement among patients undergoing alcohol detoxification. J Consult Clin Psychol. 2004;72(4):736–41.
33. Maude-Griffin PM, Hohenstein JM, Humfleet GL, Reilly PM, Tusel DJ, Hall SM. Superior efficacy of cognitive-behavioral therapy for urban crack cocaine abusers: main and matching effects. J Consult Clin Psychol. 1998;66(5):832–7.

34. Roland EJ, Kaskutas LA. Alcoholics Anonymous and church involvement as predictors of sobriety among three ethnic treatment populations. Alcohol Treat Q. 2002;20(1):61–77.
35. Taylor RJ, Chatters LM. Religious life. In: Jackson JS, editor. Life in Black America. Newbury Park, CA: Sage; 1991. p. 105–23.
36. Knox DH. Spirituality: a tool in the assessment and treatment of Black alcoholics and their families. Alcohol Treat Q. 1985/1986;2(Special issue):31–44.
37. Walitzer KS, Dermen KH, Barrick C. Facilitating involvement in Alcoholics Anonymous during out-patient treatment: a randomized clinical trial. Addiction. 2009;104(3):391–401.
38. Nowinski J, Baker S. The twelve-step facilitation handbook. A systematic approach to early recovery from alcoholism and addiction. San Francisco: Jossey-Bass; 1998.
39. Project MATCH Research Group. Project MATCH: rationale and methods for a multisite clinical trial matching patients to alcoholism treatment. Alcohol Clin Exp Res. 1993;17 (6):1130–45.
40. Stinchfield R, Owen P. Hazelden's model of treatment and its outcome. Addict Behav. 1998;23(5):669–83.
41. Brook DW, Spitz HI. The group therapy off substance abuse. New York: The Haworth Medical Press; 2002.
42. Weiss RD, Jaffee WB, de Menil VP, Cogley CB. Group therapy for substance use disorders: what do we know? Harv Rev Psychiatry. 2004;12(6):339–50.
43. Flores PJ, Georgi JM. Substance abuse treatment: group therapy. Rockville, MD: Center for Substance Abuse Treatment, Substance Abuse and mental Health Services Administration; 2005.
44. Brown TG, Seraganian P, Tremblay J, Annis H. Matching substance abuse aftercare treatments to client characteristics. Addict Behav. 2002;27(4):585–604.
45. Wells EA, Peterson PL, Gainey RR, Hawkins JD, Catalano RF. Outpatient treatment for cocaine abuse: a controlled comparison of relapse prevention and twelve-step approaches. Am J Drug Alcohol Abuse. 1994;20(1):1–17.
46. Kaskutas LA, Subbaraman M, Witbrodt J, Zemore SE. Effectiveness of Making Alcoholics Anonymous Easier (MAAEZ), a group format 12-step facilitation approach. Journal of Substance Abuse Treatment 2009;37(3):228–239.
47. Cooney N, Anton RF, Carbonari J, Carroll KM, Randall C, Roberts J. Matching clients to alcoholism treatment based on psychopathology. In: Longabaugh R, Wirtz PW, editors. Project MATCH Hypotheses: Results and Casual Chain Analyses. Bethesda, MD: Natinal Institute on Alcohol Abuse and Alchoholism; 2001. p. 82–97.
48. American Psychiatric Association. Practice guideline for the treatment of patients with substance use disorders: alcohol, cocaine, opioids. Am J Psychiatry. 1995;152 Suppl 11:1–59.
49. Noordsy DL, Schwab B, Fox L, Drake EE. Role of self help programs in the rehabilitation of persons with severe mental illness and substance use disorders. Community Ment Health J. 1996;32(1):71–81.
50. Morgenstern J, Kahler CW, Epstein E. Do treatment process factors mediate the relationship between Type A-Type B and outcome in 12-step oriented substance abuse treatment? Addiction. 1998;93(12):1765–76.
51. Ouimette PC, Gima K, Moos RH, Finney JW. A comparative evaluation of substance abuse treatment IV. The effect of comorbid psychiatric diagnoses on amount of treatment, continuing care, and 1-year outcomes. Alcohol Clin Exp Res. 1999;23(3):552–7.
52. Morgenstern J, Bux Jr DA, Labouvie E, Morgan T, Blanchard KA, Muench F. Examining mechanisms of action in 12-step community outpatient treatment. Drug Alcohol Depend. 2003;72(3):237–47.
53. Alcoholics Anonymous. Comments on AA's triennial surveys. New York: Alcoholics Anonymous World Services, Inc.; 1990.
54. Book SW, Randall CL. Social anxiety disorder and alcohol use. Alcohol Res Health. 2002;26(2):130–5.

55. Winzelberg A, Humphreys K. Should patients' religiosity influence clinicians' referral to 12-step self-help groups? Evidence from a study of 3,018 male substance abuse patients. J Consult Clin Psychol. 1999;67(5):790–4.
56. Tonigan JS, Miller WR, Schermer C. Atheists, agnostics and Alcoholics Anonymous. J Stud Alcohol. 2002;63(5):534–41.
57. Ajzen I. From intentions to actions: a theory of planned behavior. In: Kuhl J, Beckmann J, editors. Action control: from cognition to behavior. New York: Springer; 1985. p. 11–40.

Chapter 4
Processes that Promote Recovery from Addictive Disorders

Rudolf H. Moos

Abstract This chapter describes four related theories about the social processes that shield individuals from developing substance use disorders and foster the long-term process of stable remission and recovery. These theories are (1) social control theory, which focuses on the provision of support, goal direction, and monitoring; (2) social learning theory with its emphasis on abstinence-oriented norms and models, (3) stress and coping theory, which highlights the importance of self-efficacy and coping skills, and (4) behavioral economics and behavioral choice theory and its focus on the role of engagement in rewarding activities other than substance use. The discussion illustrates how the social processes associated with these four theories are reflected in the active ingredients that underlie how community contexts, especially family members, friends, and self-help groups, promote recovery. A concluding section highlights some issues that need to be addressed to enhance our understanding of the social processes involved in recovery.

Keywords Addiction recovery management · Social control theory · Social learning theory · Stress and coping theory · Behavioral economics

Introduction

A number of theory-based social processes appear to protect youngsters and young adults from initiating substance use and progressing toward misuse. These processes involve bonding and obtaining goal direction and monitoring from family, friends, religion, and other aspects of traditional society; selecting and emulating individuals who model conventional behavior and shun substance use; building

R.H. Moos (✉)
Stanford University and Department of Veterans Affairs, Center for Health Care Evaluation,
795 Willow Rd. (152-MPD), Menlo Park, CA 94025, USA
e-mail: rmoos@stanford.edu

J.F. Kelly and W.L. White (eds.), *Addiction Recovery Management: Theory, Research and Practice*, Current Clinical Psychiatry, DOI 10.1007/978-1-60327-960-4_4,
© Springer Science+Business Media, LLC 2011

self-confidence and coping skills; and participating in rewarding activities that preclude or reduce the likelihood of substance use [1, 2]. The perspective espoused here is that these processes, which protect individuals from developing substance use disorders, also help individuals who have these disorders to initiate and maintain stable remission and recovery.

A considerable body of research has identified predictors of remission and recovery from substance use disorders. Although studies of treatment are often theory-based, most of the research on remission and recovery has not been guided by theory; nevertheless, many of the key findings in this literature can be conceptualized in light of specific theories. In this regard, four related theories have identified social processes that shield individuals from developing substance use problems and may facilitate their resolution: social control theory, social learning theory, stress and coping theory, and behavioral economics and behavioral choice theory [3].

Theoretical Perspectives

The four theories to be described have been employed to identify the social processes that protect individuals from initiating and developing substance use/ misuse. For example, consistent with social control theory, parental support and monitoring enhances youngsters' and young adults' bonding with family and social values and lessens the likelihood that they will develop deviant attitudes and use substances [4]. As predicted by social learning and behavioral choice theories, friends' involvement in conventional pursuits and disapproval of substance use tends to enhance prosocial modeling and participation in activities that protect youngsters and young adults from exposure to and use of substances [5, 6]. The four theories also encompass social processes that may underlie effective treatments for substance use disorders, such as cognitive–behavioral treatment, 12-step facilitation treatment, and contingency management [7].

Social Control Theory

Social control theory assumes that a network of strong bonds with family, friends, work, religion, and other aspects of traditional society serves an important regulatory function that motivates individuals to engage in responsible behavior and refrain from substance misuse and other risky pursuits [8, 9]. These bonds help to direct behavior toward acceptable goals and pursuits and encompass monitoring or supervision. When such social bonds are weak or absent, individuals are less likely to adhere to conventional standards and tend to engage in undesirable behavior, such as the misuse of alcohol and drugs. The factors underlying strong attachments to existing social standards are adequate monitoring and shaping of behavior, including cohesive and well-organized families, friends who espouse conventional values and engage in normative behavior, and reasonable goal direction and supervision in work and social settings.

Social Learning Theory

According to social learning theory, substance use develops and is maintained by specific attitudes and behaviors of an individual's social network members and role models. Modeling effects begin with observation and imitation of substance-specific behaviors, continue with social reinforcement for and expectations of positive consequences from substance use, and culminate in substance use and misuse [10, 11]. The theory proposes that substance use is a function of positive norms and expectations about substances and family members and friends who engage in and model substance use. In contrast, a social network composed of individuals who espouse abstinence, reinforce negative expectations about the effects of substances, and provide models of effective sober living can enhance the recovery process.

Stress and Coping Theory

Stress and coping theory posits that stressful life circumstances, such as interpersonal conflict, work and financial problems, and physical and sexual abuse, arouse distress and alienation and may diminish individuals' motivations to refrain from substance use. The theory assumes that life stressors are most likely to impel substance use among impulsive individuals who lack adaptive coping skills and are motivated to avoid facing problems or negative affect [12, 13]. For these individuals, substance use is a form of avoidance coping that involves self-medication to reduce depression and anxiety, which, if successful, reinforces substance use. Consistent with social learning theory, stress and coping theory assumes that enhanced self-esteem and effective coping responses can circumvent this process and contribute to stable remission and recovery.

Behavioral Economics and Behavioral Choice Theory

Behavioral economics or behavioral choice theory focuses specifically on involvement in protective activities. According to the theory, the key element of the social context is the alternative rewards provided by activities other than substance use. These rewards can protect individuals from exposure to substances and opportunities to use them, as well as from escalating and maintaining substance use. Consistent with the social control perspective, the theory posits that the provision of effective access to rewards through involvement in educational, work, religious, and social/recreational pursuits reduces the likelihood of choosing alternative rewards, such as those that may accrue from substance use [14]. For example,

Table 4.1 Key processes of social control, social learning, stress and coping, and behavioral economics and behavioral choice theories

Theory	Processes
1. Social control	Bonding or cohesion/support
	Goal direction (from family, friends, school, work, religion)
	Structure or monitoring
2. Social learning	Observation and imitation of family/peer/community norms and models
	Expectations of positive and negative consequences
3. Stress and coping	Building self-efficacy and self-confidence
	Developing effective coping skills
4. Behavioral economics/ behavioral choice	Involvement in protective activities (effective rewards from family, friends, school, work, religion, physical activity)

physical activity can elevate mood and lessen anxiety, which may make it functionally similar to and substitutable for substance use. Involvement in physical activities also often encompasses social affiliation with individuals who do not use alcohol or drugs and reinforces the decision to refrain from using these substances.

The key elements of social control theory involve bonding or support and the provision of goal direction and structure or monitoring (Table 4.1). The most important aspects of social learning theory are observation and imitation of family and social norms and models and the formation of expectations about substance use. Stress and coping theory focuses heavily on the development of self-confidence and coping skills to manage high-risk situations and general life stressors. The salient elements of behavioral economics and behavioral choice theory are fostering involvement in traditional activities that provide relevant rewards and protect individuals from temptation to use and misuse substances.

In the following sections, a review of literature focuses on the associations between the protective resources that flow from these social processes and stable remission and recovery from substance use disorders. The vast majority of the existing literature on these protective resources has involved their influence on abstinence and remission from substance use. More information is needed about how these resources enhance the broader domains involved in recovery, such as individuals' functional abilities, well-being, and overall quality of life.

Active Ingredients of Community Contexts

Support, Goal Direction, and Structure

Family Processes

Strong bonds with family members, especially a spouse or partner, who provide general support, goal direction, and supervision are associated with less substance use and a higher likelihood of abstinence. Most generally, a supportive partner, a cohesive and well-organized family, and family members' monitoring of the designated patient's substance use have been associated with stable remission from both alcohol and drug use disorders [15, 16]. In one long-term follow-up, it was found that patients in more cohesive and well-organized or structured families were more likely to be stably remitted and that they reported fewer physical symptoms and less depression at 2-year and 10-year follow-ups [17].

Patients whose relationships with a partner lasted through the first year after an episode of acute treatment had better substance use outcomes than patients whose relationship ended, perhaps due to the increased bonding and monitoring associated with a stable relationship [18]. When family members participate in treatment and/ or provide goal direction and supervision by monitoring the patient's compliance with behavioral contracts or prescribed medication, the likelihood of remission rises. In fact, continued long-term supervision by a supportive family member may be a more important determinant of remission than the pharmacological properties of a medication such as Antabuse [19]. Moreover, when a family member or partner is involved in treatment, there is a stronger association between social support and good alcohol-related outcomes [15].

The model that guides behavioral couple therapy posits that the nature and quality of the couple's marital interactions and the partner's response to alcohol-related situations influence the designated patient's alcohol consumption. McCrady and colleagues [20] followed men with alcohol problems and their wives for 6 months after marital treatment. When women confronted their husband's alcohol and marital problems by relying more on goal-directed problem solving and monitoring and less on avoidance strategies such as self-blame and wishful thinking, their husbands drank less during treatment. When the partners experienced a better relationship at treatment intake and more marital happiness at the end of treatment, the husband drank less after treatment.

Married status itself has also been associated with stable remission from alcohol and drug use, most likely because it is a proxy for increased support, goal direction, and structure. However, indices of perceived support are more strongly associated with better outcomes than is marital status per se [15]. In addition, the association between married status and better outcomes may be more robust for men than for women [21]. Married men often rate their relationship with their wives more positively than married women rate their relationship with their husbands. Women appear to provide their husbands with more general and abstinence-specific support than men provide their wives.

Friends and Broader Social Contexts

Support, goal direction, and supervision from friends and participation in traditional social contexts, such as work and religion, can enhance the process of remission. The key factors associated with remission and recovery reflect bonding or a cohesive and supportive social network, and goal direction and monitoring, that is, a social network that is clear and direct about the importance of setting and progressing toward recovery goals [16]. Accordingly, individuals who have more supportive friends and coworkers are more likely to achieve and sustain remission from substance use [22, 23].

Religious and spiritual involvement, which also provides support and supervision from concerned individuals, and goal direction as reflected in developing a stronger purpose in life have also been associated with remission from substance use, as well as more resilience and less anxiety. Recovering individuals may benefit from religious faith and spirituality, which provide a way to attribute meaning to life stressors, to confront and overcome depression and distress, and to develop a more optimistic orientation to life [24, 25]. In this regard, opioid-dependent patients in recovery describe spirituality as a source of personal strength and self-protection in that it helps them maintain abstinence and face mortality [26, 27].

General support and specific support for reducing or eliminating substance use are independently associated with short-term abstinence after treatment. Emotional and instrumental support may enhance self-confidence and provide general resources to help individuals overcome their addictive problems; as such, it tends to be more closely associated with well-being outcomes. However, the goal direction and monitoring associated with abstinence-specific support tends to be more closely associated with better substance use outcomes [28].

More broadly, there is an integral connection between these two related sources of support. Abstinence-specific support may be more helpful in improving substance use when it occurs in the context of a generally supportive relationship; the beneficial influence of general support on remission may be due to its association with abstinence-specific support. There also may be a substitution effect in that general support may be more strongly related to remission when there is less specific encouragement for abstinence [28, 29].

Abstinence-Oriented Norms and Models

Family Norms and Models

Individuals whose partners and other close family members do not have a substance use problem or espouse positive norms and model substance are much more likely to remain abstinent from alcohol and drugs after treatment than are individuals whose partners or other close family members have a substance use problem or espouse substance use [30–32]. More specifically, in one study, patients with partners who did not have a substance use problem were about twice as likely to be abstinent at a 1-year follow-up as were patients whose partners had a substance use problem [18]. In a long-term follow-up, patients whose spouse consumed less alcohol consumed less alcohol themselves and had fewer physical and depressive symptoms at a 2-year follow-up; they also consumed less alcohol at a 10-year follow-up [17].

More broadly, husbands and wives influence each other's substance use patterns. In a 9-year follow-up of men with alcohol use disorders, men married to women who did not have an alcohol use disorder were more likely to recover. Men whose wives had alcohol use disorders were more likely to continue to have alcohol use disorders themselves, as were women whose husbands continued to have alcohol-related problems. The wives of men in recovery were integrated into a social network that might have enabled them to provide more support to help reduce their husband's drinking [33].

Friend and Peer Norms and Models

Friends and peers who have abstinence-oriented norms and refrain from using substances stabilize the process of remission. With respect to alcohol use, more nondrinking friends at baseline and an increase in nondrinking friends after treatment are associated with less heavy alcohol consumption at follow-up [34]. Individuals whose social networks are composed of fewer heavy or problem drinkers and more individuals who encourage abstinence tend to drink less themselves and are likely to sustain remission over intervals as long as 5 years [22, 23, 35, 36].

Turning to drug use, individuals who have a social network composed of members who are against substance use and who report more support for maintaining abstinence are more likely to achieve and sustain remission [31, 37]. Similarly, compared with individuals who have one or more drug users in their social network, individuals who do not have a drug user in their network are more likely to refrain from drug use [38]. For example, Gogineni and colleagues [39] showed that 83% of individuals whose partner and friends did not use substances stopped using drugs, as compared to only 34% of individuals whose partner and friends used substances.

These findings apply to both treated and untreated remission. In this vein, the presence of fewer drug users and heavy drinkers in a social network has been associated with a higher likelihood of 1-year and 5-year remission among both treated and untreated individuals [35, 40–42]. In addition, recovery-oriented social networks that support individuals' efforts to abstain have been associated with the continued maintenance of abstinence at a 5-year follow-up among individuals who were abstinent 6 months after treatment, and with the reinitiation and maintenance of abstinence among patients who had relapsed 6 months after treatment [43].

Self-Efficacy and Coping Skills

There is substantial evidence that individuals' resistance self-efficacy or confidence to avoid substance use in high-risk situations is a key factor that sustains remission and contributes to stable recovery [21, 44]. More specifically, high resistance self-efficacy at intake to treatment [45], during treatment [46], and at or after discharge from treatment [31, 47, 48] is a stable predictor of better alcohol and drug use outcomes. These findings tend to hold among both women and men [21, 46] and among untreated individuals in recovery [41].

Two broad domains of coping responses have been associated with stable remission and recovery. Substance-specific coping is directed toward managing craving or temptation to use substances, whereas general coping is directed more toward coping with diverse life stressors. Substance-specific coping skills, such as focusing on the benefits of abstinence, staying away from high-risk situations, and self-reinforcement for maintaining abstinence, help to manage substance-related temptations and are associated with remission [21, 49].

More reliance on general approach coping (such as positive reappraisal and problem solving), and less on general avoidance coping (such as cognitive avoidance and emotional discharge), helps to manage stressors and tends to foreshadow stable remission and recovery [49, 50]. In a long-term follow-up, more reliance on general approach coping and less on general avoidance coping was associated with stable remission at a 2-year follow-up and less alcohol consumption and fewer physical symptoms and depressive symptoms at a 10-year follow-up [17].

Individuals in recovery perceive substance-specific strategies, such as focusing on the problems of heavy drinking and the benefits of sobriety, and general approach strategies, such as seeking support and talking with a spouse or partner, as important ways to cope with the threat of relapse [51]. In managing diverse life stressors, reliance on approach coping tends to be more effective than reliance on avoidance coping; however, when individuals are trying to manage temptation and craving for substances, cognitive avoidance and distraction may help fend off a relapse [45, 52].

Self-efficacy and coping can augment each other. According to Litt and coworkers [45], higher baseline self-efficacy predicted more improvement in coping during treatment, suggesting that self-efficacy helped individuals benefit from treatment. In turn, increased coping skills predicted better outcomes, including a higher likelihood of stable abstinence. Improvement in self-efficacy and coping skills tends to strengthen individuals' abilities to maintain stable remission and recovery despite severe stressors.

Rewarding Activities

Consistent with behavior economic and behavior choice theory, engagement in rewarding activities other than substance use is one of the key predictors of long-term recovery. Specifically, more social participation and integration in conventional pursuits, such as regular employment, alcohol-free recreational activities, and involvement in helping other people is associated with a higher likelihood of stable remission and recovery [16, 17, 53]. Religious affiliation may be associated with recovery in part because it provides intrinsic rewards and enhances the likelihood of participation in pleasurable social and altruistic activities [24, 26].

Compared with individuals who favor short-term substance-related rewards, those who expend more effort in obtaining rewards that do not involve substance use are more likely to achieve stable remission. Successful resolution of substance use problems likely involves a change in the allocation of behavior toward activities that provide rewards that can take the place of the rewards that have accrued from substance use [54]. In this vein, recovering individuals who help their peers maintain long-term sobriety after treatment are themselves better able to maintain sobriety, probably because of the social rewards that accrue from providing support for others [55].

Active Ingredients of Self-help Groups

Self-help groups (SHGs), often called mutual help or support groups, are an integral component of the system of support for individuals with substance use disorders. Participation in SHGs tends to improve the likelihood of achieving and maintaining remission and to reduce the need for professional care. SHGs offer a safe, structured setting in which members can express their feelings, improve their communication and interpersonal skills, clarify the reasons for their substance use, learn self-control, and identify new activities and life goals.

The effectiveness of SHGs in fostering recovery is based largely on four key ingredients: (1) the support, goal direction, and structure of a consistent belief system that highlights the value of strong bonds with family, friends, work, and religion; (2) abstinence-oriented norms and values and the opportunity to identify with and obtain support from abstinence-oriented role models who espouse a substance-free lifestyle; (3) an emphasis on bolstering members' self-efficacy and coping skills, and (4) involvement in rewarding activities that do not involve substance use, including service to help others overcome substance use problems and lead more satisfying lives [56].

These critical factors appear to be common change factors that underlie long-term recovery from substance abuse. Active involvement in any one of a broad variety of SHGs has been associated with a higher likelihood of long-term remission irrespective of the particular group to which an individual belongs [57].

Support, Goal Direction, and Structure

SHGs provide a context of support, goal direction, and structure in the form of a shared ideology that enhances individuals' identification with the group. The shared ideology, which is reinforced by explaining group beliefs in understandable terms, specifying changes needed to maintain sobriety, and providing guiding principles for change, helps members negotiate the recovery process. SHG norms tend to establish a group climate that fosters personal and intimate self-disclosure, an egalitarian nature, and nondifferentiated member roles. In this vein, members tell life stories aligned with SHG principles and identify with other members' contributions, thereby maintaining solidarity, communicating acceptance, and reducing the potential for conflict.

The emphasis on spirituality is a key aspect of the goal direction in 12-step SHGs. For example, AA can be seen as a spiritual recovery movement that rewards compliance with its norms by engaging individuals in a supportive and structured social system that promotes new meaning in their lives [58]. In fact, spiritual change in the context of SHG involvement contributes to the recovery process. Among patients in day hospital or residential treatment, increases in 12-step involvement from baseline to a 1-year follow-up predicted a higher likelihood of abstinence at follow-up. This relationship was partially explained by an increase in religious practices and spirituality [59]. Spirituality also helped to explain the association between affiliation with Double Trouble in Recovery (DTR) and members' health-promoting behavior [60] and may increase trauma survivors' hope and purpose in life.

More broadly, SHGs can be characterized by three sets of underlying dimensions. Relationship dimensions reflect the quality of interpersonal relationships and encompass group cohesion and support. Goal orientation dimensions reflect the key areas in which the group encourages personal growth, such as responsibility and independence, self-discovery, and spirituality. System maintenance dimensions cover the extent to which the group embodies clear expectations and effectively structures or monitors individuals' beliefs and behavior. In a study that assessed these aspects of 12-step groups, Montgomery and coworkers [61] found that AA groups had moderate to high emphasis on the relationship dimensions (cohesion and expressiveness), specific aspects of goal direction (independence, self-discovery, and spirituality), and organization. In general, members of groups with these active ingredients tend to report more satisfaction and well-being and to experience better outcomes [62].

Group cohesion and goal direction tend to strengthen group members' social networks and overall support. Accordingly, individuals who are more involved in SHGs tend to have a larger number of close friends and more support from their friends [63–65]. In one example, patients with SUDs who were more involved in 12-step groups reported sharper increases between baseline and a 1-year follow-up in the size and frequency of contact with friends, and better relationships with their friends. Compared with social networks composed mostly of non-12-step members, social networks composed mostly of 12-step group members were better integrated and more supportive [66].

Social support and goal direction may be especially important active ingredients in groups for dually diagnosed individuals. In a study of DTR, members who participated in the group more regularly enjoyed higher levels of social support and were less likely to use substances during the following year. Higher levels of group support explained part of the association between participation in the group and less subsequent substance use. In addition, the goal direction provided by learning new attitudes and skills through modeling other members' behavior was associated with better substance use outcomes [60].

Abstinence-Oriented Norms and Models

SHGs are an important source of abstinence-specific norms and support and may be especially effective in counteracting the influence of substance users in a social network. SHGs provide modeling of substance use refusal skills, ideas about how to avoid relapse-inducing situations, practical advice for staying sober, and helpful hints about how to address everyday life problems. Compared with individuals who attend 12-step SHGs irregularly after treatment, those who continue to attend SHGs regularly are more likely to have friends who refrain from alcohol and drugs and support abstinence and recovery and are more likely to attain stable remission [57, 63, 64].

More important, the increase in friends' abstinence-oriented support associated with involvement in SHGs explains part of their positive influence on remission [35, 67]. In this vein, patients who attended SHGs were more likely to have a sponsor and 12-step friends and to maintain an abstinence goal; in turn, having a sponsor, 12-step friends, and an abstinence goal were associated with a higher likelihood of 1-year and 2-year abstinence [68, 69]. Similarly, Litt and coworkers [70] found that increases in behavioral and attitudinal support for abstinence were related to a higher likelihood of abstinence at a 15-month follow-up.

Abstinence-oriented support tends to shield individuals from the potential negative influence of their substance-using friends. In this vein, clients whose social networks were highly supportive of drinking at treatment entry, but who attended AA regularly, were more likely to be abstinent at a 3-year follow-up [71]. Similarly, Bond and colleagues [23] found that individuals who had fewer heavy drinkers in their social network and more AA-based support for reducing drinking were more likely to initiate and maintain abstinence over a 3-year interval. AA-based support mediated or explained part of the relationship between AA involvement and abstinence.

In a 5-year follow-up of this sample, Kaskutas and colleagues [72] found that individuals who maintained stable AA attendance were more likely to have a sponsor and about twice the number of friends who supported cutting down or quitting drinking than did individuals with low or declining attendance. Consistent with this finding, individuals in the medium and high affiliation groups had the highest abstinence rates at the 5-year follow-up. Some individuals who had AA-based support were likely to be abstinent even though they had several heavy drinkers and drug users in their social network, indicating that such support may counter long-standing friends' pro-use social influences.

Self-Efficacy and Coping

Affiliation with AA tends to be associated with increases in members' self-efficacy and motivation for abstinence. For example, in a long-term follow-up of initially untreated individuals with alcohol use disorders, a longer duration of participation in AA in the first year after initiating help-seeking was associated with more self-efficacy to resist drinking in high-risk situations at 8-year and 16-year follow-ups. In turn, self-efficacy at 1 year was associated with less alcohol consumption and fewer drinking problems at 16 years [73, 74].

Similarly, an analysis of data from Project MATCH showed that patients who participated more in AA developed more self-efficacy to avoid drinking. Self-efficacy predicted a higher likelihood of abstinence and explained part of the association between participation in AA and abstinence. In addition, AA attendance at 6 months post-treatment predicted self-efficacy at 9 months, which predicted abstinence at 15 months. Self-efficacy to avoid drinking explained part of the effect of AA attendance on abstinence for both less severe (Type A) and more severe (Type B) alcoholic individuals [75, 76]. These findings indicate that the emphasis on powerlessness in 12-step SHGs does not detract from members' development of self-efficacy to refrain from substance use.

Self-efficacy may encompass a broader domain than simply abstinence from substance use. Affiliation with DTR has been associated with more self-efficacy for mental health recovery and more well-being; self-efficacy for recovery explained the effect of DTR group affiliation on well-being [60]. In addition, youngsters who affiliated more strongly with 12-step SHGs experienced higher self-efficacy and motivation for abstinence; in turn, self-efficacy and motivation for abstinence were associated with a higher likelihood of subsequent abstinence [77, 78].

Affiliation with 12-step SHGs strengthens reliance on specific coping responses that help to reduce substance use. For example, individuals who are more involved in AA are more likely to rely on coping skills directed toward controlling substance use, such as spending time with nondrinking friends, seeking advice about how to resolve their drinking problems, and rewarding themselves for trying to stop drinking [79]. The active ingredients of SHGs that foster improvement in coping skills likely include modeling of substance use refusal skills, ideas about how to manage relapse-inducing situations, and practical advice for coping with craving.

Participation in SHGs is also associated with improvements in general coping skills; that is, increases in approach coping and declines in avoidance coping, including the use of substances to cope with distress [65]. In one example, individuals who were more involved in 12-step groups increased more in positive reappraisal and problem-solving coping; these approach coping responses explained part of the effect of involvement in these groups on the reduction of substance use [67]. More broadly, by promoting spirituality, SHGs can enhance members' acceptance-based responding, that is, their awareness of internal experience that enables them to select and rely on more adaptive coping responses [80].

SHGs also bolster dually diagnosed individuals' coping skills, in part by providing an opportunity to share information and engage in mutual learning. For example, patients with SUDs and PTSD who were more involved in 12-step groups during treatment relied more on positive reappraisal and problem-solving coping and less on emotional discharge coping at discharge [81]. In a study that focused on the active ingredients of DTR, members who engaged more in sharing information and mutual learning were more likely to be abstinent at a 1-year follow-up [60].

The emphasis on self-efficacy, commitment to abstinence, and reliance on approach coping may be especially important common change factors and active ingredients of SHGs. In this regard, Morgenstern and colleagues [82] found that more affiliation with AA in the month after treatment was associated with increases in each of these change factors and with better substance use outcomes. Moreover, these common change factors appeared to explain all of the effect of AA affiliation on better substance use outcomes.

Rewarding Activities

Another active ingredient of SHGs involves their role in engaging members in rewarding substance-free social pursuits, such as home groups, parties, and other leisure time activities. On average, individuals who participate more in meetings and other group-related activities are more likely to socialize with close friends, be involved in sports, attend cultural events, and engage in community activities, and are more likely to achieve and maintain abstinence [17, 23, 72]. Involvement in rewarding community activities, such as religious groups, health promotion agencies, and educational and other civic organizations, has been associated with a higher likelihood of initial remission and long-term recovery [83, 84].

SHGs also provide members an opportunity to engage in altruistic pro-social behavior and help other individuals in need, which tends to increase the helper's sense of purpose, personal responsibility, self-esteem and social status, and commitment to remaining sober and recovery. Individuals who engage in more helping during treatment by volunteering, providing moral support and encouragement, and sharing their knowledge about how to remain sober and resolve other problems are more likely to become involved in 12-step groups and to achieve short-term remission [85, 86].

In a prospective study based on data drawn from Project MATCH, Pagano and colleagues [55] found that recovering individuals who became sponsors or were otherwise engaged in helping other alcoholics were more likely to maintain remission. A total of 40% of individuals who were helping others remained abstinent in the year after treatment, whereas this was true of only 22% of individuals not engaged in helping. Similarly, compared with dually diagnosed individuals who were less involved in sharing at group meetings and helping other members, those who were more involved in these activities were more likely to attain abstinence [60].

Sponsors provide other members with support and direction, 12-step instruction, ideas to help promote abstinence and improve relationships, and peer counseling and crisis intervention. Engaging in these helping activities can improve the sponsor's self-esteem and social standing, strengthen the sponsor's social network, and provide a model of successful commitment to live a sober lifestyle. Accordingly, compared with SHG members who do not become sponsors, those who become sponsors are more likely to achieve stable recovery [83, 87]. The rewards obtained from becoming a sponsor and helping other members appear to be important active ingredients of SHGs.

Common Components of Stable Recovery

Consistent with social control, social learning, stress and coping, and behavior economic theories, four sets of social processes enhance the development of personal and social resources that promote stable recovery. These processes involve social bonding, goal direction, and monitoring; abstinence-oriented models and norms, building self-esteem and coping skills, and involvement in alternative rewarding activities. Family members and friends who strengthen social bonds, goal direction, and monitoring by maintaining a cohesive and well-organized social context, offer abstinence-oriented norms and support, build individuals' self-efficacy and coping skills, and promote engagement in social and recreational pursuits that protect recovering individuals from exposure to substance use raise the likelihood of stable remission and recovery. Similarly, SHGs have a positive influence on recovery because they promote these four key social processes.

These findings are consistent with the critical factors shown to aid recovery in long-term follow-ups of individuals with substance use disorders [88, 89]: (1) forming bonds and obtaining social support from new relationships, such as a new spouse or partner or a SHG sponsor; (2) supervision or monitoring, such as by a spouse or partner or a probation or parole officer, and the provision of positive consequences for continued remission; (3) affiliation with a group that provides a sustained source of goal direction, inspiration, and structure, such as a SHG or a religion, and (4) involvement in rewarding activities that do not involve substance use, such as a program of exercise, spiritual or religious pursuits, or community volunteer and service activities. A focus on helping other individuals in need can strengthen group ties and individuals' self-worth and well-being.

Most broadly, family members', friends', and self-help groups' influence on the trajectory of recovery depends on the same social processes that protect youngsters and young adults from developing substance use problems and promote the benefits of intervention programs: Supportive relationships and structure oriented toward traditional goals, models who uphold abstinence-oriented norms, building self-confidence and coping skills, and engagement in rewarding activities [3]. The curative social processes and protective factors that underlie the resolution of addictive problems appear to be common to relationships with family members and friends, mutual aid groups, and intervention programs.

Future Directions

The discussion has focused on identifying active ingredients of recovery-oriented social contexts associated with four well-known theories that help to understand the development and maintenance of substance use and misuse. These theories are closely related and overlapping. The specific mechanisms underlying the effects of family members' and friends' orientation toward abstinence may be associated with the social bonds and surveillance posited by social control theory as well as with the norms and role modeling posited by social learning theory. Similarly, the influence of spiritual or religious involvement could be a function of role modeling as well as the formation of social bonds or the provision of rewarding substance-free activities. Thus, although social control, social learning, stress and coping, and behavior economic and behavior choice theories hold promise for understanding the process of remission and recovery, more work is needed to specify the key variables involved and to understand the mechanisms by which they exert their influence.

Specifying Linkages Between Protective Resources and Recovery

As this review has shown, active ingredients and social processes involved in community contexts provide protective resources that are associated with remission; however, we know relatively little about the robustness of these findings with respect to the broader recovery-oriented outcomes of work and social functioning, well-being, and the development of meaningful and satisfying life goals. Although it is likely that these social processes are involved, specification of the determinants of broader recovery-oriented outcomes provides a future research agenda. More knowledge about these social processes is needed to strengthen our understanding of the underlying reasons for positive behavior change, develop recovery-oriented programs, and contribute to the long-term well-being and resilience of individuals with substance use problems.

Other questions are whether some protective resources are better predictors of long-term outcomes and whether some combinations of resources promote recovery over and above single resources by themselves. In an examination of this issue, resources associated with social control theory (bonding with family members, friends, and coworkers), social learning and stress and coping theory (self-efficacy and approach coping), and behavioral economic theory (good health and adequate finances) tended to predict the maintenance of abstinence and freedom from alcohol-related problems. A summary index of protective resources was a better predictor of stable remission than any of the individual resources alone [74].

Several related issues also should be addressed. We need to know whether personal resources predict remission differently for individuals in different stages of change; for example, the coping strategies of seeking support, self-reward, and stimulus control or avoidance may be especially helpful during the action and maintenance stages. Another important question is whether elevated resources in one domain can buffer the heightened risk of remission due to lack of resources in another domain, such as when abstinence-oriented support from AA appears to counteract the negative influence of substance users in a social network [23].

Clarifying Connections Between Treatment and Protective Resources

Protective resources may bolster the beneficial influence of treatment on long-term outcome; treatment may have a stronger and more lasting effect on individuals with more resources because they live in a social context that strengthens treatment-induced change. Treatment may be less beneficial for individuals who have fewer resources because the broader social context does little to help maintain short-term change. Alternatively, there may be a compensatory relationship: brief treatment may be sufficient for individuals with more personal and social resources, whereas individuals who have fewer resources may benefit more from extended treatment.

When we examined this issue in the long-term follow-up of individuals with alcohol use problems mentioned earlier [74], we found that protective resources and treatment amplified each other; that is, the combination of more protective resources and longer treatment was associated with a higher-than-expected likelihood of remission. Among individuals who had five or more protective resources at a 1-year follow-up, 83% of those who were in treatment for 26 weeks or longer were remitted at 3 years, compared with only 54% of those who did not enter treatment. In contrast, among individuals who had no protective resources at 1 year, remission rates were comparable for those who had no treatment and those who obtained treatment for 26 weeks or longer. Future questions to address include whether specific resources interact especially strongly with treatment in general or distinct types of treatment, whether individuals with different levels of resources can be matched to varied intensities of treatment, and whether some protective resources interact with participation in SHGs to influence outcomes.

Tailoring Treatment to Strengthen Resources that Promote Recovery

Treatment and continuing care need to focus more directly on strengthening the protective resources that promote recovery. In a process akin to problem-service matching, selected components of treatment could be allocated to individuals based on the areas in which they are especially lacking in protective resources. For example, 12-step facilitation treatment may be especially effective for clients whose social network members are heavy drinkers and supportive of drinking [90]. Other potentially effective matches involve targeting social contexts in which patients report low resistance self-efficacy [91], engaging clients in pleasurable activities that can offer alternative rewards to those associated with substance use [54], and providing couple or family-based services for individuals who are prone to relapse because their family members engage in substance use.

With respect to continuing care, we need to create systems, such as Recovery Management Checkups, to monitor individuals' remission status, identify warning signs of relapse, and initiate relapse prevention training or a return to treatment [92, 93]. In this vein, Bennett and colleagues [94] developed an Early Warning Signs Relapse Prevention (EWSRP) program to raise individuals' awareness of and ability to manage warning signs that occur early in the relapse process. Compared with patients in usual aftercare, EWSRP patients were more likely to maintain abstinence and, for those who consumed alcohol, were less likely to drink heavily. This type of approach is a step toward the development of a proactive system in which individuals are monitored regularly following acute treatment in order to raise the likelihood of stable remission. Ongoing monitoring of the status of key protective resources could help identify individuals who are in need of relapse prevention or step-up services.

Conclusion

Four related theories identify social processes that promote protective factors robustly associated with the process of recovery from alcohol and drug use disorders. This chapter has focused primarily on research conducted with adults; however, comparable protective factors appear to enhance the likelihood of stable remission among adolescents [95–97]. In addition, the emphasis here has been almost entirely on social causation or how social processes can influence recovering individuals, even though recovering individuals are active agents who choose certain social contexts and elicit specific responses from their social network. Better understanding of the mutual influence of social causation and self-selection is an essential future step in learning how to enhance the long-term process of recovery.

Most important, the protective factors that encourage stable remission may be comparable to those that enable individuals to resist substance use and misuse in the first place: high-quality relationships that provide a context for social bonding, a moderate level of goal direction and structure, abstinence-oriented norms and models, an emphasis on building self-efficacy and coping skills, and activities that provide alternatives to substance use, such as engagement in work, active leisure, and service and spiritual pursuits. The social contexts that underlie the initiation and maintenance of substance misuse may hold within them the potential for resolution of the problems they create.

Key Points

1. Support, goal direction, and structure or monitoring provided by family members and friends can foster the recovery process.
2. Individuals who have a social network composed of more abstinence-oriented friends who refrain from substance use are more likely to maintain remission and progress on the road to recovery.

3. The development of self-confidence to maintain abstinence and of both substance-specific and general coping skills that enable individuals to confront high-risk situations raises the likelihood of stable remission and recovery.

4. Engagement in rewarding pursuits, such as participation in substance-free social and community activities, religious and spiritual involvement, and providing service to others tends to bolster a recovering individual's self-worth and well-being.

5. Self-help groups contribute to better substance use outcomes and to the process of recovery by providing support, goal direction, and structure; exposure to abstinent role models; a venue for building self-confidence and coping skills; and a focus for engaging in rewarding substance-free activities.

References

1. Oetting ER, Donnermeyer JF. Primary socialization theory: the etiology of drug use and deviance. Subst Use Misuse. 1998;33:995–1026.
2. Petraitis J, Flay BR, Miller TQ. Reviewing theories of adolescent substance use: organizing pieces in the puzzle. Psychol Bull. 1995;117:67–86.
3. Moos R. Social contexts and substance use. In: Miller WR, Carroll KM, editors. Rethinking substance abuse: what the science shows and what we should do about it. New York, NY: Guilford; 2006. p. 182–200.
4. Erickson KG, Crosnoe R, Dornbusch SM. A social process model of adolescent deviance: combining social control and differential association perspectives. J Youth Adolesc. 2000;29:395–425.
5. Audrain-McGovern J, Rodriquez D, Tercyak KP, Epstein LH, Goldman P, Wileyto EP. Applying a behavioral economic framework to understanding adolescent smoking. Psychol Addict Behav. 2004;18:64–73.
6. Borsari B, Carey KB. Peer influences on college drinking: a review of the research. J Subst Abuse. 2001;13:391–424.
7. Moos R. Theory-based active ingredients of effective treatments for substance use disorders. Drug Alcohol Depend. 2007;88:109–21.
8. Hirschi T. Causes of delinquency. Berkeley, CA: University of California Press; 1969.
9. Rook KS, Thuras PD, Lewis MA. Social control, health risk taking, and psychological distress among the elderly. Psychol Aging. 1990;5:327–34.
10. Bandura A. Self-efficacy: the exercise of control. New York, NY: Freeman; 1997.
11. Maisto SA, Carey KB, Bradizza CM. Social learning theory. In: Leonard KE, Blane HT, editors. Psychological theories of drinking and alcoholism. 2nd ed. New York, NY: Guilford; 1999. p. 106–63.
12. Carpenter KM, Hasin DS. Drinking to cope with negative affect and DSM-IV alcohol use disorders: a test of three alternative explanations. J Stud Alcohol. 1999;60:694–704.
13. Trim RS, Schuckit MA, Smith TL. Level of response to alcohol within the context of alcohol-related domains: an examination of longitudinal approaches assessing changes over time. Alcohol Clin Exp Res. 2008;32:472–80.
14. Bickel WK, Vuchinich RE, editors. Reframing health behavior change with behavior economics. Mahwah, NJ: Erlbaum; 2000.
15. Beattie MC. Meta-analysis of social relationships and posttreatment drinking outcomes: comparison of relationship structure, function and quality. J Stud Alcohol. 2001;62:518–27.

16. McCrady BS. To have but one true friend: implications for practice of research on alcohol use disorders and social networks. Psychol Addict Behav. 2004;18:113–21.
17. Moos R, Finney J, Cronkite R. Alcoholism treatment: context, process, and outcome. Oxford: New York, NY; 1990.
18. Tracy SW, Kelly JF, Moos R. The influence of partner status, relationship quality, and relationship stability on outcomes following intensive substance use disorder treatment. J Stud Alcohol. 2005;66:497–505.
19. Krampe H, Stawicki S, Wagner T, Bartels C, Aust C, Ruther E, et al. Follow-up of 180 alcoholic patients for up to 7 years after outpatient treatment: impact of alcohol deterrents on outcome. Alcohol Clin Exp Res. 2006;30:86–95.
20. McCrady BS, Hayaki J, Epstein EE, Hirsch LS. Testing hypothesized predictors of change in conjoint behavioral alcoholism treatment for men. Alcohol Clin Exp Res. 2002;26:463–70.
21. Walitzer KS, Dearing RL. Gender differences in alcohol and substance use relapse. Clin Psychol Rev. 2006;26:128–48.
22. Beattie MC, Longabaugh R. Interpersonal factors and post-treatment drinking and subjective well-being. Addiction. 1997;92:1507–21.
23. Bond J, Kaskutas LA, Weisner C. The persistent influence of social networks and alcoholics anonymous on abstinence. J Stud Alcohol. 2003;64:579–88.
24. Pardini D, Plante T, Sherman A, Stump J. Religious faith and spirituality in substance abuse recovery: determining the mental health benefits. J Subst Abuse Treat. 2000;19:347–54.
25. Robinson EAR, Cranford JA, Webb JR, Brower KJ. Six-month changes in spirituality, religiousness, and heavy drinking in a treatment-seeking sample. J Stud Alcohol Drugs. 2007;68:282–90.
26. Arnold RM, Avants SK, Margolin A, Marcotte D. Patient attitudes concerning the inclusion of spirituality into addiction treatment. J Subst Abuse Treat. 2002;23:319–26.
27. Flynn PM, Joe GW, Broome KM, Simpson DD, Brown BS. Recovery from opioid addiction in DATOS. J Subst Abuse Treat. 2003;25:177–86.
28. Beattie MC, Longabaugh R. General and alcohol-specific social support following treatment. Addict Behav. 1999;24:593–606.
29. Goehl L, Nunes E, Quitkin F, Hilton I. Social networks and methadone treatment outcome: the costs and benefits of social ties. Am J Drug Alcohol Abuse. 1993;19:251–62.
30. Matzger H, Delucchi K, Weisner C, Ammon LM. Does marital status predict long-term drinking? Observations from a group of problem drinking and dependent individuals. J Stud Alcohol. 2004;65:244–65.
31. McKay JR, Foltz C, Stephens RC, Leahy PJ, Crowley EM, Kissin W. Predictors of alcohol and crack cocaine use outcomes over a 3-year follow-up in treatment seekers. J Subst Abuse Treat. 2005;28 Suppl 1:S73–82.
32. Tuten M, Jones HE. A partner's drug-using status impacts women's drug treatment outcome. Drug Alcohol Depend. 2003;70:327–30.
33. McAweeney MJ, Zucker RA, Fitzgerald HE, Puttler LI, Wong MM. Individual and partner predictors of recovery from alcohol-use disorder over a nine-year interval: findings from a community sample of alcoholic married men. J Stud Alcohol. 2005;66:220–8.
34. Mohr CD, Averne S, Kenny DA, Del Boca F. "Getting by (or getting high) with a little help from my friends": an examination of adult alcoholics' friendships. J Stud Alcohol. 2001;62:637–45.
35. Weisner C, DeLucchi K, Matzger H, Schmidt L. The role of community services and informal support on five-year drinking trajectories of alcohol dependent and problem drinkers. J Stud Alcohol. 2003;64:862–73.
36. Zywiak WH, Longabaugh R, Wirtz PW. Decomposing the relationships between pretreatment social network characteristics and alcohol treatment outcome. J Stud Alcohol. 2002;63:114–21.
37. Wasserman DA, Stewart AL, Delucchi KL. Social support and abstinence from opiates and cocaine during opioid maintenance treatment. Drug Alcohol Depend. 2001;65:65–75.

38. Schroeder JR, Latkin CA, Hoover DR, Curry AD, Knowlton AR, Celentano DD. Illicit drug use in one's social network and in one's neighborhood predicts individual heroin and cocaine use. Ann Epidemiol. 2001;11:389–94.
39. Gogineni A, Stein MD, Friedmann PD. Social relationships and intravenous drug use among methadone maintenance patients. Drug Alcohol Depend. 2001;64:47–53.
40. Latkin CA, Knowlton AR, Hoover D, Mandell W. Drug network characteristics as a predictor of cessation of drug use among adult injection drug users: a prospective study. Am J Drug Alcohol Abuse. 1999;25:463–73.
41. Russell M, Peirce RS, Chan AW, Wieczorek WF, Moscato BS, Nochajski TH. Natural recovery in a community-based sample of alcoholics: study design and descriptive data. Subst Use Misuse. 2001;36:1417–41.
42. Weisner C, Matzger H, Kaskutas LA. How important is treatment? One-year outcomes of treated and untreated alcohol-dependent individuals. Addiction. 2003;98:901–11.
43. Weisner C, Ray GT, Mertens JR, Satre DD, Moore C. Short-term alcohol and drug treatment outcomes predict long-term outcome. Drug Alcohol Depend. 2003;71:281–94.
44. Haaga D, Hall SM, Haas A. Participant factors in treating substance use disorders. In: Castonguay LG, Beutler LE, editors. Principles of therapeutic change that work. New York, NY: Oxford; 2006. p. 275–92.
45. Litt MD, Kadden RM, Cooney NI, Kabela E. Coping skills and treatment outcomes in cognitive-behavioral and interactional group therapy for alcoholism. J Consult Clin Psychol. 2003;71:118–28.
46. Hufford GS, MR VLM, Nuenz LR, Costello ME, Weiss RD. The relationship of self-efficacy expectancies to relapse among alcohol dependent men and women: a prospective study. J Stud Alcohol. 2002;61:345–51.
47. Ilgen M, McKellar J, Tiet Q. Abstinence self-efficacy and abstinence one year after substance use disorder treatment. J Consult Clin Psychol. 2005;73:1175–80.
48. Stephens RS, Wertz JS, Roffman RA. Self-efficacy and marijuana cessation: a construct validity analysis. J Consult Clin Psychol. 1995;63:1022–31.
49. Moggi F, Ouimette P, Finney J, Moos R. Dual diagnosis patients in substance abuse treatment: relationships among general coping and substance-specific coping and one-year outcomes. Addiction. 1999;94:1805–16.
50. Chung T, Langenbucher J, Labouvie E, Pandina R, Moos R. Changes in alcoholic patients' coping responses predict 12-month treatment outcomes. J Consult Clin Psychol. 2001;69:92–100.
51. McKay JR, Maisto SA, O'Farrell TJ. Alcoholics' perceptions of factors in the onset and termination of relapses and the maintenance of abstinence: results from a 30-month follow-up. Psychol Addict Behav. 1996;10:167–80.
52. Gossop M, Stewart D, Browne N, Marsden J. Factors associated with abstinence, lapse or relapse to heroin use after residential treatment: protective effect of coping responses. Addiction. 2002;97:1259–67.
53. Connors GJ, Maisto SA, Zywiak WH. Understanding relapse in the broader context of post-treatment functioning. Addiction. 1996;91(Suppl):S173–89.
54. Tucker JA, Vuchinich RE, Black BC, Rippens PD. Significance of a behavioral economic index of reward value in predicting drinking problem resolution. J Consult Clin Psychol. 2006;74:317–26.
55. Pagano ME, Friend KB, Tonigan JS, Stout RL. Helping other alcoholics in alcoholics anonymous and drinking outcomes: findings from project MATCH. J Stud Alcohol. 2004;65:766–73.
56. Moos R. Active ingredients of substance use focused self-help groups. Addiction. 2008;103:387–96.
57. Atkins RG, Hawdon JE. Religiosity and participation in mutual aid support groups for addiction. J Subst Abuse Treat. 2007;33:321–31.

58. Galanter M. Spirituality and recovery in 12-step programs: an empirical model. J Subst Abuse Treat. 2007;33:265–72.
59. Zemore SE. A role for spiritual change in the benefits of 12-step involvement. Alcohol Clin Exp Res. 2007;31 Suppl 3:76S–9.
60. Magura S. Effectiveness of dual focus mutual aid for co-occurring substance use and mental health disorders: a review and synthesis of the "Double Trouble" in recovery evaluation. Subst Use Misuse. 2008;43:1904–26.
61. Montgomery HA, Miller WR, Tonigan JS. Differences among AA groups: implications for research. J Stud Alcohol. 1993;54:502–4.
62. Moos R. Group environment scale manual. 3rd ed. Menlo Park, CA: Mind Garden; 1994.
63. Davey-Rothwell MA, Kuramoto SJ, Latkin CA. Social networks, norms, and 12-step group participation. Am J Drug Alcohol Abuse. 2008;34:185–93.
64. Groh DR, Jason LA, Keys CB. Social network variables in alcoholics anonymous: a literature review. Clin Psychol Rev. 2008;28:430–50.
65. Timko C, Finney J, Moos R. The 8-year course of alcohol abuse: gender differences in social context and coping. Alcohol Clin Exp Res. 2005;29:612–21.
66. Humphreys K, Noke JM. The influence of posttreatment mutual help group participation on the friendship networks of substance abuse patients. Am J Community Psychol. 1997;25:1–16.
67. Humphreys K, Mankowski E, Moos R, Finney J. Enhanced friendship networks and active coping mediate the effect of self-help groups on substance abuse. Ann Behav Med. 1999;21:54–60.
68. Johnson J, Finney J, Moos R. End-of-treatment outcomes in cognitive-behavioral and 12-step substance use treatment programs: do they differ and do they predict 1-year outcomes? J Subst Abuse Treat. 2006;31:41–50.
69. Kelly J, McKellar JD, Moos R. Major depression in patients with substance use disorders: relationships to 12-step self-help involvement and substance use outcomes. Addiction. 2003;98:499–508.
70. Litt MD, Kadden RM, Kabela-Cormier E, Petry N. Changing network support for drinking: initial findings from the Network Support Project. J Consult Clin Psychol. 2007;75:542–55.
71. Longabaugh R, Wirtz PW, Zweben A, Stout R. Network support for drinking. In: Longabaugh R, Wirtz PW, editors. Project MATCH: hypotheses, results, and causal chain analyses. Rockville, MD: NIH; 2001. p. 260–75. NIH Publication No. 01-4238.
72. Kaskutas LA, Ammon L, Delucchi K, Room R, Bond J, Weisner C. Alcoholics anonymous careers: patterns of AA involvement five years after treatment entry. Alcohol Clin Exp Res. 2005;29:1983–90.
73. Moos R, Moos B. Participation in treatment and alcoholics anonymous: a 16-year follow-up of initially untreated individuals. J Clin Psychol. 2006;62:735–50.
74. Moos R, Moos B. Protective resources and long-term recovery from alcohol use disorders. Drug Alcohol Depend. 2007;86:46–54.
75. Bogenschutz MP, Tonigan JS, Miller WR. Examining the effects of alcoholism typology and AA attendance on self-efficacy as a mechanism of change. J Stud Alcohol. 2006;67:562–7.
76. Connors GJ, Tonigan JS, Miller WR. A longitudinal model of intake symptomatology, AA participation and outcome: retrospective study of the Project MATCH outpatient and aftercare samples. J Stud Alcohol. 2001;62:817–25.
77. Kelly JF, Myers MG. Adolescents' participation in alcoholics anonymous and narcotics anonymous: review, implications and future directions. J Psychoact Drug. 2007;39:259–69.
78. Kelly JF, Myers MG, Brown SA. Do adolescents affiliate with 12-step groups? A multivariate process model of effects. J Stud Alcohol. 2002;63:293–304.
79. Snow MG, Prochaska JO, Rossi JS. Processes of change in alcoholics anonymous: maintenance factors in long-term sobriety. J Stud Alcohol. 1994;55:362–71.
80. Carrico AW, Gifford EV, Moos R. Spirituality/religiosity promotes acceptance-based responding and twelve-step involvement. Drug Alcohol Depend. 2007;89:66–73.

81. Ouimette PC, Ahrens C, Moos R, Finney J. During treatment changes in substance abuse patients with posttraumatic stress disorder: relationships to specific interventions and program environments. J Subst Abuse Treat. 1998;15:555–64.

82. Morgenstern J, Labouvie E, McCrady BS, Kahler CW, Frey RM. Affiliation with Alcoholics Anonymous after treatment: a study of its therapeutic effects and mechanisms of action. J Consult Clin Psychol. 1997;65:768–77.

83. Crape BL, Latkin CA, Laris AS, Knowlton AR. The effects of sponsorship in 12-step treatment of injection drug users. Drug Alcohol Depend. 2002;65:291–301.

84. Kurtz LF, Fisher M. Participation in community life by AA and NA members. Contemp Drug Probl. 2003;30:873–904.

85. Zemore SE, Kaskutas LA. Twelve-step involvement and peer helping in day hospital and residential programs. Subst Use Misuse. 2008;43:1882–903.

86. Zemore SE, Kaskutas LA, Ammon LN. In 12-step groups, helping helps the helper. Addiction. 2004;99:1015–23.

87. Cross GM, Morgan CW, Mooney AJ, Martin CA, Rafter JA. Alcoholism treatment: a ten-year follow-up study. Alcohol Clin Exp Res. 1990;14:169–73.

88. Biernacki P. Pathways from heroin addiction: recovery without treatment. Philadelphia, PA: Temple University Press; 1986.

89. Vaillant GE. A 60-year follow-up of alcoholic men. Addiction. 2003;98:1043–51.

90. Longabaugh R, Wirtz PW, Zweben A, Stout RL. Network support for drinking: alcoholics anonymous and long-term matching effects. Addiction. 1998;93:1313–33.

91. Gwaltney CJ, Shiffman S, Paty JA, Liu KS, Kassel JD, Gnys M, et al. Using self-efficacy judgments to predict characteristics of lapses to smoking. J Consult Clin Psychol. 2002;70:1140–9.

92. McLellan AT, McKay JR, Forman R, Cacciola J, Kemp J. Reconsidering the evaluation of addiction treatment: from retrospective follow-up to concurrent recovery monitoring. Addiction. 2005;100:447–58.

93. Scott CK, Dennis ML, Foss MA. Utilizing recovery management checkups to shorten the cycle of relapse, treatment reentry, and recovery. Drug Alcohol Depend. 2005;78:325–38.

94. Bennett GA, Withers J, Thomas PW, Higgins DS, Bailey J, Parry L, et al. A randomized trial of early warning signs relapse prevention training in the treatment of alcohol dependence. Addict Behav. 2005;30:1111–24.

95. Chung T, Maisto SA. Relapse to alcohol and other drug use in treated adolescents: review and reconsideration of relapse as a change point in clinical course. Clin Psychol Rev. 2006;26:149–61.

96. Schell TL, Orlando M, Morral AR. Dynamic effects among patients' treatment needs, beliefs, and utilization: a prospective study of adolescents in drug treatment. Health Serv Res. 2005;40:1128–47.

97. Williams RJ, Chang SY, Addiction Centre Adolescent Research Group. A comprehensive and comparative review of adolescent substance abuse treatment outcome. Clin Psychol Sci Pract. 2000;7:138–66.

Chapter 5
Recovery Management: What If We *Really* Believed That Addiction Was a Chronic Disorder?

William L. White and John F. Kelly

Abstract Severe alcohol and other drug problems typically take a chronic course and often require multiple episodes of intervention before stable recovery is achieved. The conceptualization of addiction as a chronic disorder has critical implications for the design, delivery, evaluation, and funding of addiction treatment. Yet, despite widespread acknowledgement that the nature and long-term course of addiction is similar to other chronic illnesses, such as hypertension and diabetes, it is still treated almost universally as an acute condition. This acute care model has been shaped by a number of influences, including the commercialization of addiction treatment and a system of managed behavioral health care, which have forced treatment into discrete, and ever-briefer, episodes of care. In this chapter, we address the shortfalls of the acute care model and contrast it with a model of sustained recovery management, which aims to remedy the mismatch between the chronic nature of addiction and the approaches designed to treat it. The nature of Recovery Management as a philosophy of organizing addiction treatment and recovery support services to enhance early prerecovery engagement, recovery initiation, long-term recovery maintenance, and the quality of personal/family life in long-term recovery is described. The shift to a model of sustained recovery management includes changes in treatment practices related to the timing of service initiation, service access and engagement, assessment and service planning, service menu, service relationship, locus of service delivery, assertive linkage to indigenous recovery support resources, and the duration of posttreatment monitoring and support.

Keywords Addiction recovery management · Addiction as a chronic disorder · Treatment career · Recovery

W.L. White (✉)
Lighthouse Institute, Chestnut Health Systems, Bloomington, IL, USA
e-mail: bwhite@chestnut.org

J.F. Kelly and W.L. White (eds.), *Addiction Recovery Management: Theory, Research and Practice*, Current Clinical Psychiatry, DOI 10.1007/978-1-60327-960-4_5,
© Springer Science+Business Media, LLC 2011

Introduction

The conceptualization of addiction as a chronic disorder has profound implications for the design, delivery, evaluation, and funding of addiction treatment. This chapter provides a framework for understanding the front-line service practices that accompany the shift from an acute care model of addiction treatment to a model of sustained recovery management.

Addiction as a Chronic Disorder

Alcohol and other drug (AOD) problems present in transient (developmental or situational) and prolonged patterns [1–4]. While the former are amenable to processes of natural recovery and brief, nonspecialized professional intervention, the latter consume inordinate quantities of specialty sector addiction treatment services [5]. Clinical populations (those admitted to addiction treatment) are distinguished from those in the larger community with AOD problems by greater personal vulnerability (e.g., family history of AOD problems, early age of onset of AOD use, traumatic victimization), greater problem severity and complexity (e.g., multiple drug dependence, injection drug use, and co-occurring psychiatric illness), and by lower levels of recovery capital (internal and external recovery initiation and maintenance assets) [5].

Studies of addiction and treatment careers [6, 7] reveal that prolonged years of AOD use and related problems and multiple treatment episodes can precede the achievement of sobriety and improvements in global health. The majority (64%) of persons entering addiction treatment in the USA already have one or more prior treatment episodes, including 22% with three or four prior admissions and 19% with five or more prior admissions [8]. Addiction treatment as a cultural institution promised that it could stop the "revolving door" through which those with AOD problems cycled through local jails and hospital emergency rooms. It is rapidly becoming the new revolving door. This is not to say that recovery from even the most severe AOD problems is not possible. The recovery prevalence rate for persons meeting lifetime criteria for a substance use disorder ranges between 50 and 60% [9–12], but the processes through which such recoveries are achieved are more complex and prolonged than once thought.

McLellan et al. [13] have confirmed that severe substance use disorders share numerous characteristics with type 2 diabetes mellitus, hypertension, asthma, and other chronic health disorders. Severe substance use disorders and other chronic health disorders

- Are influenced by genetic heritability and other personal, family, and environmental risk factors
- Can be identified and diagnosed using well-validated screening questionnaires and diagnostic checklists

- Are influenced by behaviors that begin as voluntary choices but evolve into deeply ingrained patterns of behavior that, in the case of addiction, are further exacerbated by neurobiological changes in the brain that weaken volitional control over these contributing behaviors
- Are marked by a pattern of onset that may be sudden or gradual
- Have a prolonged course that varies from person to person in intensity and pattern
- Are accompanied by risks of profound pathophysiology, disability, and premature death
- Have effective treatments, self-management protocols, peer support frameworks, and similar remission rates, but no known cures [14].

Characterizing addiction as a "chronic disorder" does *not* mean that (1) all AOD problems have a prolonged, progressive course, (2) all persons with AOD problems need specialized professional treatment and long-term posttreatment monitoring and support, (3) all persons suffering from substance dependence will relapse repeatedly and require multiple treatment episodes, (4) there is minimal hope for full, long-term recovery, or (5) that persons with a chronic form of substance dependence have any less personal responsibility for illness self-management than those with diabetes or hypertensive disease [14]. To avoid contributing to addiction-related professional and social stigma, communications about addiction as a chronic disorder are best accompanied by such disclaimers.

Characterizing addiction as a chronic disorder does suggest that much could be learned by studying how individuals, families, and health care professionals actively and effectively manage other chronic health conditions. Those patterns of severe AOD problems that constitute a chronic disorder should be afforded the basic supports used in the management of other chronic health conditions, including

- Mass public education, screening, and early intervention
- Continuity of contact over a sustained period of time with a primary health care management team
- Patient/family education and empowerment to self-manage the condition (including the mobilization of family resources to support recovery initiation and maintenance)
- Access to the latest advancements in medications for symptom suppression and management
- Access to peer-based recovery support groups and advocacy organizations
- Sustained monitoring (checkups), recovery coaching (to include focus on global health via diet, exercise, sleep, and coping strategies), and when needed, early reintervention.

Addiction has been characterized as a chronic disease in the USA for more than two centuries [15], but it has been professionally treated primarily within an acute care framework. If the field of addiction treatment really believed addiction was a chronic disorder, it would not, for example,

- View prior treatment as a predictor of poor prognosis (and grounds for denial of treatment admission)
- Convey the expectation that all clients should achieve complete and enduring sobriety following a single, brief episode of treatment
- Punitively discharge clients for confirming their diagnosis (becoming symptomatic via AOD use during their treatment)
- Relegate posttreatment continuing care services to an afterthought
- Terminate the service relationship following brief intervention
- Treat serious and persistent AOD problems in serial episodes of self-contained, unlinked interventions.

The emergence of a chronic disease framework to conceptualize addiction and recovery processes opens new ways to understand the treatment process. This new view contains three critical assumptions. First, a single brief episode of professionally directed treatment in the absence of posttreatment monitoring and support rarely has the potency to generate sustainable recovery for those with the most severe and complex substance use disorders (i.e., substance dependence with co-occurring medical/psychiatric illness). This view suggests that we as a culture are placing individuals in treatment modalities of low intensity/extensity whose design offers little likelihood of sustained remission and recovery and then personally blaming the client when that success fails to materialize. Second, multiple episodes of treatment, when integrated within a long-term recovery management plan, can generate cumulative effects and constitute incremental steps in the developmental process of recovery. Third, particular combinations and sequences of professional treatment interventions and peer-based recovery support services may generate synergistic effects (dramatically elevated long-term recovery outcomes).

Recovery as a Time-Sustained Process

A growing body of scientific studies suggests that addiction recovery is a stage-dependent process [16–23]. Stage theories of addiction recovery share six core ideas.

1. Addiction recovery, like the active process of addiction, is characterized by predictable stages and milestones.
2. Movement through the stages of recovery is a time-dependent process.
3. Each stage of recovery is marked by developmental tasks that must be mastered before movement to the next stage can occur.
4. Stages of recovery can vary by characteristics of the individual; the nature, intensity, and duration of drug use; and the social milieu within which recovery occurs.
5. Developmental stages of recovery, while highly similar within subpopulations, may differ widely from subpopulation to subpopulation (e.g., by gender or age of recovery initiation) and across cultural contexts.

6. Professional interventions helpful during one stage of recovery may be ineffective or pose iatrogenic risks when applied to another stage of recovery [5].

The idea that recovery is a time-dependent process draws empirical support from studies of the durability of addiction recovery (the point at which the future risk of lifetime relapse drops below 15%). Such studies have concluded that recovery stability is achieved not in the days and months following recovery initiation but at a point years into recovery – 4–5 years for recovery from alcohol dependence and even later for recovery from heroin addiction [10, 24–28].

Viewed over a life cycle perspective, long-term addiction recovery involves a process of recovery priming (destabilization of addiction and early motivational enhancement for recovery), one or more experiments in recovery initiation and stabilization, the transition from recovery initiation to successful recovery mainte- nance, and enhancement of quality of life in long-term personal and family recovery. Current models of addiction treatment focus only on the second of these four stages. We will briefly explore how approaches to long-term recovery management address all of these stages through critical changes in treatment practices.

Evolution of the Acute Care Model of Addiction Treatment

The acute care (AC) model of addiction treatment is distinguished by the following characteristics:

- Services are delivered "programmatically" in a uniform series of encapsulated activities (screening, admission, a single point-in-time assessment, a short course of minimally individualized treatment, discharge, and brief "aftercare" followed by termination of the service relationship).
- The intervention is focused on symptom elimination for a single primary problem.
- Professional experts direct and dominate the assessment, treatment planning, and service delivery decision making.
- Services transpire over a short (and historically ever-shorter) period of time – usually as a function of a prearranged, time-limited insurance payment that is designed specifically for addiction disorders and "carved out" from general medical insurance.
- The individual/family/community is given the impression at discharge ("gradu- ation") that "cure has occurred"; long-term recovery is viewed as personally self-sustainable without ongoing professional assistance.
- The intervention is evaluated at a short-term, single point-in-time follow-up that compares pretreatment status with discharge status and posttreatment status months or at best, a few years, following professional intervention.
- Posttreatment relapse and readmissions are viewed as the failure (noncompli- ance) of the individual rather than as potential flaws in the design or execution of the treatment protocol [14].

This acute care model was shaped by the medicalization, professionalization, and commercialization of addiction treatment and a system of managed behavioral health care that forced treatment into discrete, ever-briefer episodes of care. Even modalities that involved sustained contact with those being treated (e.g., therapeutic communities and methadone maintenance) were profoundly influenced by this acute care model of intervention [5].

Recovery Management: Long-Term Recovery as an Organizing Image

A confluence of interests in the past decade sparked calls to reexamine addiction treatment as a system of care and to extend the acute care model of intervention into severe AOD problems to a model of sustained recovery management. *Recovery management* (RM) is a philosophy of organizing addiction treatment and recovery support services to enhance early prerecovery engagement, recovery initiation, *long-term* recovery maintenance, and the quality of personal/family life in long-term recovery [5]. There were concurrent calls to wrap this philosophy of recovery management within recovery-oriented systems of care (ROSC) – the creation of a larger cultural and policy climate within which long-term addiction recovery could flourish in local communities.

These *systems transformation* efforts unfolded at national, state, and local levels (see chapters in Part III of this volume) and were accompanied by efforts to define recovery [29], calls for a recovery-focused research agenda [30], and growing interest in peer-based recovery support services and new recovery support institutions (recovery community centers, recovery homes, recovery schools, recovery industries, and recovery ministries) [31, 32].

The emergence of RM and ROSC as organizing frameworks reflected a broader conceptual shift in the addictions field from a traditional focus on pathology and intervention to a focus on long-term personal and family recovery [33–35]. The rapid rise of a new recovery-focused rhetoric within the addictions field led some treatment providers to question the necessity of change as they were already recovery oriented [36] and led recovery advocates to question whether this recovery rhetoric reflected anything substantially new or was simply the application of a new cosmetic to beautify a failing service system [37].

Changes in Service Practices

Efforts to define and evaluate recovery management as an organizing framework for addiction treatment involve key treatment system performance arenas. We discuss below eight such performance arenas (1) attraction/access to treatment,

(2) assessment and level of care placement, (3) composition of the service team, (4) service relationships/roles, (5) service dose, scope, and duration, (6) locus of service delivery, (7) linkage to communities of recovery, and (8) posttreatment monitoring, support, and early reintervention. For each arena, we note the current prevailing practice and how service practices within that arena would change within a recovery management model. This comparison is based on available system performance data and the authors' involvement with recovery management (RM) initiatives across the USA.

Attraction/Access to Treatment

The AC model of addiction treatment is not able to voluntarily attract and engage the majority of individuals experiencing substance use disorders. Only 10.8% of US citizens meeting DSM-IV criteria for *substance abuse* or *substance dependence* receive specialized addiction treatment each year [38], and only 25% will receive an episode of such care in their lifetime [39]. The vast majority of people currently entering addiction treatment do so under external coercion and at late stages of problem development. Attraction is compromised by problem perception (as not that bad), perception of self (I can resolve this on my own), perception of treatment (as inaccessible, unaffordable, and ineffective), and fear of perception of others (social stigma).

Treatment access and initial engagement are also of concern. There is a 50–64% dropout rate between the call for help and the first appointment at addiction treatment agencies [40]. Access to treatment for those seeking services is plagued by ambivalence about future drug use/abstinence, lack of geographically accessible treatment, waiting lists for treatment entry, personal/family/environmental obstacles to treatment participation, and high early dropout rates. Problems of treatment attraction and engagement are magnified for women, people of color, people with co-occurring disorders, and people with low-to-moderate severity of AOD problems [5].

A primary goal of RM is reaching people at early and middle stages of AOD problem development. This is achieved through public education and anti-stigma campaigns; assertive outreach programs; assertive waiting list management (interim support); lowered thresholds of engagement; use of case management to resolve obstacles to participation; and service delivery within nonstigmatized service sites. Early engagement is enhanced by "warm welcome" techniques, streamlined intake, telephone and mail prompts for service appointments, and extended clinic hours. Implementation of such strategies has been significantly enhanced by the work of the Network for the Improvement of Addiction Treatment (NIATx) [41]. RM's assertive approach to identifying and engaging those in need of treatment services is based on a simple assumption: the earlier the timing of intervention for any chronic disease, the better the prognosis for long-term recovery and the lower the disease toll on the individual, family, and community [5].

Assessment and Level of Care Placement

AC and RM models of assessment differ significantly, as indicated in Table 5.1.

The key dimensions of the assessment process within the RM model – continual, comprehensive, asset-based, family inclusive – are congruent with the principles that guide assessment of other chronic conditions, e.g., assessment must be global and continual, based on the evidence that chronic diseases have a tendency to beget other acute and chronic problems over time.

Composition of the Service Team

The prevailing AC model of addiction treatment has several anomalies related to its service workforce. First, the model is filled with medical rhetoric (*patient*, *diagnosis*, *disease*, *treatment*, *prognosis*, etc.), but most people admitted to addiction treatment in the USA spend little face-to-face time with physicians and other primary health care professionals during the course of addiction treatment, and patients' primary care physicians have little, if any, role in that treatment. Second, there is growing awareness of the psychiatric, psychological, and social dimensions of addiction treatment and recovery, but psychiatrists, psychologists, and social workers are not routinely included in addiction treatment teams, even though the role of the addiction counselor has been clinically modeled on these roles. Third, the resurgence of recovery rhetoric in addiction treatment belies the plummeting recovery representation of addiction counselors, the loss or weakening of recovery-focused volunteer programs and alumni programs, and the weakened connections between treatment organizations and local mutual aid service committees [32].

Table 5.1 Contrasting assessment procedures in AC and RM models of addiction treatment

Assessment dimension	AC model	RM model
Primary unit of assessment	Individual	Individual, family, community
Scope	Categorical (addiction-focused)	Global (comprehensive biopsychosocial)
Focus	Deficit-based (from problems list to treatment plan)	Asset-based (focus on recovery capital – assets, strengths)
Timing	Point-in-time intake activity	Continual
Level of care placement	Based primarily on problem severity and complexity	Based on problem severity and complexity as well as personal, family, and community recovery capital
Level of care decision making	Responsibility of professional	Greater participation by client and family

Fourth, there is a growing body of evidence of the importance of posttreatment family and community support in long-term recovery [32], but family involvement and the involvement of indigenous community healers (tribal elders, clergy, sponsors) continue to be the exception rather than the rule in addiction treatment. Fifth, the excessively high turnover of the addiction treatment workforce [42] renders near impossible the achievement of the continuity of contact and support over time that characterizes the service relationships of health care providers who specialize in the management of chronic health conditions.

Several aspects of the RM philosophy seek to address these issues, including the involvement of primary care physicians in early screening, acute stabilization, and ongoing recovery checkups; the increased involvement of psychiatrists, psychologists, and social workers at key points in the long-term individual/family recovery process; the reengagement of recovering people via peer recovery support service roles; the revitalization of service work through alumni associations and volunteer programs; and the formal inclusion of indigenous healers within the treatment and recovery support team. RM advocates are also adamant that the future of RM as a philosophy of care hinges on stabilization and leadership development within the addiction treatment and peer recovery support workforce.

Service Relationships/Roles

The relationship between addiction treatment professionals and those they serve has historically been modeled on the psychotherapy relationship. Such relationships are hierarchical (expert-driven), fiduciary (one party taking responsibility for the care of the other), transient and short-term (a clearly defined beginning and end), and shaped primarily by external regulatory and payment authorities [15]. In contrast, the relationships between chronic disease specialists and their patients reflect a sustained "collaborative care" or "partnership" approach in which each patient is empowered to assume responsibility for the long-term management of his or her disorder with care team members serving as consultants to the patient and family in this process [43].

Within the RM philosophy, the role of "expert" who "treats" the client similarly gives way to a teaching, consultation, and support role focused on enhanced skills in illness self-management. The relationship becomes a long-term recovery support alliance [44] through which clients define, implement, evaluate, and refine their own recovery action plans [5, 8]. The rapid transition from professionally directed treatment plans to client-directed recovery plans is a distinct quality of the RM model [45]. The RM emphasis on "philosophy of choice" is based on the conclusion of studies that clients who are more active in their treatment rate their treatment experience (services, primary counselor, and treatment organization) more positively, remain in treatment longer, and achieve better posttreatment recovery outcomes [46–49].

Service Dose, Scope, and Duration

There is a dose effect of addiction treatment participation with recovery outcomes improving as dose increases [50–52]. The ideal minimum dose of treatment below which recovery outcomes deteriorate is 90 days of service for nonmethadone residential and outpatient programs (across levels of care) and 1 year for methadone maintenance [53–55]. The acute care model of addiction treatment is characterized by a low dose and duration of services and a limited scope of services incongruent with the needs of persons with high problem severity/complexity and low recovery capital [5]. The majority of persons entering addiction treatment in the USA consistently receive less than this optimal dose [5], and less than half of those admitted successfully complete treatment [8].

Within the RM perspective, these inadequate service doses are analogous to providing suboptimal dosages of antibiotics in the treatment of a bacterial infection; the dose may be sufficient to temporarily suppress symptoms but may contribute to the return of the illness in a more virulent and treatment-resistant form. The RM model seeks to extend the dose of recovery support by wrapping traditional treatment in a longer continuum of pretreatment and posttreatment recovery support services and expanding the menu of clinical and non-clinical recovery support adjuncts – a trend consistent with research that ancillary services can enhance recovery outcomes by 25–40% [56, 57].

Locus of Service Delivery

The acute care model of addiction treatment is based on a series of encounters between addiction professionals that occur within an institutional environment. The clinical action unfolds on the professional's turf, not the client's. RM, as a philosophy of care, draws on the recognition that the family and social environment can significantly enhance or rapidly erode the effects of these brief clinical encounters [58, 59]. It calls for understanding the ecology of long-term recovery by shifting the question of how to get someone literally and figuratively "into treatment" to the question, "How can a long-term recovery process be firmly nested within each person's natural environment, or failing that, create alternative recovery-conducive living environments within the larger community?" The latter question opens the potential to "treat" families, neighborhoods, and communities as well as individuals. It also moves the focus of recovery support from a strictly intrapersonal endeavor to one of creating family and community milieus conducive to long-term addiction recovery.

At its most practical level, RM mobilizes resources within the family and community to support recovery through three processes:

1. Outreach (extending professional recovery supports from the institutional environment into the community)
2. Inreach (involving community-based recovery support resources within the treatment milieu)
3. Recovery resource development (organizing an ever-expanding menu of recovery support resources in the community and confronting environmental conditions that constitute obstacles to long-term recovery) [32].

This broadened definition of the "client" and the emphasis on the role of community in recovery are particularly apt for treatment organizations working with clients deeply enmeshed in cultures of addiction [60].

Linkage to Communities of Recovery

Recovery mutual aid societies and other recovery support institutions (e.g., recovery community centers, recovery homes, and recovery schools) have experienced substantial membership growth, geographical dispersion, and philosophical diversification [61, 62]. Numerous studies have concluded that participation in recovery mutual aid societies can enhance long-term recovery outcomes for diverse populations [63–65], as can participation in other recovery community support institutions [66, 67]. These potentially salutary effects are offset by addiction professionals' lack of knowledge of recovery mutual aid alternatives, passive (verbal encouragement only) linkage procedures, low rates of posttreatment participation, and high posttreatment dropout rates [32, 68].

Recovery management as a philosophy of addiction treatment emphasizes the importance of assertive linkage to communities of recovery. These assertive procedures include orientation to the value of recovery support group participation; an introduction to support group choices and the philosophy, language, and meeting rituals of various groups; encouragement to set a personal goal for group participation; use of a volunteer "guide" to facilitate entry into recovery support group networks and meetings; provision of transportation to meetings; and processing responses to meetings [69, 70]. Assertive linkage to recovery support groups early in addiction treatment increases posttreatment participation rates and recovery outcomes for adults [71–73] and adolescents [74]. The same assertive linkage procedures used for recovery support groups are also used to link people to other recovery support institutions. A core belief within RM-oriented programs is that there are multiple pathways and styles of long-term recovery and that all are cause for celebration. It is assumed that all frameworks for long-term recovery maintenance will have individuals who optimally respond, partially respond, and do not respond [75], and that client choice and individualized matching afford the best personal prospects for successful long-term recovery support [76].

Posttreatment Monitoring, Support, and Early Reintervention

Two themes emerge in long-term follow-up studies: treatment effects diminish over time, and relapse rates are high [77]. The majority (over 50%) of people completing specialized addiction treatment in the US resume AOD use in the year following treatment, most within 90 days of discharge from treatment [78–80]. The rate and speed of relapse is even higher for adolescents completing addiction treatment [81]. Put simply, most individuals are fragilely balanced between recovery and read-diction in the weeks, months, and early years following their discharge from addiction treatment [82]. Between 25 and 35% of all clients discharged from addiction treatment will be readmitted to treatment within 1 year, and nearly 50% will be readmitted within 2–5 years [51, 83, 84].

In the prevailing acute care model of addiction treatment, clients are discharged with referral to another level of care or encouraged to participate in "aftercare" groups and/or a recovery mutual aid group. "Stepped care" from higher to lower intensity of service contact through an integrated continuum of care and support is the aspirational ideal of the treatment system [85], but this goal is achieved for only a minority of clients. Only one in five adults in the USA receives a significant dose of continuing care [86], and only 36% of adolescents received *any* continuing care following discharge from residential or outpatient treatment [87].

There is a growing body of scientific evidence that suggests that posttreatment monitoring (recovery check-ups) and support can elevate recovery outcomes for adults [82, 88, 89] and adolescents [90–92]. Assertive approaches to continuing care are a hallmark of the RM model. Such assertive approaches

- Encompass all admitted clients/families, not just those who successfully "graduate"
- Place primary responsibility for posttreatment contact with the treatment institution, not the client
- Involve both scheduled and unscheduled contact
- Capitalize on temporal windows of vulnerability (saturation of check-ups and support in the first 90 days following treatment) and increase monitoring and support during periods of identified vulnerability
- Individualize (increase and decrease) the duration and intensity of check-ups and support based on each client's degree of problem severity and the depth of his or her recovery capital
- Utilize assertive linkage rather than passive referral to communities of recovery
- Incorporate multiple media for sustained recovery support, e.g., face-to-face contact, telephone support, and mailed and emailed communications
- Emphasize support contacts with clients in their natural environments
- May be delivered either by counselors, recovery coaches, or trained volunteer recovery support specialists
- Emphasize continuity of contact and service (rapport building and rapport maintenance) in a primary recovery support relationship over time [76]

The eight areas of service practice reviewed in this chapter underscore the dramatic changes in service philosophy and service practice that are involved in a shift from an AC to an RM model of addiction treatment and recovery support.

Summary

The addiction treatment field is shifting its conceptual center from pathology and interventions paradigms to a recovery paradigm. This shift is indicated by efforts to extend the acute care model of addiction treatment to a model of sustained recovery management comparable to approaches through which other chronic diseases are effectively managed.

Recovery management as a treatment philosophy is being embraced within larger systems transformation efforts aimed at creating ROSC. Recovery management involves substantial changes in treatment philosophies and practices and will by necessity involve significant changes in the policy and regulatory guidelines governing addiction treatment.

Key Points

The movement from an acute care to a recovery management model of addiction treatment involves:

- Community education, outreach, and expedited service access designed to identify and engage individuals and families at early stages of AOD problem development
- Assessment protocols that are comprehensive, strengths-based, family-focused, continual, and incorporate recovery capital into level of care placement decisions
- Expanding the recovery management team to include the patient, family, primary care physicians, recovery volunteers, and other culturally indigenous recovery support resources
- Shifting the service relationship from an expert–patient relationship to a sustained recovery management partnership via rapid transition from professionally-directed treatment plans to client-directed recovery plans
- A shift in emphasis from service intensity to service extensity and a broadening menu of clinical and non-clinical recovery support services
- A greater emphasis on home-based and neighborhood-based service delivery
- Assertive linkage to communities of recovery
- Posttreatment monitoring, stage-appropriate recovery coaching, and when needed, early reintervention.

Before exploring in Part III how these efforts are unfolding at state and local levels across the country, Part II will explore in greater depth the science upon which these systems transformation efforts are based.

References

1. Harford TC, Yi H, Hilton ME. Alcohol abuse and dependence in college and noncollege samples: a ten-year prospective follow-up in a national survey. J Stud Alcohol. 2006;67:803–9.
2. Karlamangla A, Zhou K, Reuben D, Greendale G, Moore A. Longitudinal trajectories of heavy drinking in adults in the United States of America. Addiction. 2006;101:91–9.
3. Murphy SB, Reinarman C, Waldorf D. An 11-year follow-up of a network of cocaine users. Br J Addict. 1989;84:427–36.
4. Schuckit MA, Smith TL, Danko GP, Bucholz KK, Reich T, Bierut L. Five-year clinical course associated with DSM-IV alcohol abuse or dependence in a large group of men and women. Am J Psychiatry. 2001;158:1084–90.
5. White W. Recovery management and recovery-oriented systems of care: scientific rationale and promising practices. Pittsburgh, PA: Northeast Addiction Technology Transfer Center, Great Lakes Addiction Technology Transfer Center, Philadelphia Department of Behavioral Health & Mental Retardation Services; 2008.
6. Hser YI, Anglin MD. Addiction treatment and recovery careers. In: Kelly JF, White W, editors. Addiction recovery management: theory, science, and practice. New York, NY: Springer; 2010.
7. Scott CK, Dennis ML. Recovery management checkups with adult chronic substance users. In: Kelly JF, White W, editors. Addiction recovery management: theory, science, and practice. New York, NY: Springer; 2010.
8. Substance Abuse and Mental Health Services Administration, Office of Applied Studies. Treatment Episode Data Set (TEDS): 2004. Discharges from Substance Abuse Treatment Services. Rockville, MD: Substance Abuse and Mental Health Services Administration; 2006. DASIS Series: S-35, DHHS Publication No. (SMA) 06-4207. Available from: http://www.oas.samhsa.gov/TEDSdischarges/2k4/tedsd2k4toc.cfm.
9. Cunningham J. Untreated remission from drug use: the predominant pathway. Addict Behav. 1999;24:267–70.
10. Dawson DA. Correlates of past-year status among treated and untreated persons with former alcohol dependence: United States, 1992. Alcohol Clin Exp Res. 1996;20:771–9.
11. Kessler R. The National Comorbidity Survey of the United States. Int Rev Psychiatry. 1994;6:365–76.
12. Ojesjo L, Hagnell O, Otterback L. The course of alcoholism among men in the Lundby Longitudinal Study, Sweden. J Stud Alcohol. 2000;61:320–2.
13. McLellan AT, Lewis DC, O'Brien CP, Kleber HD. Drug dependence, a chronic medical illness: Implications for treatment, insurance, and outcomes evaluation. JAMA. 2000;284:1689–95.
14. White W, McLellan AT. Addiction as a chronic disease: key messages for clients, families and referral sources. Counselor. 2008;9:24–33.
15. White W. Slaying the dragon: the history of addiction treatment and recovery in America. Bloomington, IL: Chestnut Health Systems; 1998.
16. De Leon G. Integrative recovery: a stage paradigm. Subst Abuse. 1996;17:51–63.
17. De Leon G. Therapeutic community treatment in correctional settings: toward a recovery-oriented integrated system. Offender Subst Abuse Rep. 2007;7:81–96.

18. Frykholm B. The drug career. J Drug Issues. 1985;15:333–46.
19. Klingemann H. The motivation for change from problem alcohol and heroin use. Br J Addict. 1991;86:727–44.
20. Prochaska J, DiClimente C, Norcross J. In search of how people change. Am Psychol. 1992;47:1102–14.
21. Shaffer HJ, Jones SB. Quitting cocaine: the struggle against impulse. Lexington, MA: Lexington Books; 1989.
22. Waldorf D. Natural recovery from opiate addiction: some social-psychological processes of untreated recovery. J Drug Issues. 1983;13:237–80.
23. Waldorf D, Reinarman C, Murphy S. Cocaine changes: the experience of using and quitting. Philadelphia, PA: Temple University; 1991.
24. Dennis ML, Foss MA, Scott CK. An eight-year perspective on the relationship between the duration of abstinence and other aspects of recovery. Eval Rev. 2007;31:585–612.
25. Hser YI, Hoffman V, Grella C, Anglin MD. A 33-year follow-up of narcotics addicts. Arch Gen Psychiatry. 2001;58:503–8.
26. Jin H, Rourke SB, Patterson TL, Taylor MJ, Grant I. Predictors of relapse in long-term abstinent alcoholics. J Stud Alcohol. 1998;59:640–6.
27. Simpson DD, Marsh KL. Relapse and recovery among opioid addicts 12 years after treatment. In: Tims F, Leukefeld C, editors. Relapse and recovery in drug abuse. Rockville, MD: National Institute on Drug Abuse; 1986. p. 86–103. NIDA Monograph 72.
28. Vaillant GE. A long-term follow-up of male alcohol abuse. Arch Gen Psychiatry. 1996;53:243–9.
29. Betty Ford Institute Consensus Panel. What is recovery? A working definition from the Betty Ford Institute. J Subst Abuse Treat. 2007;33:221–8.
30. Laudet A. Building the science of recovery. Pittsburgh, PA: Institute for Research, Education and Training; 2009.
31. Valentine P. Peer-based recovery support services within a Recovery Community Organization: The CCAR Experience. In: Kelly JF, White W, editors. Addiction recovery management: theory, science, and practice. New York, NY: Springer; 2010.
32. White W. The mobilization of community resources to support long-term addiction recovery. J Subst Abuse Treat. 2009;36:146–58.
33. Morgan OJ. Extended length sobriety: the missing variable. Alcohol Treat Q. 1995;12:59–71.
34. White W. Recovery: its history and renaissance as an organizing construct. Alcohol Treat Q. 2005;23:3–15.
35. White W. Recovery: old wine, flavor of the month or new organizing paradigm? Subst Use Misuse. 2008;43:1987–2000.
36. Kirk T. Creating a recovery-oriented system of care. In: White W, editor. Perspectives on systems transformation: how visionary leaders are shifting addiction treatment toward a recovery-oriented system of care. Chicago, IL: Great Lakes Addiction Technology Transfer Center; 2008. p. 19–36.
37. Huffine C. Supporting recovery for older children and adolescents. Focal Point Res Policy Pract Child Ment Health. 2005;19:22–3.
38. Substance Abuse and Mental Health Services Administration. Results from the 2002 National Survey on Drug Use and Health: National Findings. Rockville, MD: Substance Abuse and Mental Health Services Administration; 2003. NHSDA Series H-22, DHHS Publication No. SMA 03-3836.
39. Dawson SA, Grant BF, Stinson FS, Chou PS, Huang B, Ruan WJ. Recovery from DSM-IV alcohol dependence: United States, 2001–2002. Addiction. 2005;100:281–92.
40. Gottheil E, Sterling RC, Weinstein SP. Pretreatment dropouts: characteristics and outcomes. J Addict Dis. 1997;16:1–14.
41. McCarty D, Gustafson DW, Wisdom J, et al. The Network for the Improvement of Addiction Treatment (NIATx): strategies to enhance access and retention. Drug Alcohol Depend. 2007;88:138–45.

42. Kaplan L. Substance abuse treatment workforce environmental scan. Rockville, MD: Center for Substance Abuse Treatment; 2003.
43. Bodenheimer T, Lorig K, Holman H, Grumbach K. Patient self-management of chronic disease in primary care. JAMA. 2002;288:2469–74.
44. White W, Boyle M, Loveland D. Alcoholism/addiction as a chronic disease: from rhetoric to clinical application. Alcohol Treat Q. 2002;20:107–30.
45. Borkman T. Is recovery planning any different from treatment planning? J Subst Abuse Treat. 1998;15:37–42.
46. Hser YI, Evans E, Huang D, Anglin MD. Relationship between drug treatment services, retention, and outcomes. Psychiatr Serv. 2004;55:767–74.
47. Nagalaksmi D, Hser YI, Boles SM, Huang YC. Do patients' perceptions of their counselors influence outcomes of drug treatment? J Subst Abuse Treat. 2002;23:327–34.
48. Sanchez-Craig M. Brief didactic treatment for alcohol and drug-related problems: an approach based on client choice. Br J Addict. 1990;85:169–77.
49. Brown TG, Seraganian P, Tremblay J, Annis H. Matching substance abuse aftercare treatments to client characteristics. Addict Behav. 2002;27:585–604.
50. Moos RH, Moos BS. Long-term influence of duration and intensity of treatment on previously untreated individuals with alcohol use disorders. Addiction. 2003;98:325–37.
51. Simpson DD, Joe GW, Fletcher BW, Hubbard RL, Anglin MD. A national evaluation of treatment outcomes for cocaine dependence. Arch Gen Psychiatry. 1999;56:507–14.
52. Zhang S, Friedmann PD, Gerstein DR. Does retention matter? Treatment duration and improvement in drug use. Addiction. 2003;98:673–84.
53. National Institute of Drug Abuse (NIDA). Principles of drug addiction treatment. Rockville, MD: National Institute on Drug Abuse; 1999. NIH Publication No. 00-4180. Available from: http://www.nida.nih.gov/PODAT/PODATIndex.html.
54. Simpson DD, Joe GW, Broome KM, Hiller ML, Knight K, Rowan-Szal GA. Program diversity and treatment retention rates in the Drug Abuse Treatment Outcome Study (DATOS). Psychol Addict Behav. 1997;11:279–93.
55. Simpson DD, Joe GW. A longitudinal evaluation of treatment engagement and recovery stages. J Subst Abuse Treat. 2004;27:99–121.
56. McLellan AT, Alterman AI, Metzger DS, et al. Similarity of outcome predictors across opiate, cocaine, and alcohol treatments: role of treatment services. J Consult Clin Psychol. 1994;62:1141–58.
57. McLellan AT, Hagan TA, Levine M, et al. Supplemental social services improve outcomes in public addiction treatment. Addiction. 1998;93:1489–99.
58. Moos RH. Addictive disorders in context: principles and puzzles of effective treatment and recovery. Psychol Addict Behav. 2003;17:3–12.
59. Simpson DD. A conceptual framework for drug treatment process and outcomes. J Subst Abuse Treat. 2004;27:99–121.
60. White W. Pathways from the culture of addiction to the culture of recovery. Center City, MN: Hazelden; 1996.
61. White W. Addiction recovery mutual aid groups: an enduring international phenomenon. Addiction. 2004;99:532–8.
62. Humphreys K. Circles of recovery: self-help organizations for addictions. Cambridge: Cambridge University Press; 2004.
63. Kaskutas LA, Subbaraman M. Integrating addiction treatment and mutual aid recovery resources. In: Kelly JF, White W, editors. Addiction recovery management: theory, science, and practice. New York, NY: Springer; 2010.
64. Kelly JF. Self-help for substance-use disorders: history, effectiveness, knowledge gaps, and research opportunities. Clin Psychol Rev. 2003;23:639–63.
65. Kelly JF, Yeterian J. Mutual-help groups. In: O'Donohue W, Cunningham JR, editors. Evidence-based adjunctive treatments. New York, NY: Elsevier; 2008. p. 61–106.

66. Jason LA, Davis MI, Ferrari JR, Bishop PD. Oxford House: a review of research and implications for substance abuse recovery and community research. J Drug Educ. 2001;31:1–27.
67. Cleveland HH, Harris KS, Baker AK, Herbert R, Dean LR. Characteristics of a collegiate recovery community: maintaining recovery in an abstinence-hostile environment. J Subst Abuse Treat. 2007;33:13–23.
68. Kelly JF, Moos R. Dropout from 12-Step self-help groups: prevalence, predictors, and counteracting treatment influences. J Subst Abuse Treat. 2003;24:241–50.
69. Timko C, DeBenedetti A, Billow R. Intensive referral to 12-Step self-help groups and 6-month substance use disorder outcomes. Addiction. 2006;101:678–88.
70. Kaskutas LA, Subbaraman M, Witbrodt J, Zemore S. Effectiveness of Making Alcoholics Anonymous Easier (MAAEZ), a group format 12-step facilitation approach. J Subst Abuse Treat. 2009;37(3):228–39.
71. Sisson RW, Mallams JH. The use of systematic encouragement and community access procedures to increase attendance at Alcoholics Anonymous and Al-Anon meetings. Am J Drug Alcohol Abuse. 1981;8:371–6.
72. Timko C, DeBenedetti A. A randomized controlled trial of intensive referral to 12-Step self-help groups: one-year outcomes. Drug Alcohol Depend. 2007;90:270–9.
73. Walitzer KS, Dermen KH, Barrick C. Facilitating involvement in Alcoholics Anonymous during out-patient treatment: a randomized clinical trial. Addiction. 2009;104:391–401.
74. Passetti LL, Godley SH. Adolescent substance abuse treatment clinicians' self-help meeting referral practices and adolescent attendance rates. J Psychoactive Drugs. 2008;40:29–40.
75. Morgenstern J, Kahler CW, Frey RM, Labouvie E. Modeling therapeutic response to 12-Step treatment: optimal responders, nonresponders, partial responders. J Subst Abuse. 1996;8:45–59.
76. White W, Kurtz E. Linking addiction treatment and communities of recovery: a primer for addiction counselors and recovery coaches. Pittsburgh, PA: IRETA/NeATTC; 2006.
77. McKay JR, Weiss RV. A review of temporal effects and outcome predictors in substance abuse treatment studies with long-term follow-ups: preliminary results and methodological issues. Eval Rev. 2001;25:13–161.
78. Anglin MD, Hser YI, Grella CE. Drug addiction and treatment careers among clients in the Drug Abuse Treatment Outcome Study (DATOS). Psychol Addict Behav. 1997;11:308–23.
79. Institute of Medicine. Bridging the gap between practice and research: forging partnerships with community-based drug and alcohol treatment. Washington, DC: National Academy Press; 1998.
80. Hubbard RL, Flynn PM, Craddock G, Fletcher B. Relapse after drug abuse treatment. In: Tims F, Leukfield C, Platt J, editors. Relapse and recovery in addictions. New Haven, CT: Yale University Press; 2001. p. 109–21.
81. Brown SA, Ramo DE. Clinical course of youth following treatment for alcohol and drug problems. In: Liddle HA, Rowe CL, editors. Adolescent substance abuse: research and clinical advances. Cambridge, NY: Cambridge University Press; 2006. p. 79–103.
82. Scott CK, Foss MA, Dennis ML. Pathways in the relapse–treatment–recovery cycle over 3 years. J Subst Abuse Treat. 2005;28:S63–72.
83. Grella CE, Hser YI, Hsieh SC. Predictors of drug treatment re-entry following relapse to cocaine use in DATOS. J Subst Abuse Treat. 2003;25:145–54.
84. Simpson DD, Joe GW, Broome KM. A national 5-year follow-up of treatment outcomes for cocaine dependence. Arch Gen Psychiatry. 2002;59:539–44.
85. Sobell LC, Sobell MB. Stepped care as a heuristic approach to the treatment of alcohol problems. J Consult Clin Psychol. 2000;68:573–9.
86. McKay JR. Effectiveness of continuing care interventions for substance abusers: implications for the study of long-term treatment effects. Eval Rev. 2001;25:211–32.
87. Godley SH, Godley MD, Dennis ML. The assertive aftercare protocol for adolescent substance abusers. In: Wagner E, Waldron H, editors. Innovations in adolescent substance abuse interventions. New York, NY: Elsevier; 2001. p. 311–29.

88. Dennis ML, Scott CK, Funk R. An experimental evaluation of recovery management checkups (RMC) for people with chronic substance use disorders. Eval Program Plann. 2003;26:339–52.
89. McKay JR. Is there a case for extended interventions for alcohol and drug use disorders? Addiction. 2005;100:1594–610.
90. Godley MD, Godley SH, Dennis ML, Funk RR, Passetti LL. The effect of assertive continuing care on continuing care linkage, adherence, and abstinence following residential treatment for adolescent substance use disorders. Addiction. 2006;102:81–93.
91. Brown SA, Ramo DE, Anderson KG. Long-term trajectories of adolescent recovery. In: Kelly JF, White W, editors. Addiction recovery management: theory, science, and practice. New York, NY: Springer; 2010.
92. Godley MD, Godley SH. Assertive continuing care for adolescents. In: Kelly JF, White W, editors. Addiction recovery management: theory, science, and practice. New York, NY: Springer; 2010.

Part II
Research Approaches and Findings

Chapter 6
Recovery Management Checkups with Adult Chronic Substance Users

Christy K. Scott and Michael L. Dennis

Abstract Models of ongoing monitoring and early reintervention occupy a central role in the long-term management of several chronic medical conditions. Such models require adaptations to address additional challenges that are common in addiction management, such as social isolation, alienation, residential instability, and multiple co-occurring problems. While the addiction field has historically been plagued by high attrition rates, utilizing a standardized tracking model (Scott, Drug Alcohol Depend 74:21–36, 2004) demonstrates the feasibility of providing ongoing monitoring via quarterly checkups. This chapter describes the Tracking, Assessing, Linking, Engaging and Retaining (TALER) protocol that was used to successfully implement Recovery Management Checkups (RMC) in two experiments involving approximately 900 participants. Results from the two experiments also demonstrate that random assignment to RMC (1) *reduces* both the time to readmission and the time spent in the community using and (2) *increases* both levels of treatment participation and rates of abstinence. In addition, the size of the effects was larger, depending on (a) the modifications made to the second experiment and (b) the length of time that RMC was used in the second experiment. Several potential benefits from adapting the RMC approach have been identified. They include better linkage to recovery support services, greater frequency of monitoring, expansion of the protocol to address co-occurring problems; and replication in other communities or subgroups such as offenders and adolescents.

Keywords Addiction recovery management · Recovery management checkups · TALER protocol

C.K. Scott (✉)
Lighthouse Institute, Chestnut Health Systems, 720 W. Chestnut Street,
Bloomington, IL 61701, USA
e-mail: cscott@chestnut.org

J.F. Kelly and W.L. White (eds.), *Addiction Recovery Management: Theory, Research and Practice*, Current Clinical Psychiatry, DOI 10.1007/978-1-60327-960-4_6,
© Springer Science+Business Media, LLC 2011

Introduction

Historically, health care systems including addiction treatment have been organized around an episodic relationship in which a person seeks treatment, receives an assessment, is treated and presumed cured – all in a relatively short period of time. When it comes to recovery from addictions, policy makers, clinicians, patients and their families as well as the general public cling to the expectation that those entering addiction treatment should, and will, maintain lifelong abstinence following a single episode of specialized treatment. The hard facts tell a different story: 50–70% of persons leaving addiction treatment will likely resume alcohol and drug use in the first year following treatment, most within the first 30–90 days [2–6]. In fact, over half the people entering treatment have been in treatment before [7], and 3–4 admissions to treatment usually are necessary before 50% or more are able to sustain abstinence for a year or more [8]. Studies conducted in a wide range of countries including Australia [9, 10], Sweden [11], Spain [12], Thailand [13], UK [14–16], and the USA [17–19] unfortunately indicate that there is a 6–11 times higher risk of death consistently associated with people who continue using in the community. Posttreatment relapse rates, multiple admissions and increased risk of mortality demonstrate the need for multiple treatments over long periods of time, invalidate the traditional assumption that a single episode of treatment should result in immediate and long-lasting positive outcomes, and challenge the adequacy of an acute care model of treatment for individuals suffering from chronic substance use. To that end, over the past decade, the addiction field has been transitioning from an acute care model toward a chronic care model.

Challenges for Managing Addiction as a Chronic Condition

Models of Ongoing Monitoring and Early Reintervention

These models occupy a central role in the long-term management of several chronic medical conditions. Some of the common objectives of these models include (a) proactively tracking patients and providing regular "checkups," (b) screening patients for early evidence of problems, (c) motivating people to make or maintain changes, (d) negotiating access to additional formal care and potential barriers to it, and (e) emphasizing early formal reintervention when problems do arise. The core assumption of these approaches is that earlier detection and reintervention will improve long-term outcomes.

When considering ways to implement monitoring and early reintervention as a mechanism for managing addiction, characteristics of the condition posed significant and unique challenges. For example, the transient, chaotic, and clandestine lifestyle that accompanies addiction often results in physical and social mobility [20–23], which generally leads to residential instability and makes it difficult to provide ongoing monitoring. Furthermore, the nature of substance-abusing lifestyles contributes not only to unstable living arrangements, but also to alienation from friends and family members [23–25]. A common feature of programs designed to help manage other chronic medical conditions is to garner the support of friends and family to help manage the patient's condition; however, the social isolation that often accompanies years of addictive substance use may prohibit this approach. The high rates of multimorbidity such as homelessness, acute psychiatric illness, and criminal justice involvement concomitant with substance abuse remain a significant barrier to the successful implementation of a chronic care model over time. Effective strategies for managing addiction as a chronic condition will need to address these difficult issues.

Tracking, Assessing, Linking, Engaging, and Retaining

TALER is defined by the research team as "a protocol for managing addiction as a chronic condition." Over the past decade, the research team has identified and tested a potentially ground-breaking protocol which comprises five components or "objectives" to be achieved [26, 27] in order to successfully manage recovery for chronic substance users. The components are: (a) *T*racking, (b) *A*ssessing, (c) *L*inking, (d) *E*ngaging, and (e) *R*etaining (TALER). Collectively, these objectives are named the *TALER Protocol*. To provide ongoing monitoring, participants' whereabouts must be "tracked." Second, valid and reliable instruments are needed to objectively "assess" which individuals need early reintervention. Third, "linkage" assistance helps motivate and physically link the participants to formal treatment or other recovery support services. Fourth, assertive follow through helps ensure that after the assessment, participants actually "engage" in the services that are recommended. Fifth, support for "retention" is needed to prevent early dropout, a common and major risk factor for relapse. The core assumption underlying the value of the TALER Protocol is that long-term monitoring and early reintervention indeed facilitate early detection of relapse, reduce the time to treatment reentry, and consequently, improve long-term participant outcomes.

The TALER Protocol provided the platform for testing one approach to managing addiction as a chronic condition – Recovery Management Checkups (RMC). These checkups do not rely on participants to self-identify their symptoms and return to treatment; instead, RMC promotes a proactive approach that includes ongoing assessments, as well as personalized feedback, which employ such techniques as motivational interviewing (MI) to involve participants in the decision-making process related to their care. The RMC intervention relies on components that identify and address barriers, and proactively supports linkage to, and retention in, more formal services. The remainder of this chapter focuses on research efforts across three studies intended to develop an effective intervention guided by the TALER protocol and evaluate the feasibility and impact on treatment outcomes.

Study Overview

The first study, Drug Outcome Monitoring Study (DOMS), was a statewide outcome study and was conducted between August 1996 and December 1997 [1]. This study tested the feasibility of successfully implementing the first two components of the TALER Protocol – tracking and assessment. The study design focused on tracking and assessing patients' progress 3 months after discharge from substance abuse treatment. Through the late 1990s, studies in the addiction field suffered from such high attrition rates that the feasibility of providing ongoing monitoring with this population was questionable. DOMS included a total of 410 (65%) adults and 222 (35%) adolescents drawn from a total of 21 treatment units across Illinois. Staff interviewed participants at baseline and again 3-month postdischarge, using the global appraisal of individual needs (GAIN) [28]. Ranging in age from 12 to 63 (mean of 27 years), the cohort was 30% female, 57% African-American, 31% Caucasian, and 6% Hispanic; 5% belonged to other racial or ethnic groups. Based on self-report, past-year criteria were met by 78% for dependence, 53% for internalizing disorders, 35% for externalizing disorders, and 54% for violence/crime problems. Most had a history of addiction treatment (78%), had been involved with the criminal justice system (83%), and were being referred to residential treatment (81%). The research team successfully located and completed assessments with 93% of the total sample (with 92% completed within 14 days). This study was a critical building block for the next two studies because it demonstrated clearly the feasibility of tracking and assessing clients in postdischarge monitoring.

The next two studies, both randomized experiments, were designed to test the feasibility of implementing additional components of the TALER Protocol and their relative effectiveness in terms of treatment outcomes via quarterly RMC. Experiment 1 started in 2000 and involved quarterly checkups for 2 years; its design and main findings have been described at length elsewhere [2, 29]. Experiment 2 began in 2004 and involved quarterly checkups over 4 years; its design and 2-year findings are described in Scott and Dennis [30]. *The 36-month findings are being reported for the first time in this chapter.*

Both experiments used the DOMS follow-up protocol [1] for tracking, the GAIN [28] for assessment, targeted the same population (people presenting for publicly funded addiction treatment), recruited from the same central intake on Chicago's west side, and included participants regardless of the level of care that had been initially recommended for them. The Experiment 1 cohort was significantly more likely than that of Experiment 2 to be younger (36 vs. 38 mean years of age), female (59 vs. 46%), African-American (85 vs. 80%), and to meet past-year criteria for dependence (87 vs. 76%), internalizing disorders (75 vs. 53%), externalizing disorders (45 vs. 33%), and violence/crime problems (60 vs. 54%). The Experiment 1 cohort was also more likely than the Experiment 2 cohort to have a history of addiction treatment (68 vs. 62%), and less likely to have had involvement with the criminal justice system (75 vs. 83%) or to be referred to residential treatment (65 vs. 81%).

Half of the participants in each experiment were randomly assigned to the experimental RMC condition. The goals of this intervention were to identify participants who were both living in the community and using, and provide them with an immediate linkage to treatment in order to expedite the recovery process. Consistent with TALER, RMC involved the following key steps: (1) locating the person for the check-up, (2) completing and assessment to determine eligibility for the intervention, (3) linking the participant to the treatment agency, (4) engaging the participant in treatment, and (5) retaining participation in treatment for at least 14 days in residential or 7 days in intensive or regular outpatient treatment. During the intervention, "Linkage Managers" (1) used motivational interviewing techniques to provide personalized feedback to participants about the status of their condition and related problems, (2) helped participants resolve ambivalence about their dependence and move toward a commitment to change by accessing additional care, (3) addressed existing barriers to treatment, (4) scheduled an assessment, and (5) facilitated reentry.

Evolution of the RMC Protocol from Experiments 1 to 2

During and after Experiment 1, it became evident that certain aspects of the TALER Protocol needed to be improved; thus the protocol was revised. As will be discussed later, the research team was easily able to replicate the tracking model from DOMS. In terms of the "assessment" objective of TALER, however, yearly lab-based urine tests revealed high rates of "false" negatives (a positive urine test for which the individual denies past-month use); furthermore, false-negative rates increased from 15 to 19% between the 12- and 24-month follow-up waves. A related problem involved participants who reported substance use in earlier interviews, but who later maintained they had never tried a given substance. The assessment protocol in the second experiment was modified to include a reminder to the participant about which drugs they had already reported using; further, it utilized on-site urine tests with the results provided to the participant prior to his or her being asked detailed questions about recency of use, drug use combinations, "recall issues," and other drug use "inconsistencies." The false-negative rate on urine tests dropped to 5% at month 12, and the rates consistently fell further during each quarter (3% at month 24, 2% at month 36).

Regarding the TALER "linkage" objective, data from Experiment 1 indicated that providing transportation increased the chances that participants would complete the intake and first treatment appointments. Therefore, starting in month 9 of Experiment 1, and throughout Experiment 2, transportation was provided. While linkage rates to treatment were good, only 39% of the people were retained in treatment for 14 days or more in Experiment 1; this time frame is important because participants who dropped out during the first 14 days were much more likely to be using at the next interview than those who did not (62 vs. 35%, odds ratio = 3.12, $p < 0.05$). To address this weakness in the protocol, highly specified treatment "engagement" and "retention" procedures were implemented in Experiment 2. These procedures included a tele-phone and face-to-face contact schedule, including an agreement between treatment and research staff that the "Linkage Manager" would have the opportunity to conduct an intervention with any and all participants who either wanted to leave treatment early or for whom staff recommended premature release. Results that discuss the feasibility of implementing the TALER Protocol and improving outcomes from the two experiments are described below.

The TALER Protocol: A Platform for Implementing RMC

To evaluate the success of implementing RMC, Table 6.1 shows the percentage of people who completed each of the five successive "steps" or objectives in the TALER Protocol: Tracking, Assessment, Linkage, Engagement, and Retention. The top section shows the results for Experiment 1 over 2 years, and the bottom section shows the results for Experiment 2 over 3 years. In both cases, this time period is shortened by 3 months, both in the beginning (the first opportunity to receive the RMC intervention) and at the end (allowing 90 days to assess the performance). For each experiment, the results are presented by wave and summar-ized at the bottom of Table 6.1. The percentage in the first column consists of "randomized" participants. Thereafter, the percentages consist of those completing the prior TALER Protocol objective. In the final row of the table, the research team has summarized the results from the two experiments and quantified the differences between waves using Cohen's d; the latter is positive when Experiment 2 is better (e.g., more people retained) and negative when Experiment 1 does better. A value (in either direction) of 0.2 will be considered as "small," 0.4 as "moderate," and 0.8 as "large." Where applicable, the problems encountered as well as the methods undertaken in the second experiment for addressing them are described in detail. Also discussed is the level of successful outcomes achieved.

Tracking: High follow-up rates were consistently achieved across waves in each experiment (93% in experiment 1 vs. 95% in experiment 2, $d = 0.13$, n.s.d.). In both cases, there was less than a 5% variation by wave in the tracking performance rate.

Assessment: Relative to Experiment 1, the assessment in Experiment 2 was more likely to identify people in need of treatment (30 vs. 44%, $d = 0.30$, $p < 0.05$). The improvement in identification was likely due to the reduced rates of false negatives associated with the on-site urine test and immediate feedback protocol discussed earlier.

Linkage: Relative to the Experiment 1, clients in need were more likely to be linked to treatment in Experiment 2 (30 vs. 42%; $d = 0.26$, $p < 0.05$). This is probably due to the addition of transportation. In the first experiment, the transpor-tation variable as well as the practice of remaining with participants throughout the duration of the intake process, was not initiated until the 9-month wave. Notice how the linkage rate soars from 11 to 18% in the first 6 months to 34–39% thereafter. This upward movement in linkage rates also helped to reduce the quarter-to-quarter

Table 6.1 Implementation of recovery management checkups

Wave	Tracking[a]	Asessment[b]	Linkage[c]	Engagement[d]	Retention[e]
Experiment 1					
3 Months	96%	32%	18%	67%	38%
6 Month	94%	27%	11%	67%	25%
9 Months	94%	29%	34%	100%	52%
12 Months	93%	37%	36%	86%	29%
15 Months	91%	31%	37%	78%	44%
18 Months	91%	26%	34%	89%	38%
21 Months	92%	27%	39%	86%	53%
Min	91%	26%	11%	67%	25%
Average	93%	30%	30%	82%	40%
Max	96%	37%	39%	100%	53%
Experiment 2					
3 Months	96%	48%	42%	86%	53%
6 Month	95%	48%	42%	79%	53%
9 Months	97%	41%	41%	81%	77%
12 Months	96%	42%	48%	77%	64%
15 Months	95%	43%	40%	75%	56%
18 Months	96%	43%	42%	77%	50%
21 Months	93%	47%	38%	86%	63%
24 Months	95%	40%	42%	75%	52%
27 Months	95%	45%	35%	88%	60%
30 Months	95%	44%	46%	86%	78%
33 Months	93%	39%	41%	79%	81%
Min	93%	39%	35%	75%	50%
Average	95%	44%	42%	81%	62%
Max	97%	48%	48%	88%	81%
Cohen's d on difference in averages[f]	0.13	**0.30***	**0.26***	−0.03	**0.53***

*$p < .05$

[a] The n completing checkup divided by the number originally randomized to RMC (224 in Experiment 1 and 223 in Experiment 2), without any discount for those who have died

[b] The number determined to be in need of treatment divided by those completing checkup

[c] The number completing treatment intake divided by those assessed as in need of treatment

[d] The number showing to first treatment session divided by those linking to intake assessment

[e] The number staying in treatment (at least 7 days for outpatient or 14 days of residential) divided by those attending first treatment session

[f] Cohen's d calculated as 2*ARCSIN (Experiment 2 average %) − 2*ARCSIN (Experiment 1 average %)

variation seen in Experiment 1 (11–39%) to half as much in Experiment 2 (35–45%).

Engagement: Once assessments were complete, the average rate of attendance at the first session of formal treatment was very similar between the experiments (81 vs. 82%, $d = −0.3$, n.s.d.). While there was more quarter-to-quarter variability in Experiment 1 (67–100%) than in Experiment 2 (75–88%), this included both the worst and best quarters between the two experiments and the differences are not statistically significant.

Retention: Relative to Experiment 1, the rate of being retained in formal treatment (staying at least 7 session days in outpatient or 14 days in residential) was
significantly higher in Experiment 2 (40 vs. 62%, $d = 0.53, p < 0.05$). In fact, the
rates in all the quarters in Experiment 2 were above the average for Experiment 1,
and all but one of the Experiment 2 quarters were "equal" or "better than" the "best"
quarter in Experiment 1. The research team attributes these improvements to the new
Engagement and Retention procedures, including working with treatment providers
to avoid discharging of any participant prior to a specialist having had the opportunity to try to address the problem.

Impact of RMC on the Course of Addiction

Within both experiments, it was hypothesized that relative to participants assigned
to the control group, RMC participants would (1) be more likely to return to
treatment sooner, (2) reenter treatment at some time, (3) reenter treatment more
times, (4) receive more total days of treatment, (5) attend more self-help group
meetings, (6) experience more days of abstinence, and (7) have fewer successive
quarters needing treatment while living in the community. The outcomes for both
experiments are shown in Table 6.2. Differences between RMC and the control
group within experiments will be described using Cohen's effect size d. For the

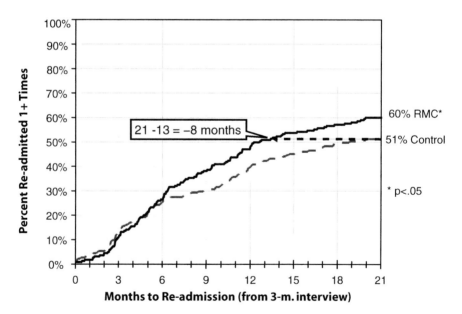

Fig. 6.1 Months to re-admission to substance treatment by condition in Experiment 1

Table 6.2 Relative effectiveness of recovery management checkups by experiment and time

Outcome variable	Recovery management checkups	Control (monitoring only)	Cohen's d
Experiment 1 (3–24 months)			
Any treatment reentry	60%	51%	**0.21***
Times reentered treatment	1.8	1.6	0.15
Total days of treatment	63	40	**0.27***
Total days of self help meetings	155	167	(0.07)
Total days of abstinence	497	490	0.04
Successive quarters needing Tx	1.9	2.3	(0.19)*
Experiment 2 (3–24 months)			
Any treatment reentry	55%	37%	**0.40***
Times reentered treatment	1.1	0.7	**0.46***
Total days of treatment	53	36	**0.23***
Total days of self help meetings	140	117	**0.26***
Total days of abstinence	480	430	**0.29***
Successive quarters needing Tx	2.6	3.4	**(0.32)***
Experiment 2 (3–36 months)			
Any treatment reentry	65%	46%	**0.46***
Times reentered treatment	1.6	0.9	**0.60***
Total days of treatment	80	58	**0.21***
Total days of self help meetings	189	163	0.12
Total days of abstinence	751	681	**0.24***
Successive quarters needing Tx	4.4	5.5	**−0.29***

*$p < 0.05$, Effect size $|d|$ of 0.2 or more is bolded

second experiment, the results are presented through year 2 (to facilitate comparison between experiments) and then again through year 3.

Experiment 1 Outcomes: Figure 6.1 illustrates the time from the 3-month interview (point of randomization and the first opportunity for RMC) to the first subsequent readmission for RMC and control participants in Experiment 1. RMC participants were significantly more likely than the control group participants to return to treatment sooner ($21-13 = 8$ months earlier, $d = +0.22, p < 0.05$). The impact on outcomes of the changes made in month 9 is best illustrated in Fig. 6.1, where one can observe that the effect on the time to reentry clearly does not start until month 9. As shown in the first section of Table 6.1, RMC participants were also significantly more likely than control participants to (1) reenter treatment at any time (60 vs. 51%, $d = 0.21, p < 0.05$), (2) receive more days of treatment, and (3) spend fewer successive quarters in the community needing treatment (1.9 vs. 2.3, $d = -0.19, p < 0.05$). There were no significant differences in the number of times they reentered treatment, the number of days of self-help meetings they attended, or the total number of days they abstained.

Experiment 2 Outcomes: Figure 6.2 shows the time from the 3-month interview (point of randomization and the first opportunity for RMC) to the first subsequent readmission for RMC and control participants in Experiment 2. RMC participants

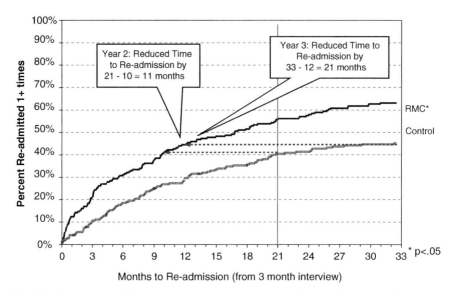

Fig. 6.2 Months to re-admission to substance treatment by condition in Experiment 2

were significantly more likely than control group participants to return to treatment much sooner during the first 2 years ($21-10 = 11$ months earlier, $d = +0.43$, $p < 0.05$) and during the first 3 years ($33-12 = 21$ months earlier, $d = 0.40$, $p < 0.05$). Note that the rate of reentry to treatment decreases over time in the control group (with very few admitted in year 3) and that the size of RMC's effect increases over time.

As shown in the second section of Table 6.1, RMC participants were also significantly more likely than control participants to reenter treatment at any time (55 vs. 37%, $d = 0.40, p < 0.05$), return to treatment more times (1.1 vs. 0.7 times, $d = 0.46$, $p < 0.05$), receive more days of treatment (53 vs. 36 days, $d = 0.23$, $p < 0.05$), have more days of abstinence (480 vs. 430 days, $d = 0.29, p < 0.05$) and spend fewer successive quarters in the community needing treatment (2.5 vs.3.4, $d = -0.19, p < 0.05$). While there was a trend for more days of self-help meetings attended, the differences were not significant (140 vs. 177 days, $d = 0.26$, n.s.d.).

As shown in the third section of Table 6.1, at year 3, the effects generally were similar or had a greater impact than at year 2. RMC participants were also significantly more likely than control participants to reenter treatment at any time (65 vs. 46%, $d = 0.46$, $p < 0.05$), return to treatment more times (1.6 vs. 0.9 times, $d = 0.60$, $p < 0.05$), receive more days of treatment (80 vs. 58 days, $d = 0.21, p < 0.05$), have more days of abstinence (751 vs. 681 days, $d = 0.24$, $p < 0.05$) and spend fewer successive quarters in the community needing treatment (4.4 vs. 5.5, $d =-0.19, p < 0.05$). There were no significant differences in days of self help-meetings attended.

Discussion

Together, the results from these studies clearly address questions related to the feasibility of using ongoing monitoring and early reintervention as a mechanism for helping individuals manage their recovery over time. By adopting the TALER Protocol, these checkups successfully addressed the duration and cyclical nature of dependence via quarterly monitoring and linkage to treatment. RMC provides a proactive approach to help participants learn to identify symptoms and resolve ambivalence about their substance use; offers the opportunity for assertive multiple episodes of care in the context of chronic care management; and includes an engagement and retention component to retain participants in treatment.

While the TALER Protocol guided the development and implementation of RMC, TALER could easily serve as a platform for managing addiction over time, using other types of approaches such as telephone counseling, recovery coaching, and case management. Furthermore, it provides a common language or performance indicator as the field transitions from an acute care model toward a long-term care model.

The feasibility of utilizing quarterly checkups as one mechanism for managing addiction over time seems well supported by these studies and others. As Orford [31] has aptly noted however, while this body of work addresses some of the shortcomings in the addiction treatment field, it also raises several other issues, not the least of which is "In what ways should the model be adapted for different populations of substance users"? Identifying the individual and environmental circumstances under which the frequency and duration of the monitoring should be adapted is an obvious place to start.

The three studies reported in this chapter focus on individuals who accessed publicly funded substance abuse treatment, reported significant levels of use, and were mostly unemployed. Given that the samples were similar, it is not known whether similar monitoring procedures would be necessary for other populations. The intensity and duration of the monitoring schedule may need to be modified as individuals progress in their recovery and/or if the regular check-up monitoring is initiated with an individual who has a less severe substance problem. Another likely adaptation might involve the entity in charge of the monitoring. Once again, individuals further into their recovery may take responsibility for their own monitoring, or they may invite family members to participate. In contrast, individuals with long, complex, and severe substance use histories may be more socially isolated and family involvement would not be a likely option. Finally, given the advances in telephone and Internet communication, testing various modes of delivery for the checkups may yield excellent results. To that end, the research team is currently surveying participants to determine the prevalence of stable access to telephone and Internet communication.

While the service options offered to participants in the second experiment were somewhat expanded as compared to the first, treatment was always presented as a first option. Given the array of continuing care, self-help, and other recovery support services, the options offered during the checkups should undoubtedly be expanded. Furthermore, improving linkages to self-help and other recovery support services, even when individuals are progressing in their recovery, enhances the opportunity to *maintain* recovery. Another significant modification to the current checkup model pertains to the mechanism used to make decisions about dealing with non-responders and on the other end of treatment, how to determine when to end a service type. In a comprehensive review, McKay [32] does an excellent job of discussing various ways to adapt current models and to develop new ones.

Implications

Addiction, like other chronic conditions, is often marked by cycles of relapse, multiple treatments, and intermittent periods of abstinence over many years before sustained recovery is reached. The implications of shifting to a chronic care model are significant and require a radical redefinition of the "continuum-of-care," as well as new service philosophies, new service delivery technologies, and a fundamental re-thinking of systems of reimbursement for addiction treatment and recovery support services.

Such a shift will also require stakeholders to address a number of critical issues. The first relates to the manner in which posttreatment monitoring, support, and early reintervention services can be integrated into the current continuum-of-care models. The next issue concerns how these services can be made readily accessible to all participants who enter treatment with high problem severity, complexity, and chronicity. The final consideration involves the organizational structure of these posttreatment recovery support services,and by whom they will be best delivered.

While the field has made solid progress in the development and testing of models for managing recovery between formal episodes of care, there remains a serious need to incorporate formal care into a chronic care model of addiction. Moreover, as the field moves forward it would be helpful to have a set of performance indicators to help communicate the success of the various approaches. For example, given the chronic nature of addiction, it is important to report the number of participants with whom the intervention was able to maintain contact, record the time period involved, note the type of assessment used to help select services, and discuss the efforts used to link, engage, and retain participants in the type of intervention offered. In the case of RMC, the TALER Protocol provided a monitoring mechanism and standardized performance indicators that focused our efforts on this long-term approach to managing addiction.

Summary of Key Points

- Models of ongoing monitoring and early reintervention occupy a central role in the long-term management of several chronic medical conditions. Such models require adaptations to address additional challenges that are common in addiction management, such as unstable living arrangements, social isolation, alienation, residential instability, and multiple co-occurring problems.

- While the addiction field has historically been plagued by high attrition rates, utilizing a standardized tracking model [1] demonstrates the feasibility of providing ongoing monitoring via quarterly checkups.
- The Tracking, Assessing, Linking, Engaging and Retaining (TALER) protocol suggests that approaches to managing addiction and long-term recovery will need to successfully achieve five distinct objectives: (a) *T*racking, (b) *A*ssessing, (c) *L*inking, (d) *E*ngaging, and (e) *R*etaining.
- The TALER Protocol was used to successfully implement RMC in two experiments involving approximately 900 participants.
- Results from the two experiments also demonstrate that random assignment to RMC: (1) *reduces* both the time to readmission as well as the time spent in the community using and (2) *increases* both levels of treatment participation as well as rates of abstinence. In addition, the size of the effects was larger depending on: (a) the modifications made to the second experiment and (b) the length of time that RMC was used in the second experiment.
- Several potential further benefits from adapting the RMC approach have been identified. They include: better linkage to recovery support services, greater frequency of monitoring, expansion of the protocol to address co-occurring problems; and replication in other communities or subgroups such as offenders and adolescents.

Acknowledgments This work was completed with support provided by the National Institute on Drug Abuse (NIDA) Grant No. DA 11323. The authors would like to thank Rod Funk and Joan Unsicker for their assistance in preparing the manuscript. The opinions are those of the authors and do not reflect official positions of the government. Any requests or comments may be sent to Dr. Christy K Scott, Chestnut Health Systems, 221 West Walton, Chicago IL 60610, 312-664-4321, cscott@chestnut.org.

References

1. Scott CK. A replicable model for achieving over 90% follow-up rates in longitudinal studies of substance abusers. Drug Alcohol Depend. 2004;74:21–36.
2. Scott CK, Foss MA, Dennis ML. Utilizing recovery management checkups to shorten the cycle of relapse, treatment reentry, and recovery. Drug Alcohol Depend. 2005;78:325–38.
3. Scott CK, Foss MA, Dennis ML. Pathways in the relapse, treatment, and recovery cycle over three years. J Subst Abuse Treat. 2005;28:S63–72.
4. Simpson DD, Joe GW, Broome KM. A national 5-year follow-up of treatment outcomes for cocaine dependence. Arch Gen Psychiatry. 2002;59:538–44.
5. Hser YI, Grella CE, Chou C-P, Anglin MD. Relationships between drug treatment careers and outcomes: findings from the National Drug Abuse Treatment Outcome Study. Eval Rev. 1998;22:496–519.
6. Godley MD, Godley SH, Dennis ML, Funk RR, Passetti LL. The effect of Assertive Continuing Care on continuing care linkage, adherence, and abstinence following residential treatment for adolescents with substance use disorders. Addiction. 2007;102:81–93.

7. Office of Applied Studies Treatment Episode Data Set – Discharges (TEDS-D), 2006. ICPSR24461-v1. Ann Arbor, MI: Inter-University Consortium for Political and Social Research [distributor]. 2009; 2009-06-22. doi:10.3886/ICPSR24461.

8. Dennis ML, Scott CK, Funk R, Foss MA. The duration and correlates of addiction and treatment careers. J Subst Abuse Treat. 2005;28:S51–62.

9. Darke S, Ross J, Teesson M. The australian treatment outcome study (ATOS): what have we learnt about treatment for heroin dependence? Drug Alcohol Rev. 2007;26(1):49–54.

10. Gibson AE, Degenhardt LJ, Hall WD. Opioid overdose deaths can occur in patients with naltrexone implants. Med J Aust. 2007;186:152–3.

11. Kristenson H, Osterling A, Nilsson JA, Lindgärde F. Prevention of alcohol-related deaths in middle-aged heavy drinkers. Alcohol Clin Exp Res. 2002;26:478–84.

12. Brugal MT, Domingo-Salvany A, Puig R, Barrio G, Garcia DO, de la Fuente L. Evaluating the impact of methadone maintenance programs on mortality due to overdose and aids in a cohort of heroin users in Spain. Addiction. 2005;100:981–9.

13. Quan VM, Vongchak T, Jittiwutikarn J, Kawichai S, Srirak N, Wiboonnatakul K, et al. Predictors of mortality among injecting and non-injecting HIV-negative users in northern Thailand. Addiction. 2007;102:441–6.

14. Copeland L, Budd J, Robertson JR, Elton RA. Changing patterns in causes of death in a cohort of injecting drug users, 1980–2001. Arch Intern Med. 2004;164:1214–20.

15. Farrell M, Marsden J. Acute risk of drug-related death among newly released prisoners in England and Wales. Addiction. 2008;103:251–5.

16. Gossop M, Stewart D, Treacy S, Marsden J. A prospective study of mortality among drug misusers during a 4-year period after seeking treatment. Addiction. 2002;97:39–47.

17. Saitz R, Gaeta J, Cheng DM, Richardson JM, Larson MJ, Samet JH. Risk of mortality during four years after substance detoxification in urban adults. J Urban Health. 2007;84:272–82.

18. Scott CK, Dennis ML, Laudet A, Funk RR, Simeone RS. Surviving drug addiction: Do treatment and adstinence reduce mortality? Am J Pub Health, in press.

19. Smyth B, Hoffman V, Fan J, Hser YI. Years of potential life lost among heroin addicts 33 years after treatment. Prev Med. 2007;44:369–74.

20. Cohen EH, Mowbray CT, Bybee D, Yeich S, Ribisl K, Freddolino PP. Tracking and follow-up methods for research on homelessness. Eval Rev. 1993;17:331–52.

21. Hansen WB, Tobler SN, Graham JW. Attrition in substance abuse prevention research. A meta-analysis of 85 longitudinal followed cohorts. Eval Rev. 1990;14:677–85.

22. Inciardi JA, Lockwood D, Pottieger AE. Women and crack-cocaine. New York: MacMillan; 1993.

23. Ziek K, Beardsley M, Deren S, Tortu S. Predictors of follow-up in a sample of urban crack users. Eval Program Plann. 1996;19:219–24.

24. Goldstein PJ, Abott W, Paige WI, Sobel I, Soto F. Tracking procedures in follow-up studies of drug abusers. Am J Drug Alcohol Abuse. 1977;4:21–30.

25. McCoy HV, Nurco DN. Locating subjects by traditional techniques. In Followup fieldwork: AIDS outreach and IV drug abuse: DHHS Publication No. 91-1736. Rockville, MD; 1991:31-73, National Institute on Drug Abuse.

26. Scott CK, Dennis ML. Recovery Management Checkups: An Early Re-Intervention Model. Chicago: Chestnut Health Systems; 2003. Available from author.

27. Dennis ML, Scott CK. Managing substance use disorders (SUD) as a chronic condition. J Addic Sci Clin Prac. 2007;4:45–55.

28. Dennis ML, Titus JC, White M, Unsicker J, Hodgkins D. Global appraisal of individual needs (GAIN): administration guide for the GAIN and related measures. Version 5. Bloomington, IL: Chestnut Health Systems; 2003.

29. Dennis ML, Scott CK, Funk R. An experimental evaluation of recovery management check-ups (RMC) for people with chronic substance use disorders. Eval Program Plann. 2003;26:339–52.

30. Scott CK, Dennis ML. Results from two randomized clinical trials evaluating the impact of quarterly recovery management checkups with adult chronic substance users. Addiction. 2009;104:959–71.
31. Orford J. Let's keep in touch: you know it makes sense. Addiction. 2009;104:972–3.
32. McKay JR. Treating substance use disorders with adaptive continuing care. Washington, DC: American Psychological Association; 2009.

Chapter 7
Assertive Continuing Care for Adolescents

Mark D. Godley and Susan H. Godley

Abstract Substance use disorders among adolescents, even treated adolescents, are perhaps more likely to result in relapse–remission cycles than among the adult population. Providing additional services for youth following discharge from treatment for substance use disorders is historically well-established and known as "aftercare" or more currently better understood as "continuing care" and viewed as a critical component of recovery management. In practice, continuing care is often a set of recommendations (relapse prevention plan) and referrals provided adolescents at the time of discharge. Unfortunately, research findings reveal relatively low rates of formal continuing care for adolescents who complete their index treatment episode and worse rates for those who leave treatment against staff advice or at staff request. Complicating matters further, adolescent patients are not as likely as their adult counterparts to attend 12-step or other mutual aid meetings. Assertive approaches to continuing care recognize that many, perhaps most, treated adolescents do not follow through with traditional referral recommendations, even if prescheduled appointment times are provided. Assertive approaches shift the responsibility for service linkage from the adolescent and his or her caregiver to a provider, care advocate (e.g., recovery coach), or other personnel who will assure continuity of care. This chapter provides a detailed description and findings from a face-to-face approach to assertive care, evaluates this approach against the Washington Circle performance measure for Continuity of Care, and ends with descriptions of several additional assertive approaches to continuing care that will be tested in the future.

Keywords Addiction recovery management · Assertive continuing care · Step-down care · Adolescent · Readiness to change

M.D. Godley (✉)
Lighthouse Institute, Chestnut Health Systems, 448 Wylie Drive,
Normal, IL 61761, USA
e-mail: mgodley@chestnut.org

J.F. Kelly and W.L. White (eds.), *Addiction Recovery Management: Theory, Research and Practice*, Current Clinical Psychiatry, DOI 10.1007/978-1-60327-960-4_7,

Introduction

Among those who treat substance use disorders, there is little debate that most adult or adolescent patients require continuing care beyond the initial care episode. Common forms of continuing care recommended after intensive outpatient or residential care are for patients to attend less-intensive outpatient aftercare groups or mutual aid meetings such as Alcoholics or Narcotics Anonymous. These types of continuing care have commonly been described as step-down care [1, 2]. Most treatment programs attempt to provide these "step-down" services, so that patients can continue to build on treatment gains. However, the more we understand about adolescents' responses to treatment, the clearer it becomes that the traditional step-down model is applicable to only a small percentage of treated adolescents. Clinical and health services research follow-up studies show that most adolescents entering treatment will experience relapse [3, 4] and many eventually return to the same or a more intensive level of treatment [5]. Complicating matters further is the low likelihood that treated adolescents initiate continuing care within the optimum time period. An examination of Fig. 7.1 shows the percentage of continuing care initiation for all adolescents discharged from a residential treatment in a Midwestern state. Only 36% of the adolescents actually received any additional treatment during the 90-day period following discharge from their index residential care episode. Of these, 20% linked with step-down care, while 15% reentered residential treatment.

These linkage data and similar findings from other state data sets suggest that the adolescent treatment system is falling substantially short of implementing the step-down care model. Research over the last decade by McLellan et al. [6], as well as others [7], makes a compelling case that the step-down model of care is at best

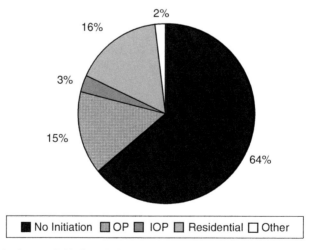

Fig. 7.1 Continuing care initiation within 90 days following residential treatment for adolescents

viable for only a small segment of patients admitted to substance abuse treatment. A more flexible model of continuing care promulgated by the American Society of Addiction Medicine [8] is based on the following definition:

> The provision of a treatment plan and organizational structure that will ensure that a patient receives whatever kind of care he or she needs at the time. The treatment program thus is flexible and tailored to the shifting needs of the patient and his or her level of readiness to change. (p. 361)

This definition better reflects the realities of a chronic condition and how it is best treated by healthcare professionals with its attendant remission–relapse cycle and the need for reintervention, than does the traditional substance abuse treatment system's linear, step-down model. McKay [2] is currently testing an adaptive continuing care model, which holds the promise of responding to patient need consistent with the ASAM continuing care definition. Adaptive continuing care includes (1) long-term monitoring; (2) flexible treatment that changes in response to information from monitoring findings; (3) attention to patient preference for choice of treatment component; (4) a reduction of patient burden over time through the use of nontraditional care settings (e.g., teletherapy); and (5) an emphasis on the role of self-care.

While the ASAM continuing care definition and adaptive care approaches appear to be a more realistic fit with the nature and course of substance use disorders and recovery for most patients, the current treatment system has limited success in providing continuity of care to adolescents entering treatment. We believe that a number of barriers in the treatment system adversely affect linkage to continuing care after a primary treatment episode. We also suspect that often more than one barrier will exist for adolescents, thus increasing the difficulty of accessing continued care.

Treatment System Barriers to Continuing Care

In our developmental work on assertive approaches to continuing care, we have identified a number of potential barriers to participation in continuing care through examination of empirical data or observation. These barriers are described below.

Discharge type and location of patient's residence. One investigation into reasons why adolescents failed to initiate continuing care was based on an examination of data from four organizations receiving grant funds under the Adolescent Residential Treatment grant initiative funded by SAMHSA's Center for Substance Abuse Treatment. In this initiative, grantees were required to develop continuing care services so that adolescents leaving residential treatment were well served and supported with continuing care outpatient services when they returned to their community. Participating treatment programs were selected because their data provided the type of discharge from residential treatment and the date of the first continuing care service.

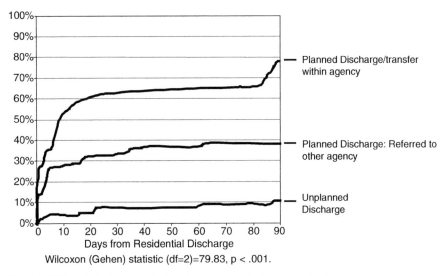

Fig. 7.2 Effect of discharge and referral type on continuing care initiation

Figure 7.2 shows that successful initiation of continuing care was most likely to occur for patients who successfully completed residential treatment and transferred to continuing care within the same organization. Under this set of criteria, nearly 60% initiated continuing care within 2 weeks. The initiation rate dropped by 50% for those who had completed treatment and needed to be transferred to another organization (presumably because they were in another treatment provider's catchment area). For those who left treatment against staff advice or were asked to leave, their rate of initiating continuing care was 5% at 2 weeks and 10% after 90 days. In the USA, most residential treatment for adolescents is regional, thus making it likely that adolescents returning home will be asked to seek continuing care from a different treatment provider. It is clear, however, that another barrier is the circumstances under which an adolescent leaves residential treatment. Those who have a less than favorable discharge are less likely to initiate continuing care. The extent to which favorable or planned discharges from treatment occur is likely to vary widely depending on treatment approach, case mix, organizational and clinical staff, and a host of other factors. However, research conducted in the USA indicates that across all treatment modalities, the median length of treatment is 50 days and 53% of admitted adolescents experience unfavorable discharges [9].

Medical model. Substance abuse outpatient treatment follows a medical model in the sense that like physicians, substance abuse treatment therapists see patients in their outpatient clinics. In their practices, physicians diagnose, prescribe, and treat trauma or illnesses that cause physical complications and pain, and if left untreated, may become life threatening. In general, people with medical issues do what it takes to attend their medical appointments, including enduring unfavorable appointment times and long waits to see their doctor. The clinic-based service delivery model works reasonably well in medicine. But do the same assumptions apply to those referred for treatment of a substance use disorder? In the case of adolescents, the vast majority are referred to treatment against their wishes by juvenile justice referrals, followed by school or other community resource. Family referrals are relatively few, and self-referrals are almost nonexistent. While it seems reasonable to assume that juvenile justice consequences would be severe for failure to show, the consequences appear to be uneven at best. Within juvenile justice, the greatest source of referrals is from juvenile probation officers. Unfortunately, juvenile probation officers are few and their caseloads large, making it very difficult to monitor, and harder yet to provide timely consequences for missed appointments. This problem can become further complicated in promoting continuing care if the adolescent has already attended an initial treatment episode (e.g., residential), and the probation officer does not fully appreciate the need for extended monitoring, support, or treatment. Drug courts for adolescents stand as an exception, but they are few in number in the USA. Where they do exist, such drug courts have reasonable patient loads and can provide almost immediate court-ordered sanctions for missed appointments. In summary, the physical symptoms of pain or life threatening illness that lead people to attend outpatient medical clinics are not present among adolescents with substance use disorders and adolescents have notoriously low levels of intrinsic motivation for treatment, thus reducing the likelihood that they will regularly attend treatment appointments at a clinic.

Resource issues. Even if there was sufficient external (e.g., school, juvenile justice), family, or self-motivation to attend treatment, resource barriers exist for a large segment of the adolescents referred for treatment. In a national sample of adolescents in treatment, almost half reported that they lived in single-parent households [9, 10], thus reliance on a parent for transportation to weekly or daily treatment attendance may conflict with work schedules or other child-care responsibilities. Moreover, most adolescents in treatment either lack a driver's license, an automobile, or both [11]. Traveling by public transportation may be feasible in major metropolitan areas, but there could be barriers associated with public transportation (e.g., fare costs, transit times and routes, and gang concerns) as well.

Family or personal crises. Many adolescent patients are members of families where one or more siblings or caregivers may be involved in legal, medical, employment, or relationship crises, and these problems may occur with some frequency. Such problems may command family members' attention and time to be focused elsewhere such that the adolescent and their caregiver(s) either forget about attending treatment appointments or no longer see it as a priority, given the crisis occurring in the present.

Treatment fatigue or demoralization. By definition, a continuing care episode means that the adolescent has already participated in a prior treatment episode. Many adolescent patients appear to become weary of treatment and want to finish it.

To the extent that treatment programs do not give patients a clear expectation for how long the acute phase of treatment will last, this may be especially true. Demoralization as a response to a relapse may also contribute to patients failing to attend continuing care appointments. Failing to appreciate or understand the need for long-term clinic monitoring and support to succeed at making significant lifestyle changes is by no means unique to those with substance use disorders. McLellan et al. [6] report that for adults, sustaining lifestyle changes that could dramatically improve the quality of life and prevent symptom exacerbation is difficult whether the chronic condition is hypertension, diabetes, or a substance use disorder.

Clinician change. For those adolescents who do initiate continuing care, there is a reasonably good chance that the counselor they start with will resign, be reassigned, or promoted. Treatment programs have clinical staff turnover rates of 50% [12]. In a recent federally sponsored implementation of an evidence-based treatment at over 30 adolescent treatment sites, annual turnover rates were 34% during the first year of the project [13], and such turnover may have a cascading effect on those who remain. For example, if a supervisor leaves or gets promoted, the likelihood of promotion for one of the counselors is quite high, but this means a new counselor must be hired and many patients will be transferred. Such transfers create barriers to continuity of care and may result in loss of patients. Although the problem of clinician turnover is not easily studied, it is likely to play a significant role in care discontinuity for many patients.

Treatment reimbursement mechanisms. The most common form of payment for medical and behavioral treatment is the fee-for-service model. Under this form of reimbursement, treatment provider organizations are paid a fee based on seeing patients in face-to-face counseling sessions. Missed individual appointments result in staff time that is not compensated. Thus, if clinics have a steady flow of new referrals, there are financial disincentives to reach out to those who miss appointments. The fee-for-service model also appears to have played a role in shaping providers toward the use of group therapy as the predominant treatment approach because this model is still financially viable even if some of the expected patients do not attend. By following this pragmatic model, the clinic is assured of seeing some patients and getting reimbursed, but there is no incentive for same-patient retention, which is necessary to optimize treatment effectiveness for many patients presenting for the treatment of substance use disorders, especially those with co-occurring disorders [14].

Summary. It is possible, perhaps likely, that multiple barriers factor into disrupted or discontinued care episodes. Difficulty arranging transportation to attend clinic appointments may interact with a period of no appointments due to the resignation of a counselor, or with treatment fatigue or demoralization, resulting in several weeks of missed appointments. At some point, clinics cease attempts to reschedule (often after two missed appointments), the case file is closed with an unknown disposition, and the patients are now lost to the treatment system and on their own, although some will enter the system again after experiencing additional problems. Continuing care approaches should be designed to address these barriers in order to effectively overcome them.

Assertive Approaches to Continuing Care

Beginning in the mid-1990s, the Chestnut Health Systems research group began studying the issue of continuing care for adolescents discharged from residential treatment. A survey of the literature found no controlled trials of aftercare/ continuing care. Instead, such research was limited to single-group follow-up studies of youth discharged from residential treatment [15–18]. These studies revealed better clinical outcomes for those adolescents participating in structured activities to promote recovery, including 12-step groups, outpatient groups, and other activities. Findings from these studies suggested the importance of continuing care and have served to heighten its importance among public funders and clinicians. However, since these studies were correlational, it was not possible to conclude that the youth had better clinical outcomes due to their participation in structured recovery-oriented activities. The field needs randomized controlled trials to test the effectiveness of continuing care for adolescents after residential treatment. We decided to test an assertive approach to continuing care that brought the intervention to the adolescent because we knew that most adolescent outpatient treatment episodes fall considerably short of the recommended 90-day length of stay for the majority of patients [19]. Also, given the barriers noted above, the likelihood of extended care [20] or continuing care occurring in community-based outpatient clinics following residential treatment seemed doubtful. Additionally, for those adolescents with a substance use disorder living in rural areas where travel distances to clinics could be 30 miles or more, we were even less optimistic that outpatient clinics would serve as a reliable option for ongoing care.

For some clinicians, the idea of traveling to a patient's home or another location close to where the patient lives is in conflict with their desire for an "office-based" practice, and others may see such outreach as "enabling" irresponsible behavior. Indeed, we have seen many clinicians complain about unmotivated patients who fail to show for clinic appointments, sometimes saying, the patient "is not ready" or has yet to "hit bottom," and "I am not going to work harder than my patient." We were influenced by the work of Marx, Test, and Stein published in the early 1970s [21] who designed a comprehensive approach for providing support and assistance to patients with severe and persistent mental health disorders to help them participate in the benefits of independent community living and avoid readmissions to state institutions. This approach was known as Assertive Community Treatment (ACT) and over time, the descriptor, "assertive approaches to continuing care" came to include the following attributes [22].

- Clinicians rather than adolescents are responsible for making sure sessions occur.
- Face-to-face sessions are conducted in settings (e.g., home and school) that are convenient for the adolescent and increase the likelihood for service continuity/ retention.
- Low patient to clinician ratios are maintained to support case management functions as well as counseling.

- Case management functions include advocacy, barrier reduction, and follow-up to assure participants link to needed services.

A central defining feature of Assertive Continuing Care (ACC) is that it shifts the responsibility for session attendance from the patient to the clinician. However, another key feature of this model is its reliance on the Adolescent Community Reinforcement Approach (A-CRA) during sessions with the patient. A-CRA helps structure how a clinician interacts with a patient about his or her ongoing substance use and recovery. These procedures are used in addition to the usual case management activities, but ensure that clinicians have a "good therapeutic toolbox" to accompany their case management work. A-CRA derives from operant learning theory and uses a positive, nonconfrontational approach to help the patient and his/her family restructure social and recreational activities to compete with the time spent using alcohol and other drugs. By learning 17 different A-CRA therapeutic procedures (see Table 7.1), the ACC clinician achieves these prosocial aims through improving relationship skills, improving decision making by learning problem solving, learning how to work through barriers or obstacles to goals, returning to satisfying social and leisure activities that do not involve the use of alcohol or other drugs, or sampling new activities to see which ones should be increased more.

Most adolescents in treatment have become involved with the juvenile justice system, are having problems with school, or both. Thus, a major focus of both ACC and A-CRA is to increase compliance with court orders, homework completion, and other legal and educational activities, to help the adolescent transition to a situation free from problems with these authorities. In home-based sessions, the clinician helps the adolescent learn and practice the A-CRA procedures most helpful in these situations including problem solving, communication skills, and breaking down compliance into small achievable goals (see Goals of Counseling procedures). Using the A-CRA procedures to teach these skills is the preferred intervention because it increases the likelihood of self-efficacy and skill generalization to other life situations. Relying on an A-CRA procedure to train adolescents to solve their problems, while desirable, is not always possible or may fail to achieve the desired result. When such failure might lead to serious negative consequences for the adolescent, including prison time or school expulsion, the ACC clinician relies on case management activities such as advocacy, transportation, and service linkage. These services result in more "doing for the adolescent," then building skills through A-CRA. Common examples of clinician advocacy on behalf of adolescent patients include speaking to the probation officer on behalf of a patient who has missed reporting in, but who has taken positive steps toward fulfilling his/her continuing care goals (e.g., started a part-time job, tried out for athletic sport). Adolescents might forget to call or check in with their probation officer as these new activities conflict with their probation appointment. Conversely, the adolescent may have relapsed and smoked marijuana, leading to a fear of reporting to the probation officer and testing positive for cannabis. In this situation, a clinician might reinforce communication skills training and role-play with the adolescent

Table 7.1 A-CRA procedures and rationales

Procedure	Rationale
Overview of A-CRA	Helps the adolescent understand what will happen during the therapy, sets positive expectations, and begins the assessment of reinforcers
Functional analysis of using behavior	Helps the adolescent examine patterns that are associated with substance use and begin to understand how to incorporate healthier ways to access the positive consequences associated with his/her substance use
Functional analysis of prosocial behavior	Clearly shows the adolescent that the therapist cares about the adolescent's happiness in important life areas, that substance use is NOT the only topic that can/will be addressed, and thus helps set a positive tone
Happiness scale	Helps the adolescent know that the therapist cares about the adolescent's happiness in important life areas, and the adolescent get a feel for how his/her life is going
Goals of counseling/treatment plan	Allows the adolescent to set goals in areas important to him/her based on the Happiness Scale, which are monitored and changed as needed
Increasing prosocial recreation	Provides the opportunity to discuss the importance of replacing substance use with healthy, rewarding, and nonusing behaviors, how this might help achieve abstinence and help increase desired reinforcers
Systematic encouragement	Helps the adolescent try out new skills by breaking them down in small steps and allowing him/her to try out a first step during the therapy session, and then take small steps between therapy sessions
Drink/drug refusal	Helps the adolescent identify people who would support his/her abstinence, identify high-risk situations, and practice assertive refusal skills
Relapse prevention	Helps the adolescent understand the behavioral chain of events that led to a relapse, generate alternative responses, and describe and set up an early warning system
Sobriety sampling	Successful completion of a short period of abstinence is easier to attain, helps the adolescent see what abstinence is like, shows caregivers that the adolescent is attempting to change and elicits their support, and lets the adolescent take control of an important goal
Communication skills	Increases the likelihood that an individual will get what he/she asks for and increases positive responses to the adolescent
Problem solving skills	Helps the adolescent develop skills to problem solve more effectively and increases his/her success in solving problems, which helps increase life satisfaction and may decrease triggers for substance use
Caregiver overview, rapport building, and motivation	Provides an overview of the therapy for caregivers, sets positive expectations, reviews research regarding positive parenting practices and enhances engagement in the therapy

(continued)

Table 7.1 (continued)

Procedure	Rationale
Adolescent–caregiver relationship skills	Provides an opportunity for adolescents/caregivers to share what they like about each other, practice communication and problem solving skills under the therapist's guidance, and set goals to work on together regarding their relationship based on a "Relationship Happiness Scale"
Homework	Ensures that skills learned "in session" are used outside of session to increase generalization
Job seeking skills (optional)	Provides the adolescent skills and encouragement to pursue a job if this is something he/she desires
Anger management (optional)	Provides the adolescent an opportunity to learn and practice effective anger management skills to reduce negative consequences of losing control
Overall/general clinical skills	Therapist skills, which ensure that they are faithful to the behavioral approach, using A-CRA procedures frequently and at appropriate times, and using good clinical skills that facilitate engagement and retention

how to speak to the probation officer about what happened. However, if the adolescent has had difficulty implementing communication skills in less stressful situations, the clinician may decide to discuss the circumstances of the missed appointment or relapse directly with the probation officer, and what the adolescent is doing to avoid these problems in the future.

The ACC manual includes chapters on case management activities that outline how clinicians can provide direct assistance to the patient and his or her family in order to obtain a needed service, comply with a legal mandate, and so on. Case management activities have long been used with the severely mentally ill, and over the past 20 years have been used with homeless alcoholics [23], and adults with chronic substance use disorders [24]. However, relatively little has been written about the use of case management services with adolescents who have substance use disorders.

Additional Key Features of ACC

As we implemented ACC, we developed specific practices that we believe increase the likelihood that clinicians will engage and retain adolescents in continuing care and these are described below.

Obtain consent to participate early. Similar to McKay's "advanced directives" [2], a critical feature of ACC is to obtain permission from patients at the beginning of their initial treatment episode to participate in continuing care sessions initiated by an ACC clinician after discharge (from residential or outpatient treatment). We realized several years ago that the single most important reason for obtaining this consent was because many patients left treatment without completing it. In practice, many treatment providers require that a patient return to treatment and successfully complete it prior to receiving aftercare or continuing care different from the type of treatment they failed to complete. ACC took a different approach, one that recognized that failure to complete treatment suggests the need to make it less difficult, more accessible, or a combination of the two. By sending the ACC clinician into the community to meet with the adolescent (with his/her prior consent), we are able to provide continuing care scaled to a level that may make it easier for the patient to accept and participate in. While not exactly the same thing as offering individual choice of treatment as recommended by McKay [2], it recognizes that patients regularly exercise their choice to leave residential or clinic-based outpatient services prior to successful completion. By bringing services to the patient where they live, go to school, or other convenient location, the ACC clinician begins to repair relationships with treatment that may have led to a premature discharge and furthers the hope and possibility for extending treatment, albeit in a nontraditional setting. Adolescents and their families who found it difficult to comply with regular attendance or felt intimidated and powerless in the clinic setting often experience such an action positively. One of the advantages of obtaining consent to provide ACC services early in the index treatment episode is that we have been able to test through randomized controlled trials whether ACC can make a difference with adolescents who fail to complete their index treatment episode, and we will discuss our findings later in this chapter.

Rapid initiation into ACC. Relapse following discharge from treatment is common and there have been multiple studies showing that approximately 60% of adolescents have relapsed by 90 days after discharge from treatment [3, 4, 25]. The ACC approach requires that clinicians work closer with treatment programs referring patients to them in order to set up a regular system of communication. One of the lessons learned early in our ACC trial was the futility of asking residential treatment clinicians to notify us the day of discharge so that we could begin ACC immediately. We quickly learned that we needed to become as assertive with referring treatment programs as we were bringing ACC to our patients and adopted a routine of checking daily with referral providers to see if patients had been discharged. In the future, electronic record systems may be more widely available and allow multiple providers with appropriate consents to learn promptly when patients are discharged (either planned or unplanned) who had consented to participate in ACC.

Homework and mid-week check-ins. In ACC, we strive to meet face-to-face with patients once per week. This frequency may be increased or decreased depending on need, but in our clinical trials, we hoped to average weekly face-to-face meetings at their home, school, or other community setting. One of the methods used to increase the likelihood that adolescents were available to meet with us at the scheduled time was to communicate with them by phone (text, email, IM) to remind them of their scheduled appointment time. These communication opportunities can also be used to check-up on their progress toward accomplishing "homework" they agreed to do from the previous session. Like most behavioral and cognitive-behavioral approaches, A-CRA and ACC seek to improve functioning by finding opportunities outside of a treatment session to apply skills practiced during session. Assigned homework usually involves either the application of a new behavioral skill (e.g., communication skills), trying out a new social/recreational opportunity, reinitiating an old one, or accessing a needed service.

Characteristics of successful ACC staff. In previous adolescent outpatient treatment research, we observed a significant predictive relationship between working alliance (i.e., the relationship between clinician and patient) and clinical outcomes at 3 and 6 months post-intake [26]. In our experience with ACC, we believe that clinicians who optimize their relationship with adolescent patients appear to have several characteristics in common. First, they are enthusiastically optimistic about the possibility of change for their adolescent patients. Second, clinicians who have the capacity to empathize and appreciate the difficulties their patients face are less likely to personalize a relapse or other setback in treatment. Third, clinicians who are flexible and tolerant are more likely to maintain optimism, enthusiasm, and empathy through some trying times with patients. It is our belief that these core characteristics help enhance therapeutic alliance and thus, the relationship with the patients. It does not appear to be important if clinicians acquired these characteristics through general life experience, personal experience with addiction and recovery, or had them as part of their genetic inheritance. Furthermore, it is doubtful that advanced degrees and clinical specialties offset the absence of one or more of these characteristics. However, the combination of these characteristics and strong clinical training may well lead to the best clinical outcomes.

Research on Assertive Continuing Care

Assertive Continuing Care: Initial Study

The first randomized field study of Assertive Continuing Care was funded by the National Institute on Alcoholism and Alcohol Abuse and implemented with adolescents from an 11-county area comprising rural and small urban communities throughout central Illinois. Youth aged 12–17 who met DSM IV criteria for current alcohol or other drug dependence and were admitted to Chestnut Health System's residential treatment program were eligible to participate. Overall, 183 adolescents enrolled, with the majority being male (71%), Caucasian (73%), and aged 15–18 (89%). Most participants had juvenile justice involvement (82%), met dependence criteria for alcohol (54%), and marijuana (87%), followed by cocaine (15%), and had one or more co-occurring mental health disorders (MDD 38%; GAD 41%; ADHD 55%; and CD 70%).

After 1 week of residential treatment, participants were randomized to attend either ACC or usual continuing care (UCC) following their discharge. To our knowledge, this was the first randomized trial of aftercare/continuing care that did not require participants to successfully complete treatment in order to be eligible to participate in the continuing care phase of the study. Only 51% of the UCC and 53% of the ACC groups did complete residential treatment, while the remainder were discharged against staff advice or at staff request. All study participants were given referrals to community clinics (typically outpatient or intensive outpatient programs) closest to their home; however, those leaving unsuccessfully had their referral information mailed to their home, while those leaving successfully were referred by their residential counselor. In addition, youth assigned to the ACC condition either left residential treatment with an appointment time that the ACC clinician would visit them at their home (usually within the first week of discharge), or if they left residential treatment unsuccessfully, they received a phone call from the ACC clinician to set up a home visit. When clinicians were not able to reach the youth by phone, they mailed cards and dropped by the adolescent's home to begin ACC (usually within 2 weeks of discharge). ACC clinicians were trained to implement both the A-CRA protocol and case management services as necessary and endeavor to maintain at least weekly face-to-face contact throughout the first 90 days post-discharge.

At the 90-day post-residential research interview (conducted by research assistants not associated with either continuing care approach), initiation rates for continuing care were significantly better for the ACC group (94 vs. 54%) as were continuing care session attendance rates (18.1 vs. 6.3 sessions). The good implementation of the intervention produced medium to large effect sizes ($d = 0.64$ for initiation; $d = 0.90$ session attendance); however, we learned that it was quite difficult to initiate ACC with many adolescents and maintain their attendance at sessions. For example, dropping by a participant's home without an appointment to have an unscheduled, impromptu session was routine if the clinician was not able to reach the participant by phone or the adolescent or family missed scheduled appointments. Oftentimes, scheduling difficulty was apparent with adolescents whose residential treatment episode ended badly and the adolescent, the family, or both had negative feelings toward the residential treatment staff. Working through this resistance required perseverance and a nondefensive and nonjudgmental approach on the part of the ACC clinician. One of the lessons learned was that even though from the same organization, the ACC clinician quite often was able to overcome the resistance by working within the A-CRA approach, which included an emphasis on the adolescent's strengths and remaining positive. Seeing adolescents and their family on "their turf" seemed to be an important action that underscored our stated intentions that we wanted to help them make a fresh start and respected that it would be difficult for them to attend clinic appointments for one or more of the reasons described earlier. This approach also probably helped diffuse anger or a sense of failure after an unsuccessful treatment experience. In summary, those adolescents seen by ACC clinicians who did not successfully complete residential treatment (approximately 50%) contributed disproportionately to the challenges in reaching the ACC group, and significantly increased the need to be assertive in outreach and case management activities such as advocacy and linkage.

After establishing that ACC clinicians could initiate and retain adolescents in continuing care services, it was important to examine whether these contacts made a difference in clinical outcomes. Tests of intermediate and longer term outcomes revealed a pattern that seemed to be related in part to dosage or amount of services received, but was actually broader and included a combination of dosage and compliance measures. Specifically, results of analyses showed that certain measures of continuing care activities appeared to cluster together and were predictive of abstinence. The 12 items included receiving a variety of behavioral skills training items, case management activities, compliance with probation and school requirements, urine testing, and follow through with referrals (Cronbach's alpha = 0.90). We found that independently of condition assignment, higher scores on the General Continuing Care Adherence (GCCA) scale significantly increased the odds of abstinence at 3 months and that ACC was significantly better than UCC in producing higher GCCA compliance scores (OR = 3.35). Thus, ACC indirectly predicted improved short-term outcomes, but also directly predicted significantly greater abstinence from marijuana at the 9-month follow-up. These results suggested that GCCA should be further evaluated to check for replication of these findings and its meditational effect on clinical outcomes. If GCCA's promise for mediating improved outcomes can be confirmed, it would provide guidelines for designing best practice guidelines for continuing care clinicians.

Assertive Continuing Care: Second Study

Results of the first ACC study increased confidence that an assertive approach to continuing care with adolescents could produce relatively stable and large effects for initiation and retention. Further, abstinence from substance use outcomes trended in the right direction, even if they did not reach statistical significance. The Chestnut research group designed a second study that would further test whether ACC augmented by motivational incentives [27] would further improve substance use outcomes, particularly in the first 90 days. The importance of maintaining abstinence during the first 90 days has been shown to be a significant predictor of abstinence at 9 months [28] and 12 months [29]. Because of prior successes of motivational incentive approaches in previous research with adults [30], we believed it would be a good pairing with ACC. In previous outpatient treatment studies with adults, Higgins and his colleagues [31, 32] paired motivational incentives with the Community Reinforcement Approach (CRA) and found that this combined intervention led to greater improvement than either CRA or motivational incentives alone. Again, with funding from the National Institute on Alcoholism and Alcohol Abuse, we designed a study that differed from the first ACC trial in the following ways: (1) adolescents were recruited from two different Chestnut Health Systems' residential treatment programs in geographically distinct parts of Illinois and (2) regardless of type of discharge, adolescents were provided referrals to their community clinics as in ACC1, but participants were randomized to either (a) UCC only, (b) motivational incentives, (c) ACC, or (d) motivational incentives plus ACC. As in the first ACC study, the active continuing care phase occurred during the first 3 months after their residential discharge, and follow-up interviews were conducted at 3, 6, 9, and 12 months postresidential discharge. The motivational incentive condition was developed in consultation with Dr. Nancy Petry and closely followed her protocol for prize drawing contingent upon completing verifiable prosocial activities [33] and abstinence [34]. For negative urine tests or completion of verified activities, adolescents earned prize drawings. The prize bowl contained 510 slips of paper, which were allocated as follows: (a) 150 or 30% of the slips showed a smiling face; (b) 324 or 62.8% of the slips read "small"; (c) 35 or 7% of the slips read "large"; and (d) 1 or 0.2% of the slips read "jumbo". The smiling face indicated that no prize was won; "small" indicated a prize worth US$1 (e.g., candy bar); "large" indicated a prize worth US$25 (e.g., prepaid cell phone), and "jumbo" indicated a prize worth US$100 (e.g., gift certificates). An important difference between previous adult trials of motivational incentives and the present study was the frequency of prize drawing opportunities. In prior studies, adult patients were asked to report two to three times per week for prize drawing opportunities (contingent on clean urine tests). Because of the large geographic distances that clinicians had to travel to reach patients in the multiple-county catchment area for this study, it was not practical to provide as frequent prize drawing opportunities, and they only occurred once per week.

Over a 4-year period, 337 adolescents were enrolled in this trial and recently the last of the follow-up interviews were completed. It was feasible to implement motivational incentives with adolescents at least once per week, using itinerant clinicians who had to conduct urine test verifications of self-report in adolescents' homes. A recent analysis of 86 participants who had completed participation in one of the motivational incentive conditions found that it was feasible to verify and reinforce prosocial activities across ten goal areas: (a) treatment/recovery work (19% of activities); (b) education (4% of activities); (c) employment (7% of activities); (d) family/friends (4% of activities); (e) health (2% of activities); (f) legal (4% of activities); (g) personal improvement (1% of activities); (h) social/recreational (54% of activities); (i) household (5% of activities); and (j) miscellaneous (<1% of activities). Overall, participants agreed to 1,739 verifiable activities (mean 20 activities/participant) and completed 64% [35]. Clinical outcome analyses of main findings for this trial are in preparation at the time of this writing. We do know, however, that the initiation and retention outcomes are similar to those in the first ACC study.

ACC Research to Validate Continuing Care Performance Measure

There is an increasing recognition on the part of policymakers, treatment providers, and health service researchers that performance measures to monitor and improve the quality of care for those with substance use disorders hold potential for elevating the overall performance of the system by defining key indicators associated with improved practice and clinical outcomes [36, 37]. Eventually, benchmarking provider performance on key indicators may provide both a report card for the public and funders and develop achievable goals for provider improvement. In 1998, the Washington Circle (WC) group was formed with the task of developing and disseminating performance measures for the substance abuse treatment field [38]. The WC group has promulgated performance measures for identification (diagnosis), treatment initiation (attending treatment once after diagnosis/referral), and treatment engagement (attending at least two additional treatment sessions within 30 days after initiation) [39]. More recently, the WC group has developed and begun testing a post-residential continuity of care measure, defined as the percentage of individuals who receive another treatment service within 14 days of discharge from residential treatment [40]. A feature of this definition is the inclusion of all patients admitted to residential treatment: those who completed and those who failed to successfully complete residential treatment. This is a sharp break with the more traditional step-down model of care and is more inclusive in the manner suggested by the ASAM definition of continuing care [41], McKay's adaptive continuing care approach [2], and as continuing care has been studied in the ACC trials. The ACC studies offer one of the few existing data sets that have the potential to help validate the WC continuity of care measures based on (a) continuing care initiation rates and (b) improved clinical outcomes as a result of meeting the WC performance measure. Thus, our group recently partnered with WC investigators to study these research questions [42].

Using the continuing care initiation rates and 3-month clinical outcomes from the ACC2 study (described above), we recoded participants into two conditions: (a) those who received an assertive approach (i.e., motivational incentives, ACC, and the combination of ACC + motivational incentives group) or (b) those who were assigned to UCC only. We analyzed initiation to continuing care following discharge based on the WC definition (initiation of a new treatment service within 14 days of discharge from residential treatment). As expected, results of this analysis showed a significant advantage for the assertive condition (78%) compared to those assigned to UCC (56%), and these findings remained significant after controlling for substance-related problems and number of days in residential treatment. Results of logistic regression testing also demonstrated that meeting the continuity of care performance measure significantly increased the odds of being abstinent and in the community as opposed to incarcerated or back in residential treatment (OR 1.92). Thus, meeting the WC criterion for continuity of care resulted in a 92% higher likelihood of being in recovery at the end of the 3-month follow-up than adolescents who did not meet the WC criterion.

By attending to the details necessary to achieve rapid initiation, a built-in feature of ACC, providers may be able to make an important difference in clinical outcomes for adolescents. Indeed, the assertive approaches were able to achieve the WC performance criterion with more than three-quarters of the adolescents assigned to those conditions. Although the UCC condition performed reasonably well (because over half of the adolescents assigned to the UCC conditions also initiated continuing care), it should be noted that prior research by our group and others found initiation rates to continuing care that were typically in the 20–36% range [1, 20, 43]. It is important to acknowledge that these findings need to be replicated with other clinical samples, but it is also reasonable to recommend that providers pay closer attention to the details of initiating continuing care within 14 days of residential discharge by identifying strategies to address the obstacles to rapid initiation.

Does Rapid CC Initiation Improve Outcomes for Residential Treatment Noncompleters?

The above findings provide encouragement that clinician assistance to enhance rapid initiation to continuing care helps to improve clinical outcomes. As seen in Fig. 7.2, rapid initiation of continuing care is most likely to occur for adolescents who have successfully completed residential treatment and been transferred within the same organization for service, while noncompleters were the least likely to initiate continuing care. In the study below, we focused on whether residential noncompleters (i.e., those who dropped out or were asked to leave) benefitted from rapid initiation of continuing care. Prior to examining the relationship of rapid initiation with substance use outcomes, we first undertook an analysis with the combined data (assertive approaches combined vs. usual approaches combined) from the two ACC studies to determine whether we could replicate the differential rates of continuing care initiation for residential completers vs. noncompleters as in the previous study [42]. Figure 7.3 shows that while the assertive conditions led to significantly higher rates of continuing care initiation (84%), the UCC conditions also resulted in a relatively high rate of continuing care for residential completers (71%).[1] With respect to noncompleters, we found that of those who participated in the UCC conditions, only 33% met the WC continuity of care performance measure, while 64% of those in the assertive condition initiated. Although the noncompleter initiation rates for the assertive condition did not match those of the completers, they were nearly double the rate for their UCC counterparts.

Having shown that assertive approaches are effective in meeting the WC continuity of care performance measure regardless of discharge type, the question remains as to whether rapid initiation improves longer-term clinical outcomes. Alternatively stated, are those adolescents who fail to complete residential treatment likely to relapse, perhaps returning to pretreatment usage, regardless of whether or not they rapidly initiate continuing care services? Using the combined

---

[1] We did not measure time to initiation of continuing care for the UCC condition in the ACC1 study. Since most people who initiate continuing care after residential treatment do so within the first 14 days after discharge, we coded all who received continuing care as initiating within 14 days.

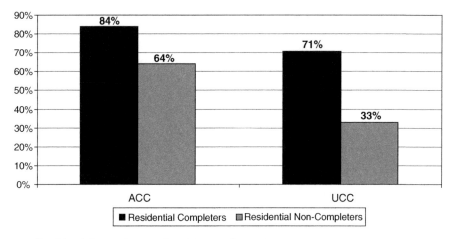

Residential completers: $x^2 = 6.51$, $p < .01$, d=.31
Residential non-completers: $x^2 = 17.71$, $p < .001$, d=.59

Fig. 7.3 Percentage meeting WC continuity of care performance standard by completion status and condition assignment

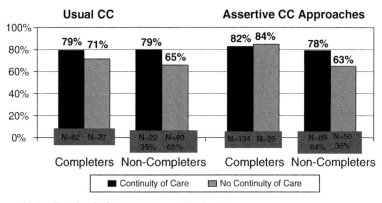

Main effect for CoC: $F = 5.18$, $p < .05$, d=.42
Interaction for completion by CoC: $F = 5.90$, $p < .05$, f-index=.14

Fig. 7.4 Percentage of days abstinent from alcohol

ACC studies, participants were recoded into one of two conditions: UCC or an Assertive Approaches group. Each participant was also coded as (a) a residential completer who initiated continuing care within 14 days of residential discharge; (b) a completer who did not initiate continuing care within 14 days of his or her discharge; (c) a residential noncompleter who initiated continuing care within 14 days; or (d) a noncompleter who did not initiate continuing care within the 14 days. Figure 7.4 shows results from an analysis of the subgroups based on alcohol use data from their 3-month follow-up interviews after residential discharge. We conducted a 2 (completers vs. noncompleters) × 2 (continuity of care vs. no continuity of care) analysis of variance within the UCC and assertive condition separately. The results indicated a main effect for initiating continuing care, regardless of residential completion status within the UCC condition. However, within the assertive condition, a significant interaction effect revealed that three subgroups (both residential completer groups – irrespective of whether they met the WC performance standard of initiating within 14 days of discharge – and the noncompleter subgroup that met the WC initiation criterion) were significantly more likely to be abstinent from alcohol than were those from the noncompleter group that did not meet the WC initiation criterion. These results confirmed that participants who met the WC performance measure for continuing care were more likely to have superior alcohol abstinence outcomes even if they failed to successfully complete residential treatment. This finding was consistent whether participants were in the UCC condition or one of the assertive conditions (see Fig. 7.4). However, nearly twice as many of the noncompleters in the assertive approaches initiated continuing care compared to UCC noncompleters. Moreover, this same pattern of results was evident for the 3-month marijuana use outcomes.

In addition to producing a much higher initiation rate among residential noncompleters, the assertive approaches produced an additional advantage, which might explain why some of the completer subgroup did not meet the WC initiation criteria but still had good outcomes. An examination of the 25 adolescents in the assertive approach completer subgroup who failed to meet the 14-day initiation criterion revealed that 23 or 93% of these participants actually received continuing care *after* the 14-day period compared with 22% of the same subgroup in the UCC condition. As ACC clinicians were instructed to continue efforts to initiate continuing care throughout the 90-day postresidential period, they were successful in eventually initiating care with nearly all youth assigned to them. An inspection of survival analyses regarding time to first use/relapse following discharge from residential treatment [3, 25] makes a compelling clinical argument for rapid initiation; however, it is possible that through a combination of preexisting and treatment-acquired recovery capital [43], some adolescents may benefit from continuing care, even if initiation is delayed beyond 2 weeks. Future research should consider the time to initiation threshold for diminishing clinical effectiveness as well as characteristics of those who will benefit from the added expense of "assertive" continuing care vs. those who may benefit from UCC only. For example, it appears that most noncompleters need a more assertive approach in order to initiate continuing care, while most residential completers do not; however, there are individuals within each of these subgroups that are exceptions to this rule.

Current and Future Research on Assertive Approaches to Continuing Care

Since there has been little examination of the use of continuing care combined with outpatient treatment, and since most adolescents in the USA attend outpatient treatment, we recently completed an outpatient trial to evaluate the effectiveness and cost-effectiveness of two types of outpatient treatment with and without ACC [22].

Results of this study found that both outpatient conditions with ACC had more days abstinent than the outpatient conditions without ACC, but this finding did not reach statistical significance [44]. An outpatient trial by Kaminer and colleagues [45] did find a significant effect for an active aftercare component. Additional studies of ACC following outpatient treatment are currently underway. Our research group has also begun to develop and test less costly assertive approaches to continuing care. For example, in the second ACC trial, we introduced mid-week telephone calls by the ACC clinician to check with adolescents on their progress toward accomplishing "homework" from the last session, to help reduce barriers to accomplishing homework, and to remind the patient of his/her next appointment time. In a recent trial with adults, we evaluated the effectiveness of using trained volunteers to initiate telephone calls to monitor, support, and if necessary, encourage additional intervention services during the first 90 days after residential treatment [46]. This randomized controlled trial demonstrated that it was feasible for para-professional staff and volunteers to initiate supportive calls to recently discharged patients. Short-term clinical outcomes from this study revealed significant improvements for the telephone support group but suggested that extending calls beyond the initial 90-day post-discharge period was both necessary and acceptable to participants.

Currently, with support from the United States SAMHSA's Center for Substance Abuse Treatment, we are developing assertive approaches for testing a telephone and short message service (SMS) texting intervention and a social networking recovery website for youth leaving treatment. Initially, these interventions will be tested in four distinct geographic areas in the USA (northwest, southwest, northeast, and midwest). The social networking site was developed based on focus group tests with adolescents in treatment, and initially it will be monitored and available only by assigned logins for 200 youth leaving treatment. It will include recovery videos and music, personal profile pages, youth-to-youth messaging, online polls, forums, and a chat room. Adolescent survey data collected from several locations throughout the USA suggested that over 90% of youth in treatment have MySpace profiles and that most of these youth have regular broadband access to the internet. Further, most youth in treatment have access to a landline, mobile phone, or both. Pilot testing of these new assertive approaches to continuing care began in late 2009.

Summary

Assertive approaches to continuing care have primarily been studied with adolescents who have been discharged from residential treatment. ACC, in particular, is increasingly being studied following an acute care episode of outpatient treatment [14]. This chapter has described our research findings regarding actual practice of continuing care in contemporary treatment programs as well as our controlled ACC research in continuing care. The following is a brief recapitulation of these findings and implications for future research and practice.

1. Post-acute care services for those discharged from treatment are widely accepted in clinical practice as a clinical necessity – historically, as aftercare (step-down care) to maintain therapeutic gains by deliberately decreasing the intensity of treatment, but more recently, to provide continuity of care that includes the level of service necessary to meet the therapeutic needs of the patient. Research shows that a relatively small percentage of patients treated for substance use disorders will meet the assumptions for, and comply with, step-down aftercare.

2. Almost all past clinical trials research on aftercare or continuing care excluded patients who failed to complete their index or acute treatment episode, which severely limits the extent to which research has tested our current understanding of continuing care as defined by the American Society on Addiction Medicine [9]. Future research should consent research participants early in their acute episode of care to participate in continuing care.

3. Our research of contemporary practice settings suggests that those who fail to successfully complete acute treatment are the least likely to initiate continuing care. This chapter described several potentially interacting factors that serve as barriers to this large segment of patients. Because of this, treatment providers are likely to see modest rates of continuing care initiation even if they consent them early in the acute care episode.

4. Assertive approaches are designed to address the substantial gap between best practice recommendations to provide continuing care and the fact that relatively few adolescents actually receive timely continuing care. Assertive approaches to continuing care shift linkage responsibility from the patient to the provider and offer research-supported methods (e.g., clinician-initiated home visits, repeated telephone contact, etc.) for overcoming barriers to continuing care initiation.

5. Results of two randomized ACC studies demonstrated that successful initiation and retention of most participants is possible. Although clinical trial outcomes of the second study are currently being analyzed, results of the first study demonstrated superior results for ACC in terms of abstinence from marijuana.

6. Assertive care studies provided an excellent vehicle to conduct a validation study of the WC performance measure for continuity of care following discharge from residential treatment. Applying this criterion to ACC study data demonstrated that achieving continuing care initiation within 14 days of residential discharge significantly improved clinical outcomes at 3 months and that assertive care was significantly better than UCC for achieving compliance with the WC continuity of care performance measure.

7. Additional research showed that assertive care linked significantly more of the residential noncompleters to continuing care than their UCC counterparts and consistent with our previous research [41], their clinical outcomes improved to a level similar to those who link on their own in UCC. We also found that within the assertive care-residential completer subgroup that failed to achieve compliance with the 14-day initiation criteria, that almost all of these patients eventually were linked by their assertive clinician and achieved abstinence at the same or higher levels of the best performing subgroups. While this and other ACC studies should be replicated by other researchers, this is the first study of its kind

to demonstrate that, by reaching out to "treatment failures", we can reengage relatively high percentages of patients and significantly improve their substance use outcomes.

8. Additional research using assertive approaches to continuing care has been conducted with adults using telephone monitoring, support, recovery management check-ups, and, when necessary, reintervention with acute treatment [8, 46]. Results of these studies are promising and future research should test these methods of continuing care with adolescents. Future research with adolescents should employ other electronic technology such as text messaging and web-based recovery support. As adolescents have virtually "grown-up" with this technology, it may prove to be a feasible lower-cost approach to providing ongoing monitoring and support.

References

1. Godley MD, Godley SH. Continuing care following residential treatment: history, current practice, and emerging approaches. In: Jainchill N, editor. Understanding and treating adolescent substance use disorders. Kingston, NJ: Civic Research Institute (in press).
2. McKay JR. Continuing care research: what we have learned and where we are going. J Subst Abuse Treat. 2009;36:131–45.
3. Brown SA, Vik PW, Creamer VA. Characteristics of relapse following adolescent substance abuse treatment. Addict Behav. 1989;14:291–300.
4. Godley SH, Godley MD, Dennis ML. The Assertive Aftercare Protocol for adolescent substance abusers. In: Wagner E, Waldron H, editors. Innovations in Adolescent Substance Abuse Interventions. New York: Elsevier Science; 2001. p. 311–29.
5. Godley SH, Passetti LL, Funk RR, Garner BR, Godley MD. One-year treatment patterns and change trajectories for adolescents participating in outpatient treatment for the first time. J Psychoactive Drugs. 2008;40:17–27.
6. McLellan AT, Lewis DC, O'Brien CP, Kleber HD. Drug dependence, a chronic medical illness: implications for treatment, insurance, and outcomes evaluation. J Am Med Assoc. 2000;284:1689–95.
7. White WL. Recovery management and recovery-oriented systems of care: scientific rationale and promising practices. Pittsburgh, PA: Northeast Addiction Technology Transfer Center; 2008.
8. Dennis ML, Scott CK. Managing substance use disorders (SUD) as a chronic condition. NIDA Sci Clin Pract. 2007;4(1):45–55.
9. Mee-Lee D, Shulman GD, Fishman M, Gastfriend DR, Griffith JH. ASAM patient placement criteria for the treatment of substance-related disorders. 2nd ed. Chevy Chase, MD: American Society of Medicine; 2001.
10. Office of Applied Studies (OAS). Treatment episode data set (TEDS): 2002. Discharges from Substance Abuse Treatment Services [DASIS Series S-25 DHHS Publication No. (SMA) 04-3967]. Rockville, MD: Substance Abuse Mental Health Services Administration. 2005. http://www.dasis.samhsa.gov/teds02/2002_teds_rpt_d.pdf.
11. Dennis ML, Dawud-Noursi S, Muck RD, McDermeit (Ives) M. The need for developing and evaluating adolescent treatment models. In: Stevens SJ, Morral AR, editors. Adolescent substance abuse treatment in the United States: exemplary models from a National Evaluation Study. Binghamton, NY: Haworth Press; 2003. p. 3–34.

12. Dennis ML, (2009). [Data analysis from Chestnut Health Systems' GAIN Coordinating Center 2008 CSAT Adolescent Treatment Data Set provided by Dr. Michael Dennis on 10/7/2009]. Unpublished raw data.
13. McLellan AT, Carise D, Kleber HD. Can the national addiction treatment infrastructure support the public's demand for quality care? J Subst Abuse Treat. 2003;25:117–21.
14. Godley SH, Garner BR, Smith JE, Meyers RJ, Godley MD. A large-scale dissemination and implementation model. Clin Psychol Sci Prac. (in press).
15. Chan YF, Godley MD, Godley SH, Dennis ML. Utilization of mental health services among adolescents in community-based substance abuse outpatient clinics. J Behav Health Serv Res. 2009;36:35–51.
16. Alford GS, Koehler RA, Leonard J. Alcoholics Anonymous-Narcotics Anonymous model inpatient treatment of chemically dependent adolescents: a two-year outcome study. J Stud Alcohol. 1991;52:118–26.
17. Hoffmann NG, Kaplan RA. One-year outcome results for adolescents: key correlates and benefits of recovery. St. Paul, MN: CATOR/New Standards; 1991.
18. Jainchill N, Hawke J, De Leon G, Yagelka J. Adolescents in therapeutic communities: one-year posttreatment outcomes. J Psychoactive Drugs. 2000;32:81–94.
19. Norbert R, McNenamy C. Treatment outcomes in an adolescent chemical dependency program. Adolescence. 1996;31:91–107.
20. McKay JR. Is there a case for extended interventions for alcohol and drug use disorders? Addiction. 2005;100:1594–610.
21. Marx AJ, Test MA, Stein LI. Extrohospital management of severe mental illness: feasibility and effects of social functioning. Arch Gen Psychiatry. 1973;29(4):505–11.
22. Godley SH, Godley MD, Karvinen T, Slown LL, Wright KL. The assertive continuing care protocol: a clinician's manual for working with adolescents after residential treatment of alcohol and other substance use disorders. 2nd ed. Bloomington, IL: Lighthouse Institute; 2006.
23. Orwin RG, Sonnefeld LJ, Garrison-Mogren R, Smith NG. Pitfalls in evaluating the effectiveness of case management for homeless persons: lessons from the NIAAA Community Demonstration Program. Eval Rev. 1994;18(2):153–207.
24. Vanderplasschen W, Rapp RC, Wolf J, Broekaert E. Comparative review of the development and implementation of case management for substance use disorders in North America and Europe. Psychiatr Serv. 2004;55(8):913–22.
25. Godley MD, Godley SH, Dennis ML, Funk RR, Passetti LL. Preliminary outcomes from the assertive continuing care experiment for adolescents discharged from residential treatment. J Subst Abuse Treat. 2002;23:21–32.
26. Tetzlaff BT, Kahn JH, Godley SH, Godley MD, Diamond GS, Funk RR. Working alliance, treatment satisfaction, and patterns of posttreatment use among adolescent substance users. Psychol Addict Behav. 2005;19:199–207.
27. Petry NM, Martin B, Cooney JL, Kranzler HR. Give them prizes and they will come: contingency management for treatment of alcohol dependence. J Consult Clin Psychol. 2000;68:250–7.
28. Godley MD, Godley SH, Dennis ML, Funk RR, Passetti LL. The effect of Assertive Continuing Care (ACC) on continuing care linkage, adherence and abstinence following residential treatment for adolescents. Addiction. 2007;102:81–93.
29. Higgins ST, Badger GJ, Budney AJ. Initial abstinence and success in achieving longer term cocaine abstinence. Exp Clin Psychopharmacol. 2000;8:377–86.
30. Higgins ST, Petry NM. Contingency management: incentives for sobriety. Alcohol Res Health. 1999;23(2):122–7.
31. Higgins ST, Budney AJ, Bickel WK, Foerg FE, Donham R, Badger GJ. Incentives improve outcome in outpatient behavioral treatment of cocaine-dependence. Arch Gen Psychiatry. 1994;51(7):568–76.

32. Higgins ST, Budney AJ, Bickel WK, Hughes JR, Foerg F, Badger G. Achieving cocaine abstinence with a behavioral approach. Am J Psychiatry. 1993;150(5):763–9.
33. Petry NM, Tedford J, Martin B. Reinforcing compliance with non-drug-related activities. J Subst Abuse Treat. 2001;20:33–44.
34. Petry NM. A comprehensive guide to the application of contingency management procedures in general clinic settings. Drug Alcohol Depend. 2000;58:9–25.
35. Godley SH, Godley MD, Wright KL, Funk RR, Petry N. Contingent reinforcement of personal goal activities for adolescents with substance use disorders during post-residential continuing care. Am J Addict. 2008;17:278–86.
36. Horgan C, Garnick D. The quality of care for adults with mental and addictive disorders: issues in performance measurement. Background paper for the Institute of Medicine Institute for Behavioral Health. Waltham, MA: Schneider Institute for Health Policy, Heller School for Social Policy and Management, Brandeis University; 2005.
37. McLellan AT, Chalk M, Bartlett J. Outcomes, performance, and quality: what's the difference? J Subst Abuse Treat. 2007;32:321–30.
38. McCorry F, Garnick DW, Bartlett J, Cotter F, Chalk M. Developing performance measures for alcohol and other drug services in managed care plans. Jt Comm J Qual Improv. 2000;26:633–43.
39. Garnick DW, Lee MT, Chalk M, Gastfriend D, Horgan CM, McCorry F, et al. Establishing the feasibility of performance measures for alcohol and other drugs. J Subst Abuse Treat. 2002;23:375–85.
40. Garnick DW, Lee MT, Horgan CM, Acevedo A. Washington Circle Public Sector Workgroup. Adapting Washington Circle performance measures for public sector substance abuse treatment systems. J Subst Abuse Treat. 2009;36:265–77.
41. Garner BR, Godley MD, Funk RR, Lee MT, Garnick DW. The Washington Circle continuity of care performance measure: predictive validity with adolescents discharged from residential treatment. J Subst Abuse Treat. 2010;38(1):3–11.
42. Donovan DM. Continuing care: promoting the maintenance of change. In: Miller WR, Heather N, editors. Treating addictive behaviors. 2nd ed. New York: Plenum Press; 1998. p. 317–36.
43. Laudet AB, White WL. Recovery capital as a prospective predictor of sustained recovery, life satisfaction, and stress among former poly-drug substance users. Subst Use Misuse. 2008;43 (1):27–54.
44. Godley SH, Garner BR, Passetti LL, Funk RR, Dennis ML, Godley MD. Adolescent outpatient treatment and continuing care: main findings from a randomized clinical trial. Drug Alcohol Depend. 2010;110:44–54.
45. Kaminer Y, Burleson JA, Burke RH. Efficacy of outpatient aftercare for adolescents with alcohol use disorders: a randomized controlled study. J Am Acad Child Adolesc Psychiatry. 2008;47(12):1405–1412.
46. Godley MD, Coleman-Cowger VH, Titus JC, Funk RR, Omdorff MG. A randomized controlled trial of telephone continuing care. J Subst Abuse Treat. 2010;38(1):74–82.

Chapter 8
Long-Term Trajectories of Adolescent Recovery

Sandra A. Brown, Danielle E. Ramo, and Kristen G. Anderson

Abstract A growing literature has emerged examining long-term patterns of substance use among teens who exhibit casual and more severe use. This work evaluates treatment outcomes for teens who have substance abuse problems and identifies important developmental correlates of those outcomes as teens age into young adulthood. This research informs the development of valuable addiction recovery management models and identifies some factors that are particularly important to be considered in teens as compared to adults. This chapter reviews the literature on trajectories of substance abuse among teens who use alcohol and drugs.

We first consider patterns of substance involvement among those teens who have had an episode of alcohol or drug treatment. We then consider three domains of empirically identified factors associated with substance use after treatment, including (1) biological factors (psychiatric comorbidity, neurocognitive factors), (2) personal characteristics (e.g., demographic factors, motivation, cognition, personality traits, self-help group attendance), and (3) social/environmental factors (e.g., living environment, peer associations, parental factors).

We then examine substance use trajectories of those teens who have not entered treatment. We examine the primary substance use patterns identified in the literature and the factors associated with a "natural recovery" or with a more persistent pattern of use as these youth age into adulthood. We conclude by summarizing the key differences between teens who enter treatment and those who do not, highlighting how teen recovery patterns differ from adult recovery patterns, and discuss the importance of adolescent recovery patterns to an addiction recovery model.

Keywords Addiction recovery management · Adolescent · Trajectories of substance use · Long-term patterns of use · Treatment outcomes for adolescents

S.A. Brown (✉)
Departments of Psychiatry and Psychology, University of California, San Diego,
and Psychology Service VA San Diego Healthcare System, San Diego, CA, USA
e-mail: sanbrown@ucsd.edu

J.F. Kelly and W.L. White (eds.), *Addiction Recovery Management: Theory, Research and Practice*, Current Clinical Psychiatry, DOI 10.1007/978-1-60327-960-4_8,
© Springer Science+Business Media, LLC 2011

Introduction

Treatment of alcohol and drug problems during adolescence is important not only because of the impact on short-term recovery for youth but also because of the potential long-term impact on alcohol and drug involvement and development.

Although limited, there is a growing literature on longer term outcomes for youth. This literature informs us regarding the specific extent to which, and how, adolescent substance involvement changes with age, and the manner in which treatment is effective in arresting the deleterious effects of alcohol and substance use among youth as they mature into young adulthood. This growing literature has begun to focus on important developmental tasks of adolescence and emerging adulthood. Further, longitudinal research can demonstrate how patterns of alcohol and drug use over time influence success in the new tasks and roles of adulthood.

The present chapter focuses on long-term patterns of substance involvement of adolescents called trajectories. We describe separately these patterns for youth whose drinking and other drug use has resulted in treatment, and for those in the community.

Understanding the long-term course of adolescent and other drug involvement is critical as we develop models of recovery, as well as treatment strategies and techniques. Only by knowledge of constellations of risk that drive poorer outcomes and life tasks and transitions which accentuate risk can we optimally assist youth interested in recovery. Adolescence is a time of development during which many aspects of life are in flux. Table 8.1 demonstrates the major developmental tasks of adolescence, demonstrating the range of responsibilities involved in transitioning from adolescence into adulthood. As we describe processes by which teens use alcohol and drugs and recover from problems with these substances, the developmental tasks outlined here will serve as risk or protective factors for an individual in different ways. No doubt, knowledge of developmental milestones in adolescence has important implications for individuals, their families, and the social systems, which seek to facilitate the development of successful and productive adults.

What Happens to Teens After Drug and Alcohol Treatment?

Early work demonstrated that teens tend to relapse quickly, with approximately half of the adolescents receiving community-based treatment for substance use disorders (SUDs) relapsing within the first 3 months following treatment [1] and two thirds to four fifths of youth relapsing after 6 months [2, 3]. A growing body of research has identified patterns of substance-related outcomes for those who received substance abuse treatment as adolescents. Most of this work has classified teens into groups based on the extent of their substance use in the first year [4, 5] to 3 years [6]. For example, in a 3-year longitudinal study, Chung et al. [7] characterized patterns of alcohol dependence symptoms across 3 years in adolescents who

Table 8.1 The diversity of developmental contexts and tasks during late adolescence/early adulthood (ages 16–20)

Developmental contexts	
Contexts	Examples
Living arrangements	Alone
	In a dorm
	With parents
	With friends
	With romantic partner
Educational settings	High school
	College
	Night school
	Trade school
Work settings	Part-time versus full-time employment
	Career initiation
	Unemployment
Developmental tasks	
Tasks	Examples
Relational	Dating and sexual behavior
	Marriage
	Starting a family
	Socializing with peers
Occupational/Educational	Completion of mandatory education
	Vocational training
	College/professional education
	Starting a career
Legal	Driver's license
	Criminal responsibility
	Financial responsibility

Note: From Brown et al. [16] Copyright, American Academy of Pediatrics, reprinted with permission

had either inpatient or outpatient treatment. They identified five patterns of alcohol use, based on classification of participants as "abstainers," "nonproblem drinkers," and "problem drinkers" at 1 and 3 years after treatment: *chronic problem drinker* (37%), "*worse*" (15%), "*better*" (14%), *stable nonproblem drinker* (21%), and *abstainer/nonproblem* (12%). This classification strategy was compared to one in which alcohol symptom severity was used to classify individuals. By using diagnostic symptoms, five trajectories were identified: *Better-Low Severity* (2%), *Better-Moderate Severity* (34%), *Slow Improvers* (14%), *Moderate Severity* (40%), and *High Severity* (9%).

These studies highlight the usefulness of empirically based alcohol or drug use trajectories and the varying ways in which to categorize use among teens after substance abuse treatment, calling for longer-term follow-up periods to understand the course of substance use into early adulthood.

Longer-term substance use patterns among treated teens have tended to use clinical categorization to classify teens based on substance use after treatment.

For example, work in our lab has characterized the substance involvement, social and behavioral functioning in the years after treatment [2, 8–10]. Based on quantity/frequency of use and associated problems exhibited over multiple follow-up time points after treatment, youth were clinically categorized into five groups: *Abstainers* (7%), *Users* (8%), *Slow improvers* (10%), *Worse with time* (27%), *and Continuous heavy users* (48%) [2]. Using a similar approach, Winters et al. [11] compared substance use patterns of adolescents in a 12-step-based Treatment group, Waiting List control group, and Community Control group across five and a half years. Based on frequency of use and SUD diagnostic criteria at three follow-up time points, they found that the Treatment group had consistently better outcomes than Waiting List controls, while Community Controls demonstrated lower substance use than the other two group at all three assessed time points.

In an effort to describe teen alcohol use in the 8 years following treatment, Abrantes described four trajectories of alcohol patterns in 140 adolescents who had an inpatient treatment episode [7]. Based on these 8-year trajectories, teens were labeled as *Abstainers* (22%), *Infrequent users* (24%), *Worse with time* (36%), and *Frequent users* (18%). Worse alcohol trajectories were associated with more severe alcohol dependence symptoms, severe drug use during treatment, and poorer psychosocial functioning in late adolescence. This longitudinal work identified trajectories on the basis of alcohol outcomes and underscores the importance of extending the trajectory analysis approach beyond the 8-year period as well as incorporating the use of multiple substances (i.e., marijuana and other drugs), which are so often used in conjunction with alcohol among youth in substance abuse treatment [12]. In this study, important fluctuations in use were linked to development.

In the longest clinical outcome study to date, Anderson et al. [13] identified six longitudinal patterns of alcohol and other drug use over the decade following adolescent treatment: *Abstainers/Infrequent Users* (29%), *Late Adolescent Resurgence* (18%), *Early 20s Resurgence* (14%), *Frequent Drinkers* (16%), *Frequent Drinkers/Drug Dependent* (17%), and *Chronic* (6%). Figure 8.1 highlights the topography of alcohol, marijuana, and other drug use within each trajectory class. These trajectories reflect both the diversity of youth outcomes and dynamics of drug and alcohol involvement as adolescents transition into adulthood. Consistent with recent findings for youth in the first year post treatment [4, 5], the vast majority of this sample, approximately two thirds, dramatically improved after treatment. Two trajectory classes represented differences in the timing of accelerations in substance engagement (*Late Adolescent Resurgence and Emerging Adulthood Resurgence*). Similarly, Clark et al. [14] found six trajectory classes when modeling retrospective reports of SUD symptoms across early adolescence to mid-adulthood in SUD adults, including the presence of classes distinguished by developmental shifts in mid-adolescence, late adolescence, and emerging adulthood. These time periods correspond to important developmental transitions in emerging adulthood roles and responsibilities [15–18]. Additional measures of alcohol and other drug involvement and DSM-IV diagnosis support the characterization of distinct patterns of substance engagement and problems for teens following treatment.

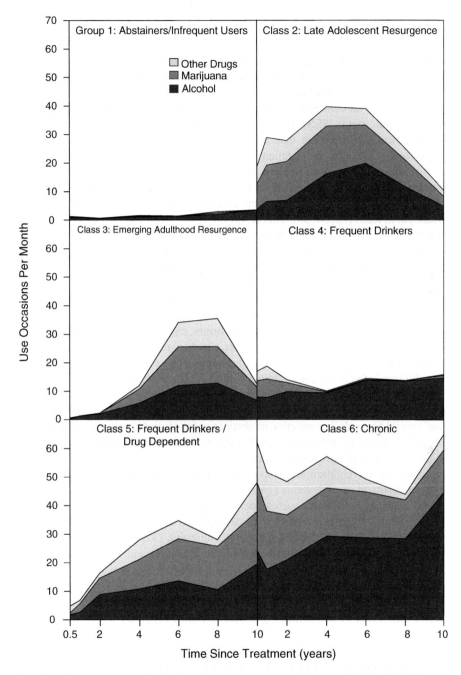

Fig. 8.1 Composite use of alcohol, marijuana, and other drugs across a decade after adolescent treatment. Units are in days per month for each type of substance (e.g., days beer + days wine + days hard liquor, eight types of drugs). *Note:* from Anderson et al. [13]

What Predicts Adolescent Recovery After Treatment?

A body of research has sought to identify factors associated with treatment outcomes. Factors can be thought of in four major categories: background variables, pretreatment substance use, environmental influences, and personal characteristics. *Background variables* focus on demographic characteristics such as age, gender, ethnicity, and socioeconomic status (SES). While studies have shown that girls are at less risk for posttreatment substance use than boys [19, 20], less consistent evidence has been found for the impact of age, ethnicity, and SES [10, 21].

Pretreatment substance use has been implicated in adult substance treatment outcomes [22, 23], but studies have shown that pretreatment substance use characteristics alone have not been predictive of relapse patterns up to 1 year following treatment in teens [20, 24, 25]. This is surprising given the diversity of substances to which youth are exposed and presumed differences in addictive potential across substances. However, one study from our laboratory has found that those youth who relapse on alcohol or marijuana progress to other substances more slowly than those who relapse on their drug of choice [26].

Environmental influences capture the interpersonal and historical factors implicated in substance use outcomes. Family environment, the extent to which youth feel supported and connected to their family of origin, can have protective influences on treatment outcomes for teens [27]. However, a body of research has shown that family history of alcoholism can convey risk for poor substance-related decision making in that children in families with alcoholics display higher levels of impulsivity than their peers [17]. While general indices of peer support suggest that poorer support exerts a detrimental impact on teen substance use [28–30], having nonusing social supports in one's social networks is predictive of abstinence for around a year after treatment [9, 25, 31]. As teens age into young adulthood, developmental milestones such as high-school graduation, professional occupations, marriage/cohabitation, and financial responsibility for children are associated with better outcomes among those who were in treatment as adolescents [13].

Personal characteristics such as personality, motivation, learning, self-esteem, and psychiatric diagnosis and symptomatology can impact youth trajectories post-treatment. For example, factors such as disinhibition [32, 33] and alcohol expectancies [34–36] have been implicated in the initiation and maintenance of use patterns across development. In addition, externalizing disorders and internalizing disorders have been associated with poorer prognosis for SUD teens [32, 37]. Entering treatment without a concurrent mental health problem is associated with greater likelihood of abstaining 1 year after treatment [9].

Recovery Without Treatment for Adolescents

In the Unites States, the vast majority of youth with harmful or disordered substance use do not receive treatment (89–94%) [38]. Such low rates of service provision are a function of lack of access to services, lack of self-awareness regarding the need for treatment, and the perception among youth that treatment is not geared to their needs [16, 39]. Irrespective of the issues underlying limited service utilization, the fact remains that youth, similar to adults, often do not receive formal treatment for alcohol and drug-related problems, and a sizable proportion recover [40–42]. As many as 15–20% of high-school students who drink make purposeful efforts to cut down or stop drinking. Studies of binge drinking among high-school students show substantial variability in drinking over time. As many as 15% of student drinkers who binge change to abstaining or nonbinge consumption each year [43]. Epidemiological research demonstrates that far more individuals cease meeting criteria for a substance use disorder than receive treatment, and consequently, it appears that many youth do not continue on a trajectory of disordered use across their lifespan [16, 44].

One issue in evaluating recovery without treatment for youth is identifying the boundary condition necessary for the onset and discontinuance of problematic engagement with alcohol and other drugs [45]. As with treated youth, a diversity of metrics has been used to identify use patterns across time in nontreated youth, ranging from quantity/frequency (or each individually), heavy use, problems, and exceeding diagnostic thresholds. Do we identify onset as meeting diagnostic criteria for alcohol- and drug-use disorders? Work by Pollack and Martin [46] and Chung and Martin [47] would suggest that the presence of *diagnostic orphans* (i.e., youth who do not meet diagnosis for SUDs but are experiencing clinically significant problems) would be overly exclusionary and fail to account for use patterns that would be of clinical concern within or outside of the treatment context [42]. Similarly, how do we determine when youth have recovered? Work by our group suggests that different outcome indices (e.g., relapse status, dependence symptoms) are predicted by different factors for youth in treatment [9]. For the purposes of this review, we describe multiple patterns of change for adolescents using alcohol or other drugs at levels associated with developmentally significant problems, abuse, or dependence, as well as a reduction in use to less intense or problematic levels.

Common Patterns of Recovery in Nontreated Youth

Most studies of youth identify four to six longitudinal patterns of substance use for teens [48]. However, some have questioned whether this represents true differences within the population or is an artifact of the modeling strategies employed [49]. Studies have examined patterns of alcohol, and to a lesser extent other drug use, in community samples of youth. While the focus of this chapter is on youth with problematic engagement with alcohol and other drugs, it is important to note that the most common use pattern endorsed by youth is that of nonuse and is the most consistent pattern identified across studies [16]. While nonusers become less frequent in community samples as youth move from early adolescence to emerging adulthood [50], many youth in the community do not engage in alcohol or drug use and most do not exhibit problematic use.

The majority of studies on adolescent use patterns have focused on alcohol, given that alcohol is the most commonly used illicit substance among adolescents [50]. In a recent integrative review, Brown et al. [16] have summarized the most common trajectories of alcohol use identified in longitudinal research on adolescents, from middle adolescence (e.g., age 16) to emerging adulthood (e.g., age 20). These six patterns include: *Abstainers/Light Drinkers* (stable, low, or nonuse of alcohol; ~20–65%), *Stable Moderate Drinkers* (stable moderate use, limited heavy use; ~30%), *Fling Drinkers* (developmentally limited use; ~10%), *Decreasers* (early onset but declining course; ~10%), *Chronic Heavy Drinkers* (early onset and stable course of heavy drinking; <10%), and *Late-Onset Heavy Drinkers* (late onset but rapid escalation to heavy drinking; <10%). Fling drinkers and Decreasers are of interest when considering recovery without treatment for alcohol-use problems. Theoretically, these groups have been typified as developmentally limited drinkers or alcoholics [51, 52], characterized by heavy or potentially disordered drinking that remits as a function of young adult development.

While these patterns might typify drinking patterns within adolescence, of interest to the study of recovery patterns is the relation between adolescent alcohol-use disorders (AUDs) and remission. Jacob et al. [53] examined trajectories of AUDs from adolescence to mid-1940s among men from the Vietnam Era Twin Registry. They identified four trajectories in those meeting diagnostic criteria for AUDs: *Severe Chronic Alcoholics (23%), Severe Nonchronic Alcoholics (11%), Young Adult Alcoholics* (37%), and *Late Onset Alcoholics* (28%). The Young Adult Alcoholics were characterized by high probabilities of early diagnosis, peaking around age 21 and declining thereafter. The authors suggest that this group represents the continued recovery of adolescents with developmentally limited alcoholism. Interestingly, the Young Adult Alcoholics were least likely to seek treatment for their alcohol use.

Less data is available for the longitudinal patterns of other drug use in nonclinical samples of adolescents. Marijuana use has been examined across time for youth ranging from late childhood to emerging adulthood, in isolation and in conjunction with alcohol. Marijuana use was monitored for 10 years beginning with a large school-based sample of early adolescents (2,000+; age 13) [54]. Abstainers (45% of the sample), the most common pattern, were excluded from the trajectory analyses. Four use trajectories were identified: *Early High Users* (5% of the sample; monthly–weekly use at age 13, decreasing use until 18 with stable moderate use afterwards [three to ten times/year]), *Stable Light Users* (17%; low level of use at 13 and beyond [no more than ten times/year]), *Occasional Light Users* (53%; no use at age 13 and low rates of use at each time point), and *Steady Increasers* (25%; no use at age 13 with increasing level across time to highest use group by age 23 [monthly–weekly use]). Early High Users seemingly "burn out" on their use of marijuana in adolescence, even though this pattern is associated with continued light use into emerging adulthood.

Polysubstance use is the norm rather than the exception for youth with SUDs [44]. Authors have examined the developmental patterns of polysubstance use among youth from late childhood to emerging adolescence. Using a sample of almost 500 community teens, Flory et al. [55] modeled alcohol and marijuana trajectories separately for girls and boys. They identified three patterns of alcohol and marijuana consumption by sex, similar in shape, if not magnitude, of use: *Nonusers, Early Onset, and Late Onset.* Most participants were assigned to the Nonusing group, followed by the Late onset, with the lowest probability of group membership for Early onset. Women were more likely to demonstrate the Early and Nonuse patterns compared to men. As to recovery, the Early-Onset group demonstrated precocious engagement with marijuana, beginning around age 11–12, peaking around age 15–16 years, and declining at the final assessment at 19–21 years. In both sexes, there was an overlap between alcohol and marijuana use trajectories, such that early-onset use of both substances occurred together. While it is tempting to consider the Early-onset group as representing "recovery," caution must be used as this group also demonstrated the highest level of psychopathology and poor functioning at study outset and also had high levels of alcohol abuse/dependence and arrests compared to low-use groups, suggesting that the reductions of use at the final assessment point might be better accounted for by external influences on use (e.g., treatment and/or incarceration) than actual recovery.

Conjoint developmental trajectories of alcohol and tobacco, bridging late adolescence through emerging adulthood (ages 18–26 years), suggest heavy drinking and smoking cigarettes should be considered concurrently [56]. Using a U.S. national longitudinal dataset (Monitoring the Future; MTF), six classes were used to describe use patterns over time: *Chronic High Drinker/Smoker* (6%), *Chronic High Drinker/Low Smoker* (14%), *Moderate Drinker/Developmentally Limited Smoker* (5%), *Nondrinker/smoker* (56%), *Low Drinker/Chronic High Smoker* (8%), *Moderate Drinker/Late Onset High Smoker* (5%), and *Moderate Drinker/ Smoker* (6%). Interestingly, while patterns suggested a general decrease in heavy drinking across development, smoking remained relatively stable. Jackson and colleagues suggest that this level of developmental comorbidity between two abused substances better elucidates the co-occurrence and mutual influences in addiction than previous modeling attempts.

Chassin et al. [17] examined AOD patterns in a mixed sample of children of alcoholics (COAs) and controls. First, they modeled trajectories integrating alcohol consumption and other drug use in youth from age 11 to 30 years. Four patterns of consumption were identified across adolescence into adulthood: *Light Drinking/Rare Drug Use* (24%), *Moderate Drinking/Experimental Drug Use* (45%), *Heavy Drinking/Drug Use* (20%), and *Abstainers* (11%). The most common illicit substances used were marijuana and amphetamines. In terms of dependence diagnoses, Chassin and colleagues identified five trajectories across development: *No Diagnosis* (identified *a priori*; 61%), *Alcohol Only* (~19%), *Drug Only* (~10%), *Comorbid* (6%; high probability of both alcohol and drug dependence), and *Persistent* (~5%; mostly persistent alcohol diagnosis). Interestingly, these investigators examined the associations between use patterns and dependency and found that consumption patterns were related to dependence status. Particularly, individuals with a high probability of being within the Heavy Drinking/Heavy Drug Use group were more likely to be diagnosed, across each type of diagnosis classification. Classification as a Light Drinker/Rare Drug User was associated with the least likelihood of dependence diagnosis (abstainers were excluded from analysis). This finding suggests that the examination of use, as depicted above, has direct implications for dependence status. Youth who moderate or reduce their use across time are less likely to meet criteria for a dependence diagnosis and, therefore, more likely to meet the definition of recovery posited at the beginning of this section.

Predictors of Recovery in Nontreated Samples

While there is utility in depicting developmental patterns of substance use and dependence across time, of particular interest both scientifically and clinically is the ability to predict what factors might impact these trajectories. For example, the studies depicted above have explored the impact of a diversity of predictors such as sex [55, 57, 58], race and ethnicity [54, 56], familial factors [17, 54–56], socioeconomics [55–57], peer and parental use [55], personality [17, 55, 56], psychopathology [17, 56], and outcome expectancies [56] on the probability of being assigned to a particular trajectory group. Unfortunately, while some studies have found these factors to differentiate between alcohol and drug patterns across time in youth, the predominant focus of this work has focused on the predictors of progression to high or problematic use in adolescence. Thus, there is often little or no attention to factors associated with recovery or reductions in use. This makes the identification of factors associated with reductions in use in community samples difficult to identify within the existent literature [16].

One area of consistency within the literature is the identification of sex differences in patterns of use, some of which are associated with reductions in use across time. While some authors have used the strategy of modeling separate trajectories as a function of sex [55, 57, 58], others have examined the relative likelihood of teenaged girls or boys falling within a particular pattern of substance use and problems. For studies that have modeled separate paths of use for girls and boys, the patterns are relatively similar for each sex, but often the intensity of use is higher for boys in comparison to girls. However, in samples where differing patterns emerged for alcohol use [57, 58], trajectories for girls seemed to include a time-limited or decreasing group, while such a pattern was not identified for boys. While these two studies represent findings from different cultures (i.e., US and East Germany) and different operationalizations of drinking behavior, this suggests a need for further examination of sex or gender effects on recovery from more intensive alcohol use in adolescent samples.

A study of natural recovery from binge drinking among college students (ages 18–29 years; mean age: ~20) suggests that a minority of college students reduce or stop binge drinking from high school to college (22%) [59]. *Natural reducers*, those who reduced binge drinking without treatment, were more likely to be older, be married, and attend church more regularly. Additionally, subtle changes were identified in alcohol expectancies and self-efficacy such that reducers had lower enhancement expectancies and greater self-efficacy to resist pressure to drink. While this study did not examine trajectories of use per se, it suggests that research into recovery without treatment for adolescents has the potential to identify modifiable, external contingencies related to reductions in use.

Conclusions and Directions for the Development of Recovery Models

The present chapter summarizes many of the current findings regarding long-term course of alcohol and drug involvement in youth. We have particularly focused on adolescence through young adulthood and made distinctions between patterns that emerge for youth in the general population and longitudinal trajectories that unfold for those teens whose alcohol or drug problems are severe enough for them to be placed in formal treatment.

It is clear that diversity in alcohol and other drug-use patterns is the norm for adolescents, regardless of the sample source. While the vast majority of youth who use illegal substances use only alcohol, and the majority never meet criteria for an alcohol or drug-use disorder, there is much diversity in use, which emerges over time among those who initiate alcohol and other drug involvement while they are still underage. There are substance involvement patterns in both community and clinical samples that appear time-limited whereas other trajectories bode poorly for the long-term involvement and development of the teen. Many of the predictors commonly considered to have prognostic value for the onset or progression of alcohol or drug involvement appear to have little utility for prediction of short-term or long-term resolution of alcohol or drug involvement. It is clear, however, that the continued heavy use of alcohol and other drugs is associated with poorer life functioning across many domains critical to development and to successful accomplishment of adult roles. Long-term recovery appears to be a more difficult outcome to predict using our current models of substance involvement. Clearly, research is needed that focuses on the key elements associated with transitions out of substance involvement and the factors that are associated with long-term recovery rather than short-term abstinence. Personal characteristics may be helpful in this process but only as they directly relate to the environmental or developmental challenges faced by youth as they progress into new stages of responsibility and take on new roles necessitated by progression into young adulthood.

Unlike the majority of adults with alcohol- or drug-use disorders who historically have entered treatment, adolescents in treatment are commonly using many substances when they enter treatment. While alcohol alone is often the precipitant of treatment for adults, youth entering treatment have typically had a history of heavy alcohol use but have progressed to concomitant use of other substances.

Consequently, the long-term outcomes and trajectories of teens in treatment can only be understood after fully considering all the substances used. One cannot assume that by knowing the use of a treatment participant's drug of choice, similar use (or abstinence) can be presumed for other drugs including alcohol. Research suggests marked variability in both nicotine and alcohol use relative to other substances, and important developmental outcomes may vary as a function of this concomitant use. Similarly, some youth with a history of polysubstance abuse may resolve into heavy use of alcohol with no concomitant use of other drugs. This clinically important information could not have been gleaned without the use of newer statistical procedures that afford the opportunity to consider the complicated longitudinal patterns of substance involvement as teens transition into adulthood.

Given the important differences in the developmental demands and expectations for girls and boys across adolescence, it is not surprising that gender differences emerge in the trajectories of use for teens in the general population as well as those who receive alcohol and drug treatment. In general, in community samples of youth, similar patterns may emerge across genders; however, boys tend to use in a more severe fashion than girls, and girls show more resolution. Several long-term studies suggest that recovery is more likely for female treatment participants than male adolescents. Of course, this is not the case when other psychopathologies are present which tends to dampen the recovery rates for both genders in both the short and long term. These research findings suggest the need for gender-focused research, which might clarify the predictors or maintaining factors operative for females, but not for males. Additionally, certain treatment strategies or processes may be more important to the recovery process of females than males. Other foci and strategies may need to be developed to optimize the recoveries of males in this age range. For example, while researchers and clinicians would agree that supports for sobriety are critical for all those in treatment, certain supports may be more critical in facing specific developmental challenges of males relative to females (e.g., employment), whereas other developmental tasks may have a stronger protective role in terms of recovery (e.g., pregnancy and childbirth for females). Such gender-specific developmentally relevant research could substantially aid in the development of more fruitful models of youth recovery.

The long-term trajectories of youth in the community and youth in treatment hold tremendous potential for building and informing models of youth recovery from alcohol- and other drug-use disorders. Community sample patterns can not only assist in defining norms and prevalence of common trajectories but also help identify the timing and context of transitions into and out of problematic substance involvement. These trajectories can guide researchers and clinicians to the major inflexion points in substance involvement. Investigation of these typical change points can help us ascertain the personal, developmental, and environmental factors involved in accelerations in use or transitions in patterns, as well as recovery timing and context. Similarly, trajectory-focused investigations of youth in treatment may not only teach us the developmental timing and context of risk but also provide the focus for recovery-oriented investigations and potential new interventions. For example, our longitudinal research found that late adolescence (around age 18) was a period of particular acceleration in use for those who had been treated but were currently abstaining [13]. By investigating the environmental changes that occurred during this period, it became clear that moving out of the family of origin changes many contingencies related to abstinence (e.g., exposure to alcohol/drugs, access and availability of substances, social supports for abstinence, consequences of use, etc.) [18]. Thus, this developmental task can become a focus for targeted intervention efforts to support recovery for youth facing this risk as they transition into adulthood. Similarly, other investigators have identified high-risk social interactions linked to developmental transitions (e.g., 21st birthday celebrations) that may trigger accelerations in use or the onset of a diagnostically significant event (e.g., blackouts, withdrawal, etc.) [13]. Trajectory research can assist in identifying these developmental events, challenges, and opportunities to build recovery rather than diminish success. Additionally, identifying points of desistance or precipitants of new abstention efforts can aid in the identification of motivations and resources youth draw upon in their successful efforts to recover.

Just as we have highlighted the diversity in trajectories of substance involvement of youth as they transition into adulthood, there are multiple trajectories of recovery. Not all youth will recover at the same rate or in the same way. Even early abstinence is attained in different ways by different youth. What a trajectory approach provides is an empirical foundation to begin to understand the personal, environmental, and developmental factors that constitute pathways to success, which are fundamental to a Recovery Management Approach to addiction treatment.

Key Points

- The long-term trajectories of youth in the community and youth in treatment hold tremendous potential for building and informing models of addiction recovery management.
- Diversity in alcohol- and other drug-use patterns is the norm for adolescents.
- There are substance involvement patterns in both community and clinical samples that appear time-limited, whereas other trajectories bode poorly for the long-term involvement and development of teens.
- Continued heavy use of alcohol and other drugs is associated with poorer life functioning across many domains critical to development and successful accomplishment of adult roles.
- Adolescents in treatment are commonly using many substances when they enter treatment; consequently, the long-term outcomes and trajectories of teens in treatment can only be understood after fully considering all the substances used.
- Gender differences emerge in the trajectories of use for teens in the general population as well as for those receiving alcohol and drug treatment.

References

1. Brown SA, Mott MA, Myers MG. Adolescent alcohol and drug treatment outcome. In: Watson RR, editor. Drug and alcohol abuse prevention. Clifton, NJ: Humana Press; 1990. p. 373–403.
2. Brown SA, D'Amico EJ, McCarthy DM, Tapert SF. Four-year outcomes from adolescent alcohol and drug treatment. J Stud Alcohol. 2001;96:381–8.
3. Cornelius JR, Maisto SA, Pollock NK, et al. Rapid relapse generally follows treatment for substance use disorders among adolescents. Addict Behav. 2001;27:1–6.
4. Chung T, Maisto SA, Cornelius JR, Martin CS. Adolescents' alcohol and drug use trajectories in the year following treatment. J Stud Alcohol. 2004;65:105–14.
5. Chung T, Maisto SA, Cornelius JR, Martin CS, Jackson KM. Joint trajectory analysis of treated adolescents' alcohol use and symptoms over 1 year. Addict Behav. 2005;30:1690–701.
6. Godley SH, Dennis ML, Godley MD, Funk RR. Thirty-month relapse trajectory cluster groups among adolescents discharged from out-patient treatment. Addiction. 2004;99 Suppl 2:129–39.
7. Chung T, Martin C, Grella CE, Winters KC, Abrantes AM, Brown SA. Course of alcohol problems in treated adolescents. Alcohol Clin Exp Res. 2003;27:253–61.
8. Abrantes A, McCarthy DM, Aarons G, Brown SA. Long-term trajectories of alcohol involvement following addictions treatment in adolescence. Symposium presented at the Research Society on Alcoholism. San Francisco, CA; June 2002.
9. Anderson KG, Ramo DE, Schulte MT, Cummins K, Brown SA. Substance use treatment outcomes for youth: integrating personal and environmental predictors. Drug Alcohol Depend. 2007;88(1):42–8.
10. Brown SA, Myers MG, Mott MA, Vik PW. Correlates of success following treatment for adolescent substance abuse. Appl Prev Psychol. 1994;3:61–73.
11. Winters KC, Stinchfield R, Latimer W, Lee S. Long-term outcome of substance-dependent youth following 12-step treatment. J Subst Abuse Treat. 2007;33:61–9.
12. Substance Abuse and Mental Health Services Administration, Office of Applied Studies. Treatment Episode Data Set (TEDS): 1995–2005. National Admissions to Substance Abuse Treatment Services, DASIS Series: S-37. Rockville, MD: Substance Abuse and Mental Health Services Administration, Office of Applied Studies; 2007.
13. Anderson KG, Ramo DE, Cummins K, Brown SA. Alcohol and drug involvement after adolescent treatment and functioning during emerging adulthood. Drug Alcohol Depend. 2010;107(2–3):171–81.
14. Clark DB, Jones BL, Wood DS, Cornelius JR. Substance use disorder trajectory classes: diachronic integration of onset age, severity, and course. Addict Behav. 2006;31:995–1009.
15. Aseltine Jr RH, Gore S. Work, postsecondary education, and psychosocial functioning following the transition from high school. J Adolesc Res. 2005;20(6):615–39.
16. Brown SA, McGue MK, Maggs J, et al. A developmental perspective on alcohol and youth ages 16–20. Pediatrics. 2008;121:S290–310.
17. Chassin L, Flora DB, King KM. Trajectories of alcohol and drug use and dependence from adolescence to adulthood: the effects of familial alcoholism and personality. J Abnorm Psychol. 2004;113:483–98.
18. Kypri K, McCarthy DM, Coe MT, Brown SA. Transition to independent living and substance involvement of treated and high risk youth. J Child Adolesc Subst Abuse. 2004;13(3):85–100.
19. Catalano RF, Hawkins JD, Wells EA, Miller J, Brewer D. Evaluation of the effectiveness of adolescent drug and alcohol abuse treatment, assessment of risks for relapse, and promising approaches for relapse prevention. Int J Addict. 1991;25:1085–140.
20. Latimer WW, Newcomb M, Winters KC, Stinchfield RD. Adolescent substance abuse treatment outcome: the role of substance abuse problem severity, psychosocial, and treatment factors. J Consult Clin Psychol. 2000;68:684–96.

21. Jainchill N, DeLeon G, Yagelka J. Ethnic differences in psychiatric disorders among adolescent substance abusers in treatment. J Psychopathol Behav Assess. 1997;18:133–48.
22. Schuckit MA, Smith TL, Daeppen J-B, et al. Clinical relevance of the distinction between alcohol dependence with and without a physiological component. Am J Psychiatry. 1998;155:733–40.
23. Scott CK, Foss MA, Dennis ML. Factors influencing initial and longer-term responses to substance abuse treatment: a path analysis. Eval Program Plann. 2003;26:287–95.
24. Brown SA, Vik PW, Creamer VA. Characteristics of relapse following adolescent substance abuse treatment. Addict Behav. 1989;14:291–300.
25. Richter SS, Brown SA, Mott MA. The impact of social support and self-esteem on adolescent substance abuse treatment outcome. J Subst Abuse. 1991;3:371–85.
26. Brown SA, Tapert SF, Tate SR, Abrantes AM. The role of alcohol in adolescent relapse and outcome. J Psychoactive Drugs. 2000;32:107–15.
27. Friedman AS, Terras A, Kreisher C. Family and client characteristics as predictors of outpatient treatment outcome for adolescent drug abusers. J Subst Abuse. 1995;7:345–56.
28. Latimer WW, Winters KC, Stinchfield R, Travers RE. Demographic, individual, and interpersonal predictors of adolescent alcohol and marijuana use following treatment. Psychol Addict Behav. 2000;14:162–73.
29. Piko B. Perceived social support from parents and peers: which is the stronger predictor of adolescent substance abuse? Subst Use Misuse. 2000;35:617–30.
30. Ashby Wills T, Resko JA, Ainette MG, Mendoza D. Role of parent support and peer support in adolescent substance use: a test of mediated effects. Psychol Addict Behav. 2004;18:122–34.
31. McCrady BS. To have but one true friend: implications for practice of research on alcohol use disorders and social network. Psychol Addict Behav. 2004;18:113–21.
32. Brown SA, Gleghorn A, Schuckit MA, Myers MG, Mott MA. Conduct disorder among adolescent alcohol and drug abusers. J Stud Alcohol. 1996;57:314–24.
33. Caspi A, Moffitt TE, Newman DL, Silva PA. Behavioral observations at age 3 years predict adult psychiatric disorders: longitudinal evidence from a birth cohort. Arch Gen Psychiatry. 1996;53:1033–9.
34. Christiansen BA, Goldman MS. Alcohol-related expectancies versus demographic/background variables in the prediction of adolescent drinking. J Consult Clin Psychol. 1983;51:249–57.
35. Stacy AW, Newcomb MD, Bentler PM. Cognitive motivation and drug use: a 9-year longitudinal study. J Abnorm Psychol. 1991;100:502–15.
36. Smith GT, Goldman MS, Greenbaum PE, Christiansen BA. Expectancy for social facilitation from drinking: the divergent paths of high-expectancy and low-expectancy adolescents. J Abnorm Psychol. 1995;104:32–40.
37. Tomlinson KL, Brown SA, Abrantes A. Psychiatric comorbidity and substance use treatment outcomes of adolescents. Psychol Addict Behav. 2004;18:160–9.
38. Substance Abuse and Mental Health Services Administration. The trends in substance use, dependence or abuse, and treatment among adolescents: 2002–7. Washington, DC: US Department of Health and Human Services Office of Applied Studies; 2008.
39. D'Amico EJ, McCarthy DM, Metrik J, Brown SA. Alcohol-related services: prevention, secondary intervention, and treatment preferences of adolescents. J Child Adolesc Subst Abuse. 2004;14(2):61–80.
40. Blomqvist J. Self-change from alcohol and drug abuse: often-cited classics. In: Klingman H, Sobell LC, editors. Promoting self-change from addictive behaviors: practical implications for policy, prevention, and treatment. New York, NY: Springer; 2007.
41. Blomqvist J. Self-change from alcohol and drug abuse: often-cited classics. In: Klingman H, Sobell LC, editors. Promoting self-change from addictive behaviors: practical implications for policy, prevention, and treatment. New York, NY: Springer; 2006.

42. Clark DB. The natural history of adolescent alcohol use disorders. Addiction. 2004;99 Suppl 2:5–22.
43. D'Amico EJ, Metrik J, McCarthy DM, Frissell KC, Applebaum M, Brown SA. Progression into and out of binge drinking among high school students. Psychol Addict Behav. 2001;15 (4):341–9.
44. Brown SA. Facilitating change for adolescent alcohol problems: a multiple options approach. In: Wagner EF, Waldron HB, editors. Innovations in adolescent substance abuse interventions. Amsterdam: Pergamon/Elsevier; 2001. p. 167–85.
45. Smart RG. Natural recovery or recovery without treatment from alcohol and drug problems as seen from survey data. In: Klingman H, Sobell LC, editors. Promoting self-change from addictive behaviors: practical implications for policy, prevention, and treatment. New York, NY: Springer; 2007. p. 59–71.
46. Pollock NK, Martin CS. Diagnostic orphans: adolescents with alcohol symptoms who do not qualify for DSM-IV abuse or dependence diagnoses. Am J Psychiatry. 1999;156:897–901.
47. Chung T, Martin CS. Classification and course of alcohol problems among adolescents in addictions treatment programs. Alcohol Clin Exp Res. 2001;25(12):61–9.
48. Wiesner M, Weichold K, Silbereisen RK. Trajectories of alcohol use among adolescent boys and girls: identification, validation, and sociodemographic characteristics. Psychol Addict Behav. 2007;21:62–75.
49. King KM. Patterns of alcohol use across adolescence: are there really four types of teenagers. Symposium Presented at the Research Society on Alcoholism Annual Meeting. San Diego, CA; June 2009.
50. Johnston LD, O'Malley PM, Bachman JG, Schulenberg JE. Monitoring the future: national results on adolescent drug use: overview of key findings, 2007. Bethesda, MD: National Institute on Drug Abuse; 2007. p. 1–70.
51. Schulenberg JE, Maggs JL. A developmental perspective on alcohol use and heavy drinking during adolescence and the transition to young adulthood. J Stud Alcohol. 2002;14 (Suppl):54–70.
52. Zucker RA, Chermack ST, Curran GM. Alcoholism: a life span perspective on etiology and course. In: Sameroff AJ, Lewis M, Miller SM, editors. Handbook of developmental psychopathology. 2nd ed. New York, NY: Kluwer Academic/Plenum; 2000. p. 569–87.
53. Jacob T, Bucholz KK, Sartor CE, Howell DN, Wood PK. Drinking trajectories from adolescence to the mid-forties among alcohol dependent males. J Stud Alcohol. 2005;66:745–55.
54. Ellickson PL, Martino SC, Collins RL. Marijuana use from adolescence to young adulthood: multiple developmental trajectories and their associated outcomes. Health Psychol. 2004;23:299–307.
55. Flory K, Lynam D, Milich R, Leukefeld C, Clayton R. Early adolescent through young adult alcohol and marijuana use trajectories: early predictors, young adult outcomes, and predictive utility. Dev Psychopathol. 2004;16:193–213.
56. Jackson KM, Sher KJ, Schulenberg JE. Conjoint developmental trajectories of young adult alcohol and tobacco use. J Abnorm Psychol. 2005;114(4):612–26.
57. Weisner M, Weichold K, Silbereisen RK. Trajectories of alcohol use among adolescent boys and girls: identification, validation, and sociodemographic characteristics. Psychol Addict Behav. 2007;21(1):62–75.
58. Windle M, Mun EY, Windle RC. Adolescent-to-young adulthood heavy drinking trajectories and their prospective predictors. J Stud Alcohol. 2005;66:313–22.
59. Vik PW, Celluci T, Ivers H. Natural reduction in binge drinking for college students. Addict Behav. 2003;28:643–55.

Chapter 9
Residential Recovery Homes/Oxford Houses

Leonard A. Jason, Bradley D. Olson, David G. Mueller, Lisa Walt,
and Darrin M. Aase

Abstract Over 10,000 people live in recovery homes called Oxford Houses throughout the USA. Among these approximately 1,400 abstinent living environments, residents are provided an unlimited period of time to gain fellowship and support for becoming productive members of society. The evolution of 17 year collaboration between this Oxford House organization and a research team at DePaul University is described. In addition, economic issues are explored including the finding that this recovery community appears to have both low costs and high benefits. Issues involving the sustainability of the Oxford Houses are also presented. The chapter also reviews gender roles and women's specific issues to highlight how Oxford Houses have the potential to be empowering. Finally, comorbid psychiatric conditions are reviewed in the context of how Oxford Houses can promote not only abstinence among this group, but also improved psychological functioning.

Keywords Addiction recovery management · Recovery homes · Abstinent living environment · Recovery community · Long-term abstinence

The Oxford House Story

This chapter focuses on the history and growth of the Oxford House Movement, and the evolution of a Participatory Action Approach collaboration between this self-help organization and researchers at DePaul University. We begin with a brief description of the origin and nature of Oxford Houses. Subsequently, we explored some of the economic benefits and costs of Oxford Houses as well as

L.A. Jason (✉)
Psychology Department, Center for Community Research, DePaul University,
990 W. Fullerton Ave., Chicago, IL 60614, USA
e-mail: ljason@depaul.edu

J.F. Kelly and W.L. White (eds.), *Addiction Recovery Management: Theory, Research and Practice*, Current Clinical Psychiatry, DOI 10.1007/978-1-60327-960-4_9,
© Springer Science+Business Media, LLC 2011

issues involving the sustainability of the Oxford Houses. The chapter also reviews gender roles and comorbid psychiatric conditions among residents of these recovery homes.

Origin and Nature of Oxford Houses

Beginning in 1975, Paul Molloy and his fellow house members created one Oxford House. Since that time, this one house has expanded to a network of over 1,400 USA Oxford Houses plus just over 30 Canadian and 8 Australian Houses, each providing support to persons with substance abuse problems. Former substance abusers now rent houses throughout the USA, with no supervision except what they provide on their own. Houses are single-sex dwellings, and some allow residents to live with minor children. Individual members are expected to pay monthly rent and assist with chores. Houses generally have functional kitchens, laundry facilities, and common areas where residents conduct business meetings and spend social time, with 7–12 individuals living in a house and usually sharing bedrooms. Houses are located in multiethnic communities with access to public transportation and employment opportunities. Unlike other aftercare residential programs, such as half-way houses, Oxford House has no prescribed length of stay for residents.

Each House operates democratically with majority rule for most policies and an 80% majority regarding membership [1]. Residents must follow three simple rules: pay rent and contribute to the maintenance of the home, abstain from using alcohol and other drugs, and avoid disruptive behavior. Violation of the above rules results in eviction from the House [1]. Each Oxford House has a President, Treasurer, Comptroller, Coordinator, Secretary, and Building Maintenance person elected to 6-month terms. This process gives all house members opportunities to exert leadership and make sure rules are being followed. The revolving leadership system helps residents inexperienced with financial issues and general management to become more skilled in these areas. Members report that it is easier to follow rules enforced by other house residents, who must also comply with these rules, than by professionals who might be more distant and removed. New members attend eight self-help meetings during this first month. During the first 2 weeks, they are also required to do a "one on one" with all members of the house. This process involves each member sitting down with the new resident to allow the new resident to tell the story of his/her addiction and what he/she is doing to avoid substance use and stay abstinent. Groups of houses in the same geographic area are placed into a chapter. Chapters have officers that are elected and include a Chapter Chairperson, a Vice Chairperson, a Treasurer, a Secretary, and a Housing Service Committee Chairperson.

In 1988, Congress passed the *Anti-Drug Abuse Act* allocating federal funds to any state for the start-up of recovery homes such as Oxford Houses. A group of recovering substance abusers, through the support of an established House, could request $4,000 from their state in an interest-free loan to begin a new Oxford House.

Repayment of loans was returned to the fund for start-up costs of additional Houses in that state. Several states also provided funds to hire Oxford House recruiters to help open Oxford Houses. These actions led to the expansion of Oxford Houses. In the late 1990s, states were no longer required to administer a state loan program, but many states continued to offer these loans to Oxford Houses.

The aspect that is most unique to Oxford House involves the high levels of abstinence-specific social support, which encourages abstinence. The self-governing policies described above help create and nurture these abstinence-specific social support networks. In the absence of professional staff, residents develop rules and policies, learn to self-govern, assume positions of leadership within their Houses, and participate in the bodies that develop, monitor, and assist individual houses.

Participatory Action Approach

In 1992, the first author saw Paul Molloy, the founder of Oxford Houses, interviewed on CBS's *60 Minutes*. Intrigued by the description of these Oxford Houses, he contacted Mr. Molloy and out of that initial conversation grew a long-term collaborative partnership between a university-based research team and a grassroots community-based organization [2]. Mr. Molloy was enthusiastic about a collaborative effort that would examine Oxford Houses.

Our work with the Oxford House organization typifies an action research perspective, one focusing on developing practical knowledge about issues of pressing concern using participatory processes [3, 4]. We used *Participatory Action Research* (PAR) methods, a community-based model that collaboratively involves multiple segments of the community in research endeavors, and uses approaches that reflect ecological theory and an empowerment agenda [5, 6]. Hill et al. [7] identified themes within an action agenda that include collaboration and action. Collaboration allows all stakeholders within the community to be represented [2].

Shortly after the first author contacted Mr. Molloy, Oxford House decided to establish Oxford Houses in the Midwest. In 1992, the first Oxford House representative, named Bill, was sent from Oxford House, Inc. to Chicago in order to begin the establishment of Oxford Houses in Illinois. Although the Illinois Department of Alcohol and Substance Abuse (DASA) awarded money from the state's revolving fund to support the opening of the first house, there were funding complications at DASA that left the Oxford House representative without necessary housing and financial support. Somewhat discouraged, Bill found temporary lodging at a local shelter where consequently he was robbed of all his personal belongings. Frustrated and dejected, he was on the verge of leaving Chicago and abandoning his task all together. Congruent with an action-oriented agenda, our research team provided Bill with free accommodations, first at the home of one of the members of the research team and then at the DePaul University priests' residence, so Bill could proceed with his venture. For several months, we also provided him with office space, a telephone, and other resources to facilitate his efforts. Because of this joint effort, Bill was able to successfully establish the first Oxford House home in Illinois. The home was located near the university and for appreciation of the support provided by our group, it was named the "DePaul House."

Over the next 7 years, pilot studies were conducted and collaborative work was continued with local and national organizations. As an example, a grant proposal was jointly written to a local foundation to provide funds to hire a recruiter to open two Oxford House homes for women and children in the area. The funded grant was jointly administered by both the DePaul University research team and the Illinois Oxford House organization. DePaul researchers also talked to reporters when members of the press wrote articles about Oxford House. Finally, the research team supplied some of their preliminary research findings to the Oxford House organization during a Supreme Court lawsuit against an Oxford House home in the state of Washington. The suit, based on a zoning law that prohibited more than five unrelated people from living in one dwelling, was representative of some communities' unwillingness to support Oxford Houses or other recovery homes for fear of reducing their property values. Fortunately, the suit against Oxford House was defeated, and the positive precedent the case set has had an important impact on other Oxford Houses, similar residences, and other halfway houses.

During this time, efforts were undertaken to obtain external federal funding to support larger and more sophisticated research studies on the process of communal living within Oxford House. We submitted multiple federal proposals, but members of a scientific review committee recommended that our team needed to evaluate the effectiveness of Oxford House through a randomized outcome study. We were hesitant to advance a methodology that could potentially upset the natural process of self-selection that occurs within Oxford House. That is, members of each Oxford House interview discuss and vote on whether an applicant should be admitted as a resident in their house. This democratic process is an important cornerstone to the Oxford House approach to recovery, and we did not want to disrupt that process; as doing so would fundamentally change the structure of how Oxford House operates.

When this dilemma was presented to Mr. Molloy, he said that he would support a random assignment design, as this would help out efforts to secure funds to assess in a rigorous way the effectiveness of the Oxford Houses. We developed a protocol that accommodated random assignment within Oxford House's democratic system of selection. In our study, individuals finishing substance abuse treatment were randomly assigned to either an Oxford House or Usual Aftercare, with follow-up assessments at 2 years. Using this design in our proposal, we secured our first Oxford House focused National Institute on Alcohol Abuse and Alcoholism (NIAAA) grant (to be described below). The prior collaborative relationship with Oxford House helped the DePaul researchers gain the approval of Mr. Molloy, who was able to provide the organizational support and technical expertise for a rigorous randomized outcome study. We later also received a National Institute of Drug Abuse (NIDA) grant to interview Oxford House residents in a national sample over a period of a year.

Community coalitions, such as the one described in this article, address the lack of various services addressing specific social problems [8]. Coalitions often employ an ecological approach and empower community members to facilitate social change. Our work employed collaborative methods throughout, and the ideas for most of our work was generated and guided by our Oxford House partners [9]. As an example of the collaborative nature of our work, at the end of one presentation at an Oxford House annual convention, an Oxford House member approached the first author and suggested that we include the issue of tolerance in our future research. He mentioned that prior to living in an Oxford House, he was very prejudiced against people who were different from him, and he pointed to a woman, who was his girlfriend, noting she was HIV positive. Before living in an Oxford House, he said that he would never even talk to her as he was so prejudiced and narrow minded, and he discriminated against people who were infected with HIV. He then mentioned that it was just as important to measure these types of changes that were occurring among residents as it was to assess abstinence. We took this feedback to our team and later began a study on the development of tolerance among Oxford House members [10].

Coalitions such as the Oxford House/DePaul collaboration foster a sense of community in those individuals within the group by promoting methods of information exchange, support for multiple perspectives, and collaborative activities [9]. This emergence of common experiences enhances the trust and awareness of each other [11]. Because of our collaboration with Oxford House, when the Oxford House organization made several presentations to officials as the US Office of National Drug Control policy, they included us in the meetings. In addition, when a new Illinois governor was elected in 2001, as part of cost saving initiatives, he ended the $100,000 loan program and support of Oxford House recruiters for the state of Illinois. When the findings from our randomized NIAAA-funded Oxford House study [12] were released, we met with the head of DASA in Illinois, and our positive findings led the state to restart both the $100,000 loan program and the recruiter support. Our data also was used in expert testimony by the first author to argue in court cases to stop communities from passing not in my backyard legislation that would prevent Oxford Houses from existing in many towns [13].

When working closely with community partners, there are also challenges to the research relationship that need to be addressed. As one example, an official from a large federal agency was asked to develop a position paper on Oxford Houses. He ultimately recommended that the houses should be substantially expanded. However, as he was finishing writing the position paper, he mentioned to the first author that the Oxford House organization was too disorganized, lacked sufficient infrastructure, and had poor leadership to expand this program. He then suggested that the first author should assume the role of training and monitoring of recruiters to expand the system. Even though such a contract would have involved millions of dollars, the first author refused this offer and informed the leadership of the Oxford House organization of this plan. This action preserved our relationship with the Oxford House organization and prevented one of the federal departments from exerting undue influence on the Oxford House model's operations. There is an appropriate role for the federal government in helping expand these Oxford Houses, in providing additional loan supports, for helping states hire additional recruiters, and for helping defray legal costs from court expenses of communities trying to prevent Oxford Houses from being established in many neighborhoods. But in providing help, the federal government needs to be wary of usurping the authority or leadership of this grass roots organization.

Economic Issues

In the following section, we will discuss some of the economic potential benefits of the Oxford House model. In Illinois, roughly 900,000 adults and 90,000 youth are candidates for substance abuse treatment services. Not all of these individuals are actually seeking treatment, but on average, 700 individuals are on waiting lists at any one time. In most states, service capacity could reasonably be doubled to fit the need. Treatment for substance abuse is as effective, adherence is greater, and relapse is lower for substance abuse-related problems than for many other serious health conditions such as diabetes and cardiovascular disease [14]. From a public health perspective, a most reasonable goal is to focus on recovery systems that have demonstrated *social and economic* benefits by providing greater access to effective recovery opportunities, and, according to a particular stage in a person's recovery.

Yearly costs for the USA associated with alcohol and drug problems are around $500 billion. The Center on Addiction and Substance Abuse (CASA) states that for every dollar spent on social harms, 96¢ is spent on "shoveling up the wreckage" and only 4¢ used to prevent and treat addiction. Studies have found that the economic benefits of treatment range from $1 saved to every dollar invested to $18 saved for every $1 invested [15]. Treatment in itself, particularly when contrasted to incarceration – the common alternative path of substance use, is well worth the amount put up front.

We are not suggesting that the mutual-help residence is the end-all in recovery options – such an argument would go against the NIDA's principles of effective treatment that suggests that no one intervention works for every individual. However, meeting the dual goals of increasing well-being and effective treatment economics requires a more integrated continuum of care, and Oxford Houses fit in such a model.

If we look at our most commonly used modalities of detoxification and inpatient treatment, we have seen average treatment durations shrink dramatically from 90 to 30 days and sometimes to simply a 3-day detoxification. They are expensive, as are almost all professional modalities. That is not to say they are unnecessary, and whether we are talking about traditional inpatient treatment, therapeutic communities, recovery homes, or individual therapy, we see advances from brief interventions, motivational interviewing, and harm reduction strategies. Randomized studies have shown that, if engaged in early enough, brief interventions can be effective, and of course, reduced time means reduced costs.

Then there are the classic 12-step options such as Alcoholics Anonymous and Narcotics Anonymous. Weekly meetings occur and sometimes individuals attend every day. Strong peer support is provided with no societal/taxpayer costs. Such an approach does quite well because it helps counter those dangerous social networks of family, friends, dealers, bars, and other forms of temptation. Even within the 12-step model, a person may end up returning to homes where these networks and temptations exist. Paul Molloy has observed that some individuals are without a home, but few of these individuals have a home that does not constantly invite drinking and using (through direct temptations and enabling).

Each modality (12-step groups and therapeutic communities) has its advantages, but the mutual-help residence has perhaps the greatest strength of having the low societal costs of the 12-step model with the duration, frequency, and intensity that most treatment providers believe is necessary to bring about effective recovery outcomes. Short treatment stays are often their number one attribution for the cycle of relapse and multiple treatment stays.

The economic advantages of Oxford House are attributable to the fact that participants pay their own rent at a low cost due to sharing rental costs. Many residents enter the house unemployed, but are continually encouraged and supported by other members to find employment. Oxford Houses are organized in chapters, which are typically geographic clusters of houses. Members throughout these chapters have many employment connections and tend to build successful relationships with various employers in a particular region.

Economics are relevant to any section of the multilevel treatment scheme provided, but it is clearly tied to federal and state policy. Our research group's first foray into studying societal costs of opening up Oxford Houses began with us obtaining federal loan information from states and Oxford House main offices in the Washington DC area [16]. This program was an amendment in the anti-drug abuse act of 1988 previously discussed in this chapter. In addition to collecting information from this program, we explored the literature for ranges of inpatient treatment and jail/prison costs to obtain per person and estimated yearly ranges of these costs. In addition, based on a procedure developed by French [17], we utilized data from our large, NIDA-funded national data set related to incarceration and treatment. This approach allowed us to use the past histories of these participants, adjusting their treatment and incarceration costs to be consistent with the Oxford House sample. Annual program costs per person were estimated for Oxford House based on federal loan information and data collected from Oxford House, Inc. In addition, annual treatment and incarceration costs were approximated based on participant data prior to Oxford House residence in conjunction with normative costs for these settings. Societal costs associated with the Oxford House program were relatively low, whereas estimated costs associated with inpatient and incarceration history were high.

In an NIAAA grant-supported study, 150 individuals who completed treatment at alcohol and drug abuse facilities in the Chicago metropolitan area were recruited, with half being randomly assigned to live in an Oxford House, while the other half received community-based aftercare services (Usual Care). A 24-month follow-up [18] found 31.3% of participants assigned to the Oxford House condition reported substance use compared to 64.8% of Usual Care participants, 76.1% of Oxford House participants were employed versus 48.6% of Usual Care participants, and days engaged in illegal activities during the 30 days prior to the final assessment was a mean of 0.9 for Oxford House and a mean of 1.8 for Usual Care participants. Two years after entering Oxford House, 14 of the women assigned to the Oxford House condition had regained custody of their children, while only one woman had lost custody. On the other hand, in the Usual Care condition, only six women regained custody of their children, while two lost custody. Oxford House participants earned roughly $550 more per month than participants in the usual care group. Annualizing this difference for the entire Oxford House sample corresponds to approximately $494,000 in additional production. The lower rate of incarceration in this study among Oxford House versus usual care participants corresponded to annualized savings for the Oxford House sample of roughly $119,000. Together, the productivity and incarceration benefits yield an estimated $613,000 in savings accruing to the Oxford House participants.

In 2007, the Oxford House organization received about $1.6 million in grants from state and local governments to pay outreach workers to develop and maintain networks of individual Oxford Houses in nine States and the District of Columbia. If the Oxford Houses had been traditional, fully staffed halfway houses, the cost to taxpayers would have been $224,388,000 [19].

We can get a better understanding of how well the start-up loan policy fits with the nature of the Oxford House model and the national growth of new houses by considering two methods. The best way to conceptualize the growth of houses is as either (a) a grassroots, house-to-house, or (b) a relatively hands-off top–down policy method.

Oxford Houses started out as a grassroots movement. Paul Molloy describes his recovery home closing down and all of the members saying, "Let's rent our own house." They did so, and instead of hiring staff they voted on everything democratically. This approach was successful, and others in recovery heard about the Oxford House success. The original members had built up a savings account, and they decided to loan money to others to open up a second house. This grassroots method continued from there.

Mutual help, in general, has a curious relationship with the obtaining of government funds. Mutual help researchers and mental health consumers alike have believed that government involvement, particularly the providing of funds, can interfere with the sovereignty of a mutual-help group. The fear has often been that once the government gets involved in opening up houses, the government will start to create new rules, standardize each house, and essentially ignore the features that have evolved that ultimately allowed the model to work. What is positive about what happened with the stipulations of the Anti-Drug Abuse Act of 1988 is that it allowed the houses to keep their self-determination and individual responsibility by allowing states to take on a revolving loan fund that would help hire people to open up houses. However, the majority of the funds were to make loans available to anyone in recovery who wanted to open up these houses and begin to pay the state back for these loans, which is exactly why it was called a "revolving loan fund."

To examine the impact of this policy on the nationwide growth of Oxford Houses – the diffusion of this innovation – we looked at house growth (either

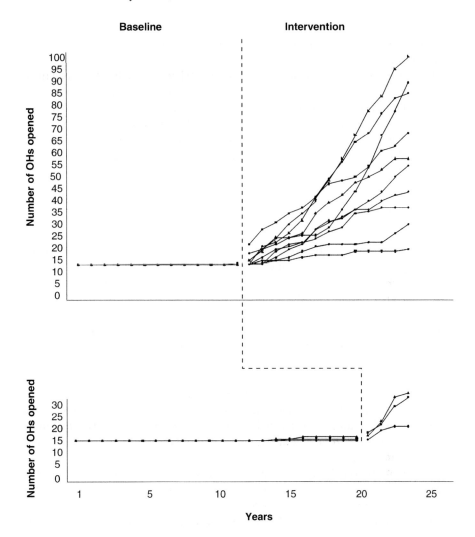

Fig. 9.1   The growth of Oxford Houses over time

grassroots growth or growth in states adopting the policy) in a state-level multiple baseline framework. We therefore essentially treated the policy as a behavioral intervention, tracing the growth of houses in 13 states. On Fig. 9.1, on the y-axis, we have the number of houses. The y-axis shows the number of houses starting at zero and going up to 100. Each line represents one of 13 states. In the top figure, the low number of houses in each state leads up to a point of dramatic growth in each of these states. This date is 1988/89 when the Anti-Drug Abuse act went into effect, and these ten states were among those that had picked up the loan funds and technical assistance involving hiring recruiters. In the figure below, we see when three other states did not use the loan fund and technical assistance, very few

Oxford Houses emerged; however, when the states utilized the loan fund and the technical assistance associated with it, growth of Oxford Housed increased with this policy initiative [20].

In some of our other examinations of this data [21], we found that these loan funds also increased the number of women's houses. Perhaps policy makers who were running these funds saw the need for and encouraged more of these types of houses. We also saw some states drop the fund, and nevertheless we still saw the grassroots method of house openings continue in these states, suggesting that the federal loan policy really increased the growth of Oxford Houses.

Sustainability

Our research team recently conducted a study to explore the longevity of Oxford Houses and find patterns of closure among houses. We examined houses that were included in a large NIDA-funded national study that concluded in 2001. We discovered that of the 214 houses included in the study, 172 were still open and 29 were closed [22]. This translates to an 86.9% sustainability rate for houses 6 years after the initial study was completed. On average, houses were open 7.28 years (SD = 3.75), suggesting that houses have considerable longevity.

Sustainability for any organization is important but it is particularly important for nonprofit self-run settings. Shediac-Rizkallah and Bone [23] have identified two important factors in the sustainability of health programs: program/project factors and organization/environment factors. Since the focus of this chapter is on Oxford House, we will continue this discussion through an examination of two important factors that have contributed to the sustainability of Oxford House: volunteers and organizational strength.

Research has found that volunteers are important for sustainability [24, 25]. Clearly, the benefits of volunteers are numerous for both the organization and the volunteer. The organization receives no cost or low-cost labor and a commitment to the project while the volunteer often enjoys self-esteem benefits [24] and develops new job skills and friendships [25]. Oxford House routinely utilizes current residents in the sustainability of the house. For instance, residents with long tenures often volunteer to move into a new house and provide experience and support for new residents [1]. Oxford House alumni often return to Oxford House and provide support or volunteer in the community. In a 2008 study, alumni reported returning to an Oxford House to be involved after moving out. They reported staying in contact and visiting several times per month for several reasons, including conventions, house meetings, and acting as a mentor to current house residents among many other reasons [26].

Organizational strength can be conceptualized in many ways. Evashwick and Ory [27], for instance, report that the number of years the organization has been in existence is one measure. Oxford House has been in existence over 30 years. As mentioned earlier, originally founded in 1975 with one house in Silver Spring,

Maryland, it has grown to over 1,400 houses. Today over 10,000 people are living in the network of houses. Alternatively, researchers have found that responding to challenges is another barometer of organizational strength [28, 29]. Oxford House has overcome several challenges including community opposition to groups of unrelated individuals in recovery living together in a home [30, 31]. Several legal cases have found in favor of Oxford House. Additional struggles included starting up new houses, finding sources of funding, and effectively managing the network of houses throughout the USA. Oxford House has overcome each one of these challenges and today stands strong as one of the more successful recovery programs in the country. The visible leadership of key figures such as Paul Molloy and the unsung local champions has significantly contributed to the sustainability of Oxford House as a solution to successful recovery from alcohol and drugs.

While the previous sections in this chapter have dealt with larger, systemic issues such as economics and sustainability, the remainder of the chapter will highlight how individual factors can interact with the Oxford House model to promote recovery. First, a discussion of etiological issues involving gender roles and women's specific issues will highlight how Oxford Houses have the potential to be empowering and effective despite many complicating societal pressures influencing substance abuse among women. Second, comorbid psychiatric conditions will be discussed in the context of how Oxford Houses can promote not only abstinence among this group, but also improved psychological functioning. While Oxford Houses are not necessarily for everyone, aspects of the model have potential to be an innovative environment for many oppressed groups that often have their specific issues neglected or unintegrated within traditional treatment settings.

Oxford House and Gender Roles

In one of our studies [32], we explored similarities and differences between women and men, particularly looking at their social support networks and their beliefs that they could remain abstinent from alcohol and drugs. For women, social support networks were directly related to their confidence in remaining abstinent, whereas for men, social support seemed to play a smaller role in determining these beliefs. Belyaev-Glantsman et al. [32] examined employment and sources of income for different genders and ethnic groups residing in our NIDA-funded national Oxford House sample. Men compared with women reported significantly higher mean income from employment as well as total income. African-Americans compared with European-Americans reported significantly more work in the past 30 days; however, the rate of pay between these two ethnic groups was not significantly different. Longer length of stay in Oxford House was related to higher incomes.

In another study [33], participants completed a survey regarding the resources they have gained or lost dealing with substance abuse. Some resources on the survey include the support of family and friends as well as skills to cope with recovery. Women tended to gain more resources then men in recovery; however, men lost less resources during stressful situations. Finally, individuals with more than 6 months in the Oxford House reported significantly less resource loss than those with less than 6 months in the Oxford House. The results of this study show that the Oxford House model may be beneficial to all residents, regardless of their ethnicity or gender.

With a national USA sample of Oxford House members [34], we investigated whether members help others inside and/or outside their community. Women compared with men reported providing more help to housemates over the past 6 months, were more likely to report that they helped others maintain their abstinence as a result of OH, and reported engaging in more reciprocal help related to abstinence in their houses. In contrast, men reported greater rates of helping strangers and acquaintances who did not live in OH than women.

Perhaps one of the most disheartening realizations is that, because women see such a need for the support a romantic relationship can provide they may willingly place themselves in situations where chances of relapse are high. These women may purposely trade an increased risk of relapse and their long-term physical health to create and maintain romantic relationships. Since the first author has been working within the Oxford House association for many years, and the other authors have worked side by side with many former substance abusers (both successful and unsuccessful in their recovery), many of us has had the chance to hear some of the stories linking romance and recovery. These stories caused us to think of two questions: "What can be done to help empower women in recovery? What can we learn from women that have been successful in their recovery?"

In order to try and answer these questions, we began talking with women in recovery that had lived in an Oxford House. When talking with these women, we found a similar storyline lurking beneath the tales of romance and addiction. Women talked about the power of romance, how the romantic relationship was their one source of social support, of comfort. Women also spoke of how their histories of drug abuse had made them "users" of everyone. The literature supports this type of mindset in the recovering substance abuser, and many studies explain that this atmosphere of manipulation places great burdens on available social supports and also causes the expectation that abusers have to watch themselves with everyone [35].

The women particularly talked of their romantic partners, of the roller coaster ride of patterns of drug use, abstinence, and eventual relapse. Many talked about past interpersonal violence and trauma, and the constant fear of victimization. Women talked of not respecting themselves, of not knowing how to respect themselves. This is where the story turns. For many, recovery involves both giving up the "right" to use others and reassuming responsibility for one's actions thus, similar to what other researchers have reported [36], the women we spoke with spoke of how the Oxford House gave them the opportunity to form new kinds of relationships, to learn new skills, to reconceptualize their ideas of friendship and sex, and to build social supports outside of and independent of romantic relationships.

Because of these anecdotal stories of former Oxford House members, we believe that the Oxford House model may provide a supportive environment that is especially helpful for women in recovery. OH members may provide one another with both general and abstinence-specific social support that can replace the unhealthy support they might each receive from nonrecovery conducive family, friends, and romantic partners. At the same time, Oxford Houses may provide opportunities for the women in recovery to build communication and reasoning skills and establish strong trusting bonds with women that have been through the same experience that they currently have. Oxford House members may serve to modulate the behavior of each other, much as the "romantic female partner modulator" discussed before. The Oxford House model may also provide valuable social support independent of the romantic relationship, and hopefully, this social support will encourage women to be more likely to leave nonrecovery conducive, or abusive partners behind. In addition, we believe the experience of living in a supportive, democratically run environment that provides opportunities to build life skills (by serving in the different positions in the house and learning from other members), women will be able to see beyond the restrictions of strict gender roles and envision sober, self-fulfilled lives in which they hold the power and ability to navigate through.

Currently, we are attempting to address these research questions in a 5-year longitudinal study funded by the National Center on Minority Health and Health Disparities. This 5-year study follows women recently involved with the criminal justice system in substance abuse recovery for 2 years, and randomly assigns them to either the Oxford House or usual aftercare condition. We have added several measures to five time point interviews that investigate the interactions between romantic relationships, different sources of social support, and living environment. We hope to understand the complex relationship between romance and recovery, and possibly be able to identify the OH as an effective self-recovery living environment that may be especially beneficial to women in recovery.

Psychiatric Comorbidity

While recovery programs have often been considered male oriented due to the era that Alcoholics Anonymous originated in and societal norms that have placed disproportionate expectations on women compared to men, they have also often not been integrative for a number of other subgroups of the general population. An organization such as an Oxford House is unique in that, aside from the three basic rules mentioned previously in this chapter, Houses are able to operate with autonomy. Such an organic approach that exemplifies nonstandardization has the potential to look very different from House to House, Chapter to Chapter, and community to community. This flexibility allows each House to establish its own identity and to empower residents to make their own choices and adaptations that promote their individual recovery. One example of a subgroup in the population that may benefit from Oxford Houses is an individual who has comorbid psychological and substance abuse problems.

Psychiatric comorbidity is often reciprocal in nature; experts often disagree about the "chicken and the egg" concept when clearly, different etiologies and interactions between these two health problems are evident. Due to the fact that 33–60% of individuals with substance abuse issues also have a mood or anxiety disorder [37] and that those estimates of comorbidity are higher for other populations such as those with Schizophrenia, the question facing treatment providers is no longer "Which came first?" but "How do we address *both* problems to avoid these devastating health consequences?". The unique aspect of Oxford Houses is that because they are organic and self-run (by individuals who are harsher critics on themselves than treatment providers are); they also are equipped to address the complexities that comorbid psychiatric conditions present to recovery. In fact, evidence from prior research and observations from our research team indicate that Oxford Houses function in ways that often prevent the very behaviors and expressions of affect that are commonly associated with relapse.

For example, many researchers have documented how substance abuse is frequently a response to negative emotions [38] (i.e., *self medication*). Within an Oxford House, individuals are not permitted to exhibit isolative behaviors such as staying in one's room all day or locking the door, as the residents are well aware that these avoidant behaviors can lead to urges to self-medicate. Furthermore, while the national Oxford House organization does not require Houses to impose external treatment demands on a resident, many local Oxford House affiliates (such as the Illinois State Board for Oxford Houses) require ongoing attendance at AA or NA and encourage individuals to seek outpatient treatment for psychiatric issues. In fact, some Oxford Houses even have developed their own medication administration systems, where psychiatric medications are kept in a lock-box to ensure that they are taken appropriately and within prescription guidelines. Such engagement in the community and attentiveness to treatment adherence helps to deconstruct the behavioral issues associated with internalizing affective problems and develop new behaviors, much like a professional treatment provider would attempt to do in therapy or a treatment setting. The difference in effectiveness, however, lies in the fact that Oxford House residents impose these regulations on each other, who have had similar experiences and share a common bond.

Beyond issues such as depression and anxiety, researchers have often suggested that underlying temperamental features such as impulsivity and "deviant" personality characteristics may be the underlying catalyst for both substance abuse and impulse-control psychiatric disorders. The organizational structure within Oxford Houses as self-governed settings has the innovative potential to subdue opposition to rules and regulations due to the fact that residents are participants in making the rules. For example, while Oxford Houses often allow more personal freedoms among residents, they are also more likely to enforce harsh penalties for disruptive behavior [39]. Penalties might consist of fines or behavioral contracts that are agreed upon by a majority of members living within the House. Furthermore, many behavioral issues are discussed at business meetings and resolutions are agreed upon by the collective group and not an external authority figure [40].

Such contingencies employed among a group of individuals living together are comparable to those that a treatment provider would attempt to internalize within a patient, but are perhaps more effective due to the fact that there is no external authority involved.

Empirical research has demonstrated that Oxford Houses, and specifically living in an Oxford House for a longer period of time, can produce psychological benefits such as improvements in both internalizing affective [41] and behavioral symptoms [42]. Furthermore, although treatment gains still suggest that those with psychiatric comorbidity do not improve as much as those with only substance abuse problems [43], randomized and within-subjects designs with Oxford House residents have suggested that those with psychiatric disorders or problems have similar beneficial outcomes for substance use abstinence compared to those without psychiatric problems [44, 45]. Such findings renew the interest in how these differences occur and not just why they do.

Mutual help as a concept has received an increasing amount of attention in recent years. In fact, dual-focused (both 12-step oriented and focusing on psychiatric issues) self-help groups have emerged that have demonstrated interesting approaches to integrating substance abuse and mental illness care. These innovative concepts rely on social networks, innovative strategies, and the ability to think beyond addiction as the only underlying problem for individuals. Oxford Houses present a unique contingency operation that is organized such that the results are partly influenced by what each individual resident invests in the system – but ultimately is successful because of what each resident gets out of the system reciprocally.

Conclusions and Future Directions

Oxford Houses are unique residential living environments that came to be out of both need and because of the dearth of empowering treatment modalities available historically and currently. These environments are both economical and effective catalysts in promoting abstinence from drug and alcohol use across the country. Despite mixed results from traditional treatment programs, the Oxford House model presents an environment that is economical, practical, and capable of being flexible for specific groups of residents that have different needs. While self-help is somewhat empowering, the Oxford House movement reminds researchers and everyone else that self-reliance and community-building are the foundation to building stronger relationships.

For the next few years, we will continue our exploration of gender issues, leadership, and individual characteristics with support from the NIAAA, the NIDA, and the National Center on Minority Health and Health Disparities. Two of our studies explore how Oxford House settings can aid individuals with substance abuse after being released from jail and prison. In one of our studies, funded by NIDA, ex-offenders are being randomly assigned to either professionally led Therapeutic Communities, Oxford Houses, or usual care postrelease settings, and we are examining program effects (i.e., substance use, criminal and health outcomes), and economic factors associated with these models. The aims of this project are important from a public health perspective as there may be treatment matching, case management, and financing factors that could be manipulated to enhance the cost-effectiveness of community-based substance abuse treatment for offenders leaving prison. Knowledge of the various environments that directly and possibly additively contribute to long-term abstinence could guide public health and criminal justice resource allocation decisions.

In a study funded by the National Center on Minority Health and Health Disparities, which was described in an earlier section with women being released from jail into either an Oxford House or Usual Aftercare, we have established a Community Advisory Board that will link with a network of existing coalitions in Chicago. The Community Advisory Board will further affect community-based changes for formerly incarcerated women by integrating and supporting service networks from which women historically have been isolated. The community advisory board is involved in all aspects of this project leading to more efficient translation of the research findings into practice.

Finally, with funding from NIAAA, we are also in the process of evaluating culturally specific Oxford Houses for Spanish speaking substance abusers. Culturally modified Oxford Houses may be a more effective option for Hispanic/Latino individuals who are Spanish-dominant, less comfortable with USA culture, or identify more strongly with their ethnic culture. Culturally modified Oxford Houses may also provide a more culturally congruent experience such as welcoming visits by extended family members. In addition, residents of culturally modified Oxford Houses are more likely to use culturally congruent communication styles, characterized by an emphasis on relationships, downplaying direct conflict in relationships in order to preserve harmony, and respect. In the present study, we are compare the outcomes of Hispanic/Latino individuals assigned to a culturally modified Oxford Houses to those assigned to a Traditional Oxford House. Within these three current NIH funded studies, we will continue to collaborate with our Oxford House partners and continue to explore the many issues that have been reviewed in this chapter.

This Oxford House model appears to promote the development of long-term abstinence skills to prevent relapse. As residents of Oxford Houses are required to self-govern and assume positions of leadership within their Houses, according to established protocols that foster consistency across houses and create a supportive milieu. This democratic feature of Oxford Houses possibly helps create the abstinence-specific supportive environment. Findings from a series of studies has demonstrated that Oxford House living represents an inexpensive aftercare model that can empower men and women through increased employment and income, and decreased rates of relapse and criminal behaviors [12, 46]. These studies suggest that the Oxford Houses have the capacity to promote personal responsibility and help substance abusers remain abstinent and maintain employment.

Key Points

1. Thousands of people exiting substance abuse treatment settings and prisons are in need of abstinent supportive community-based settings.
2. Oxford Houses represent one type of recovery home that helps integrate substance abusers back into society.
3. Researchers and community organizations have much to gain from participatory collaborations.
4. The federal government can provide support for these types of collaborative relationships.
5. We need to learn more about how natural, community-based supportive systems help substance abusers stay abstinent over long periods of time.

Authors' Notes

We appreciate the support of Paul Molloy and Leon Venable and the many Oxford House members who have collaborated with our team for the past 15 years, including also Bertel Williams, Kathy Sledge, Robin Miller, Bill Kmeck, Makeba Casey, Lester Fleming, Ron Blake, Stephanie Marez, Carolyn Ellis, LaRonda Stalling, Randy Ramirez, and Gilberto Padilla. In addition, our thanks to other colleagues and graduate students for helping us with the studies mentioned in this article including (in alphabetical order): Josefina Alvarez, Christopher Beasley, Peter Bishop, Blake Bowden, Carmen Curtis, Lucia D'Arlach, Meg Davis, Joseph Ferrari, David Groh, Annie Flynn, Gwen Grams, Ron Harvey, Elizabeth Horin, Bronwyn Hunter, Eve Kot, John Majer, Megan Murphy, Olya Rabin-Belyaev, Ed Stevens, Ed Taylor, and Judah Viola. The authors appreciate the financial support from the National Institute on Alcohol Abuse and Alcoholism (NIAAA grant numbers AA12218 and AA16973), the National Institute on Drug Abuse (NIDA grant numbers DA13231 and DA19935), and the National Center on Minority Health and Health Disparities (grant MD002748).

References

1. Oxford House, Inc. Oxford House manual. Silver Spring, MD: Oxford House, Inc.; 2006.
2. Davis MI, Jason LA, Ferrari JR, Olson BD, Alvarez JA. A collaborative action approach to researching substance abuse recovery. Am J Drug Alcohol Abuse. 2005;31:537–53.
3. Reason P, Bradbuy H. Handbook of action research. Participatory inquiry & practice. Thousand Oaks, CA: Sage; 2001.
4. Suarez-Balcazar Y, Davis M, Ferrari J, Nyden P, Olson B, Alvarez J, et al. Fostering university-community partnerships: a framework and an exemplar. In: Jason LA, Keys CB, Suarez-Balcazar Y, Taylor RR, Davis M, Durlak J, Isenberg J, editors. Participatory community

research: theories and methods in action. Washington, DC: American Psychological Association; 2004. p. 105–20.

5. Parsons M, Warner-Robbins C. Formerly incarcerated women create healthy lives through participatory action research. Holist Nurs Pract. 2002;16:40–9.
6. Riger S. Epistemological debates, feminist voices. Am Psychol. 1992;47:730–40.
7. Hill J, Bond M, Mulvey A, Terenzio M. Methodological issues and challenges for a feminist community psychology issue. Am J Community Psychol. 2000;28:759–72.
8. Berkowitz B, Wolff T. The spirit of the coalition. Washington, DC: American Public Health Association; 2000.
9. Davis MI, Olson BD, Jason LA, Alvarez J, Ferrari JR. Cultivating and maintaining effective action research partnerships: the DePaul and Oxford House collaborative. J Prev Interv Community. 2006;31:3–12.
10. Olson BD, Jason LA, Davidson M, Ferrari JR. Increases in tolerance within naturalistic, self-help recovery homes. Am J Community Psychol. 2009;44:188–195.
11. Chavis D, Florin P. Community development, community participation. San Jose, CA: Prevention Office, Bureau of Drug Abuse Services; 1990.
12. Jason LA, Olson BD, Ferrari JR, LoSasso AT. Communal housing settings enhance substance abuse recovery. Am J Public Health. 2006;91:1727–9.
13. Jason LA, Groh DR, Durocher M, Alvarez J, Aase DM, Ferrari JR. Counteracting "Not in My Backyard": the positive effects of greater occupancy within mutual-help recovery homes. J Community Psychol. 2008;36:947–58.
14. Jason LA, Olson BD, Foli K. Rescued lives: The Oxford House approach to substance abuse. New York: Routledge; 2008.
15. Olson BD, Street P, Rider P, Whitney T. Social and economic report for treatment-on-demand in Illinois. 2006. http://psychoanalystsopposewar.org/blog/wp-content/uploads/2008/01/social-and-economic-report-olson-et-al.pdf. Accessed 17 Aug 2009.
16. Olson BD, Viola JJ, Jason LA, Davis MI, Ferrari JR, Rabin-Belyaev O. Economic costs of Oxford House inpatient treatment and incarceration: a preliminary report. J Prev Interv Community. 2006;31:63–74.
17. French MT. Drug Abuse Treatment Cost Analysis Program (DATCAP): program version user's manual. 8th ed. Florida: University of Miami; 2003.
18. Jason LA, Olson BD, Ferrari JR, Majer JM, Alvarez J, Stout J. An examination of main and interactive effects of substance abuse recovery. Addiction. 2007;102:1114–1121.
19. Oxford House Inc. Annual report. 2007. http://www.oxfordhouse.org/userfiles/file/doc/ar2007.pdf. Accessed 12 July 2008.
20. Jason LA, Braciszewski JM, Olson BD, Ferrari JR. Increasing the number of mutual help recovery homes for substance abusers: effects of government policy and funding assistance. Behav Soc Issues. 2005;14:71–9.
21. Braciszewski JM, Olson BD, Jason LA, Ferrari JR. The influence of policy on the differential expansion of male and female self-run recovery settings. J Prev Interv Community. 2006;31:51–62.
22. Mortensen J, Jason LA, Aase D, Mueller D, Ferrari J. Organizational factors related to the sustainability of recovery homes. Manuscript submitted for publication. 2009.
23. Shediac-Rizkallah MC, Bone LR. Planning for the sustainability of community-based health programs: Conceptual frameworks and future directions for research, practice, and policy. Health Ed Res. 1998;13:87–108.
24. Hitlin S. Doing good, feeling good: values and the self's moral center. J Posit Psychol. 2007;2:249–59.
25. Taylor TP, Pancer SM. Community service experiences and commitment to volunteering. J Appl Soc Psychol. 2007;37:320–45.
26. Jason LA, Aase DM, Mueller DG, Ferrari JR. Current and previous residents of self-governed recovery homes: characteristics of long-term recovery. Alcohol Treat Q. 2009;27:442–452.

27. Evashwick C, Ory M. Organizational characteristics of successful innovative health care programs sustained over time. Fam Community Health. 2003;26:177–93.
28. Carmeli A, Schaubroeck J. Organizational crisis-preparedness: the importance of learning from failures. Long Range Plann. 2008;41:177–96.
29. Hunter DE. Using a theory of change approach to build organizational strength, capacity, and sustainability with not-for-profit organizations in the human services sector. Eval Program Plann. 2006;29:193–200.
30. Davis MI, Jason LA. Sex differences in social support and self-efficacy within a recovery community. Am J Community Psychol. 2005;36:259–74.
31. Jason LA, Ferrari JR. Oxford house recovery homes: Characteristics and effectiveness. Psych Services. 2010;7:92–102.
32. Belyaev-Glantsman O, Jason LA, Ferrari JR. The relationship of gender and ethnicity to employment in recovery homes. In: Jason LA, Ferrari JR, editors. Recovery from addiction in communal living settings: The Oxford House model [Special Issue]. J Groups Addict Recover. 2009;4:92–9.
33. Brown JT, Davis MI, Jason LA, Ferrari JR. Stress and coping: the roles of ethnicity and gender in substance abuse recovery. J Prev Interv Community. 2006;31:75–84.
34. Viola JJ, Ferrari JR, Davis MI, Jason LA. Measuring in-group and out-group helping in communal living: helping and substance abuse recovery. In: Jason LA, Ferrari JR, editors. Recovery from addiction in communal living settings: The Oxford House model [Special Issue]. J Groups Addict Recover. 2009;4:110–28.
35. Green LL, Fullilove MT, Fullilove RE. Remembering the lizard: reconstructing sexuality in the rooms of narcotics anonymous. J Sex Res. 2005;42:28–34.
36. MacRae R, Aalto E. Gendered power dynamics and HIV risk in drug using sexual relationships. AIDS Care. 2000;12:505–15.
37. Grant BF, Stinson FS, Dawson DA, Chou SP, Dufour MC, Compton W, et al. Prevalence and co-occurrence of substance use disorders and independent mood and anxiety disorders. Arch Gen Psychiatry. 2004;61:807–16.
38. Khantzian EJ. The self-medication hypothesis of addictive disorders. Am J Psychiatry. 1985;142:1259–64.
39. Ferrari JR, Jason LA, DaviS MI, Olson BD, Alvarez J. Assessing similarities and differences in governance among residential recovery programs: self vs. staff rules and regulations. Ther Communities Int J Ther Support Org. 2004;25:185–98.
40. Jason LA, Olson BD, Ferrari JR, Layne A, Davis MI, Alvarez J. A case study of self-governance in a drug abuse recovery home. North Am J Psychol. 2003;5:499–514.
41. Aase DM, Jason LA, Ferrari JR, Groh DR, Alvarez J, Olson BD, Davis MI. Anxiety symptoms and alcohol use: a longitudinal analysis of length of time in mutual help recovery homes. Int J Self Help Self Care. 2006–2007;4:21–35.
42. Aase DM, Jason LA, Olson BD, Majer JM, Ferrari JR, Davis MI, Virtue SM. A longitudinal analysis of criminal and aggressive behaviors among a national sample of adults in mutual-help recovery homes. In: Jason LA, Ferrari JR, editors. Recovery from addiction in communal living settings: The Oxford House model [Special Issue]. J Groups Addict Recover. 2009;4:82–91.
43. Burns L, Teesson M, O'Neill K. The impact of comorbid anxiety and depression on alcohol treatment outcomes. Addiction. 2005;100:787–96.
44. Jason LA, Olson BD, Ferrari JR, Majer JM, Alvarez J, Stout J. An examination of main and interactive effects of substance abuse recovery. Addiction. 2007;102:1114–21.
45. Majer JM, Jason LA, North CS, Ferrari JR, Porter NS, Olson BD, et al. A longitudinal analysis of psychiatric severity upon outcomes among substance abusers residing in self-help settings. Am J Community Psychol. 2008;42:145–53.
46. Jason LA, Davis MI, Ferrari JR, Anderson E. The need for substance abuse after-care: longitudinal analysis of Oxford House. Addict Behav. 2007;32:803–18.

Chapter 10
Continuing Care and Recovery

James R. McKay

Abstract Reviews of the continuing care research literature indicate that interventions that feature longer planned durations and active efforts to deliver the treatment components are more likely to show positive effects than other interventions. However, this literature has a number of limitations, including a focus on inpatient samples, treatment completers, and traditional treatment models and interventions. In addition, these studies have not attempted to identify which patients are likely to benefit the most from continuing care. Finally, there have been few tests of interventions that attempt to build strengths and other positive factors consistent with a recovery-oriented approach to continuing care. Recent findings from three addiction disease management research programs that have attempted to address many of these limitations are presented and discussed. In addition, several research-based recommendations for improving continuing care are offered, including reducing patient burden, providing incentives for participation, combining continuing care with other services, actively linking patients to other recovery supports, and making the interventions more recovery-oriented. Finally, the potential problems associated with considering abstinence as a requirement for being "in recovery" while participating in extended continuing care or other disease management interventions are discussed.

Keywords Addiction recovery management · Continuing care interventions · Treatment systems

J.R. McKay (✉)
Center on the Continuum of Care in the Addictions, University of Pennsylvania,
3440 Market Street, Suite 370, Philadelphia, PA 19104, USA
e-mail: mckay_ j@mail.trc.upenn.edu

J.F. Kelly and W.L. White (eds.), *Addiction Recovery Management: Theory, Research and Practice*, Current Clinical Psychiatry, DOI 10.1007/978-1-60327-960-4_10,
© Springer Science+Business Media, LLC 2011

Introduction

The goals of this chapter are to review evidence for the effectiveness of continuing care in addictions and to more broadly discuss the role of continuing care in the recovery process. At this point, there is a body of research on continuing care, and the findings from these studies that have been summarized in prior reviews tell a fairly consistent story [1, 2]. At the same time, there have been major changes to the addiction treatment system over the past 20 years that raise questions about how much the findings from many of these studies tell us about the effectiveness of continuing care within contemporary treatment systems or in the systems that are likely to emerge in the coming years.

Prior to 1990, continuing care was fairly simple to define. It was the outpatient phase of treatment that (hopefully) followed the completion of an inpatient or residential treatment experience, and it was consequently often referred to as "aftercare." The nature of continuing care in those days was also remarkably consistent. It was almost always weekly group counseling with a heavy 12-step focus, typically provided over 3–6 months [1]. Since 1990, the picture has gotten much more complicated. Most patients are now treated entirely in outpatient settings [3], so the distinction between the initial and continuing care phases of treatment is much less clear. Moreover, continuing care may begin at intake rather than discharge from the first treatment phase, may take any number of forms, and may be provided in settings other than a typical addiction treatment program. One might even ask whether "continuing care" will continue to exist as a separate phase of treatment or will instead become a component of disease management-oriented treatment systems.

Therefore, in addition to briefly reviewing the results of continuing care studies, this chapter closely examines the limitations of this literature with regard to determining the effectiveness of continuing care contemporary newer systems of care. Several newer studies that attempt to address the limitations in prior studies are described. The degree to which findings from continuing care studies inform our understanding of recovery is also discussed. In most cases, the endpoints in continuing care studies have been measures of alcohol and drug use, whereas current writings on recovery stress that abstinence is necessary but not sufficient, and that true "recovery" involves improvements in other important areas of functioning [4].

What Contributes to the Chronic Nature of Substance Use Disorders?

Not all individuals with substance use disorders have chronic forms of these disorders. However, at least half of the patients who enter the formal treatment system will have multiple treatment episodes [5]. In our treatment studies at the University of Pennsylvania, we found that, for example, patients have undergone an average of three or four prior treatments [6]. There are a number of biological, psychological, and social factors that appear to contribute to the chronic nature of substance use disorders. Some of these factors are themselves relatively slow to change or even permanent, including genetic vulnerability, neurocognitive deficits, dysfunctional beliefs and expectancies regarding substance use, family and social problems and lack of support for recovery, deficits in life skills, and high-risk environments [7–9]. Because these risk factors persist for long periods, it is no surprise that many individuals with substance use disorders experience multiple relapses over time. In fact, the real surprise is that so many people manage to recover.

What Are the Implications of Having a Chronic Disorder?

Chronic disorders come in different shapes and sizes. With disorders such as hypertension and type I diabetes, patients seldom achieve remission once the disorder has been diagnosed [10]. The severity of the disorder may wax and wane over time – for example, blood pressure will be higher at some points than at others – but patients usually do not achieve "normal" blood pressure or glucose levels unless they stay on their medications. In other words, these disorders are chronic and relatively constant. With substance use disorders, on the other hand, many individuals achieve complete remission following a treatment episode and may maintain that status for several months or years while not in treatment, only to eventually relapse to heavy levels of use [11]. Substance use disorders can therefore be chronic but intermittent, at least for some individuals.

Therefore, continuing care for substance use disorders must be flexible if it is to be efficacious and cost-effective. Some patients will need long-term, more highly structured continuing care, whereas others will need very little. Still others, perhaps the majority of patients who end up in the formal treatment system, will need continuing care that can be adjusted up or down in intensity and frequency over time as they go through alternating periods of abstinence and use [1, 2]. During periods of abstinence, low level monitoring may be optimal as it places minimal burden on the patient and reduces costs [12]. However, when risk levels rise or episodes of actual substance use begin, monitoring needs to be able to be ratcheted up to the level of treatment to interrupt and address whatever processes are leading to further deterioration [5].

Effective management of chronic disorders also requires that patients are able to make good use of nontreatment supports – both within themselves and in the community. The ability to learn and to practice good "self-care" is seen as a very important part of the management of chronic disorders of all types [13]. One of the key goals of treatment – particularly continuing care – is to equip patients to engage in the basic tasks of good self-care. Although these tasks vary from disorder to disorder, they generally include self-monitoring of status and symptoms, coping with stressors, and interacting effectively with service providers and other sources of support. Continuing care can also help promote strong recoveries by linking patients to sources of support in the community [14]. These might include employment and educational opportunities, parenting and childcare services, medical or psychiatric care, housing, and recovery centers.

Finally, early onset addiction can severely disrupt the development of effective life skills in many areas of functioning. Therefore, significant numbers of patients who achieve abstinence will nonetheless still face formidable challenges in their attempts to develop the kinds of meaningful and satisfying lives that can provide a buffer against relapse. This is why recovery has to be more than the achievement of abstinence.

In summary, continuing care for individuals with chronic forms of substance use disorders needs to be flexible with regard to frequency, intensity, and focus; able to provide successful linkage to other sources of professional and paraprofessional support in the community; and able to promote self-care and the development of life skills.

Research Findings on the Effectiveness of Continuing Care

Although the number of published studies of continuing care for substance use disorders is small relative to the number of published studies of initial or primary treatment, the number of such studies is steadily increasing. In fact, there are now more than 20 published controlled studies that compare various approaches to continuing care for patients who have completed some form of primary treatment. Most of these studies have been reviewed in detail elsewhere [1, 2], with the following conclusions offered:

- Half of the studies find evidence for the effectiveness of a particular continuing care intervention.
- Studies that compare an active continuing care intervention against a minimal or no continuing care condition are more likely to yield positive findings than studies that compare two or more active continuing care conditions.
- Continuing care interventions that feature longer planned durations of care and/ or active efforts to deliver the treatment to the patient are more likely to yield positive findings than interventions that do not have these features.
- More recent studies are more likely to find significant treatment effects than studies published prior to the late 1990s.

Examples of continuing care interventions that yielded significant treatment effects include home visits by psychiatric nurses [15], behavioral couples therapy [16], structured coping skills-based treatments [17, 18], telephone counseling [6, 19, 20], and comprehensive interventions that involved active linkage to community resources [21, 22].

Limitations of Published Research on Continuing Care

Unfortunately, the treatment studies that were included in these reviews have a number of limitations, which potentially reduce the amount of useful information that can be gleaned from the results and used to improve continuing care. The majority of studies were done with treatment completers drawn from inpatient samples who were participating in what could be called a traditional model of care and receiving fairly conventional treatment approaches. These studies also fail to differentiate patients who are most likely to benefit from continuing care.

Focus on Inpatient Samples

The majority of the continuing care studies included in the McKay [1, 2] reviews made use of patients who had completed inpatient or residential treatment – 75% of the studies, in fact. Although continuing care is highly recommended for such patients, they currently make up only a small percentage of people in addiction treatment. The vast majority of patients in specialty care for substance use disorders receive outpatient treatment. It is therefore important to consider whether patients completing residential or inpatient care face the same issues as those in outpatient treatment.

In most cases, patients now only end up in residential or inpatient care if they have some combination of severe addiction, co-occurring disorders, poor motivation, unsuccessful outpatient treatment experiences, or living situations that will not be supportive of abstinence [23]. While in treatment, these individuals generally do not have access to alcohol or drugs, and they do not have to confront risky situations. This combination of multiple risk factors for relapse coupled with no opportunities to practice in vivo coping behaviors makes a powerful case for continuing care upon discharge.

Patients in outpatient treatment, on the other hand, may have fewer risk factors for relapse than those who are admitted to inpatient settings, although it is not uncommon to see outpatients with some risk factors. Perhaps more important, individuals who are able to remain engaged in outpatient care long enough to complete the initial phase of care and become eligible for continuing care have already demonstrated some ability to cope successfully with ready access to alcohol and drugs as well as other risky situations that can easily lead to relapse. Therefore, these patients may not need as much continuing care to achieve good longer-term outcomes. If that were the case, studies that focus on inpatient and residential samples may overstate the effect of continuing care within an outpatient service delivery system.

Focus on Treatment Completers

Continuing care has generally been thought of as a phase of treatment that is delivered only to those patients who complete an initial phase of care. Therefore, only more successful patients have been included in studies of continuing care. This bias is likely less severe in studies of patients recruited from residential or inpatient treatment, as the majority of patients in these settings complete treatment, due to the fact that these interventions are relatively short and provided in controlled environments. However, dropout rates are much higher in outpatient treatment [24], which means that patients who receive continuing care in traditional service delivery models are clearly not representative of patients who begin treatment.

These potential biases could work in two directions. In outpatient populations, the bias toward more successful patients might result in an underestimation of the benefits of continuing care because of ceiling effects. Most of these patients will do relatively well, so there may be less room for continuing care to show an effect. On the other hand, if patients who drop out early do not benefit from efforts to engage them in continuing care, the inclusion of these patients in studies could diminish or wash out the impact of continuing care on more successful patients.

Focus on Traditional Treatment Models

Most of the controlled trials of continuing care have been done within the context of traditional treatment models, in which patients step down through discrete levels of care. Examples of these models include 4 weeks of inpatient or intensive outpatient treatment followed by weekly outpatient care. In these models, the difference between initial treatment and continuing care is very clear, and it often involved changes in treatment setting or facility as well as in frequency and intensity. In many settings, however, the distinction between these two phases of care is now much less distinct, particularly in systems that rely primarily on outpatient treatment [1]. It is not clear to what extent findings regarding the effectiveness of continuing care generated in these more traditional treatment models generalize to more contemporary models of care. This issue is of course related to the first two issues raised above.

Failure to Consider Which Patients Most Need Continuing Care

The inclusion/exclusion criteria for studies of continuing care have typically been similar to criteria used in studies of initial or primary treatment. Participants must have a substance use disorder and someone who can serve as a locator to facilitate follow-up, and they must not be too impaired with a major psychiatric disorder or cognitive deficit. In addition, as discussed earlier, they must also have completed some minimum amount of an initial treatment. Interestingly, studies almost never specify that participants must show evidence that they have a chronic form of a substance use disorder, such as some number of prior treatment experiences followed by relapse or a history of failure to complete treatment episodes.

One might argue that anyone who enters the formal addiction specialty care treatment system in fact has a chronic substance use disorder, and therefore all patients are likely to benefit from effective continuing care [10]. However, most disease management programs for other disorders focus efforts on patients who have utilized a considerable amount of treatment services over the prior year or two, which is taken as an indication that their disorders are not well managed with conventional treatment [25]. It is conceivable that results of published continuing care studies might have been different if only patients with, say, four or more prior detoxification or treatment episodes over the past 2 years were included in the study sample.

Focus on Conventional Approaches to Continuing Care

In addition to the concerns noted above with regard to which patients have been included in continuing care studies and the types of treatment systems that have been studied, several characteristics of the interventions themselves raise questions about how relevant the research findings are to recovery-oriented systems of care. Specifically, most treatments studied have (1) focused primarily on reducing deficits rather than building strengths, (2) been fixed rather than flexible, and (3) not considered patient preference to any degree.

Deficits vs. Strengths

The majority of continuing care studies included in the reviews of that literature have tested interventions designed to reduce deficits in coping skills and biases in cognitions and beliefs (CBT-type interventions) or to sustain endorsement and participation in 12-step models [2, 26]. Both kinds of interventions have elements that attempt to reduce deficits and those that try to increase strengths. In the case of 12-step interventions, for example, the treatment aims to reduce problematic behavior (e.g., self-centeredness, refusal to give up control, other character defects, and the mistaken belief that one will be able to drink normally again) and to develop strengths and prorecovery behaviors (e.g., helping others, offering amends for past transgressions, engaging in social interactions and relationships that do not involve substance use). Coping skills treatments such as CBT do attempt to reinforce strengths to some degree, but the emphasis in most components of the intervention and in most sessions is really on fixing problems and deficits in behaviors and cognitions [27]. The assumption is that more rewarding activities in recovery will be possible if the problems and deficits that sustain continued substance use are ameliorated through the identification and rehearsal of better coping behaviors and the correction of problematic or biased cognitions.

This emphasis in most continuing care treatments on addressing deficits is at odds to some degree with a more recovery-oriented approach, which focuses to a greater extent on identifying, nurturing, and further developing an individual's skills, talents, and interests [14, 28]. During a continuing care treatment session, the difference between these two orientations could be profound. For example, in a typical coping skills intervention, most sessions start with a review of any episodes of use, followed by a functional analysis to better understand what went wrong if a slip or relapse occurred. Next, upcoming high-risk episodes are reviewed, and potential coping responses are identified and rehearsed [29].

In a more recovery-oriented approach to continuing care, there is greater emphasis on the identification, monitoring, and supporting of life goals that are selected by the patient. These goals are usually framed in a positive direction – "I want to spend more time being physically active outside" – and the underlying motive for the goal is also positive – "because it is enjoyable for me." Contrast this with a typical goal in a social skills treatment – "I want to get better at refusing drinks when they are offered to me" – which follows from a deficit-based motive or explanation – "because I am impulsive and don't think through things." Writing on how best to maintain behavior change over time, Rothman [30] observed that fear of negative consequences may help someone stop smoking or using alcohol and drugs, but enjoyment of the benefits that these behavior changes might bring is probably necessary to sustain changes in these behaviors.

Little Consideration of Patients' Preference

Recovery-oriented treatment places a great deal of emphasis on the importance of patients' choice with regard to treatment goals and methods to achieve those goals [14, 28]. The importance of patients' choice has also been stressed in other areas of medicine, especially with regard to the management of chronic diseases [13, 31]. Conversely, most continuing care interventions that have been studied in controlled trials come with a set of goals and methods that patients are expected to endorse and follow through on. This is particularly true of 12-step-oriented interventions, where there is very little room for patients' choice. In fact, patients are urged to "get out of the driver's seat," surrender their will to a higher power, and follow the directives of the program to attend meetings and work the 12 steps. The point here is not that this approach does not work – there is plenty of evidence that 12-step programs can provide highly effective continuing care – but that there is little room for patient choice or preference.

Fixed vs. Flexible

Most of the continuing care interventions that have been included in reviews could be said to be relatively rigid or fixed. That is, the interventions were delivered in a standardized fashion according to guidelines provided in manuals and were not modified or adjusted to a significant degree on the basis of changes in patients' response over time.

Problems Further Upstream

We have seen that the literature on continuing care is limited in a number of significant ways, which raises questions about the true effectiveness of these interventions. An even larger problem concerns how few people receive any continuing care at all, due to problems with engagement, retention, and transition to continuing care.

The Engagement Problem

Epidemiological studies have shown that overwhelming majority of individuals with substance use disorders never enter formal treatment or self-help organizations [32]. Of these people, many recover and do not experience another episode of dependence or abuse. However, this still leaves a very sizeable number of people who do not achieve stable remission, instead either continuing to use consistently or going through repeated periods of heavy use separated by some reductions in use or abstinence. People in this group might well benefit from treatment that includes some sort of extended care phase, but something about treatment is sufficiently unappealing that they never engage in it. With regard to continuing care, the elephant in the room that no one wants to talk about has been that most people with substance use disorders do not want standard treatment, much less extended versions of it.

The Retention Problem

In order for individuals with substance use disorders to receive continuing care of any sort, they have to participate in treatment for more than a few weeks. This is particularly important in a recovery-oriented model of care, in which the goal of treatment is more than simply the initiation of abstinence. Recovery requires sustained behavior change, including longer abstinence or sharply decreased use, connection to and engagement with community supports, and progress toward meaningful social and employment goals. According to recent statistics, however, average stays in IOP and OP are 46 and 76 days, respectively [24]. This is clearly not enough time for most patients to make significant progress toward a real recovery.

The Transition Problem

Significant numbers of patients who complete a first phase of treatment fail to make the transition to step down care [33, 34]. This appears to be due to a number of reasons, including the lack of availability of continuing care at the facility, a desire on the part of the patient to be "done" with treatment, and other barriers such as distance from the facility and competing work and family responsibilities. At the very least, the shift from one phase of care to the next is a natural point for patients to reexamine whether they want to continue, and in many cases the answer appears to be "no."

What We Really Know About Continuing Care and Recovery

Limitations in the body of research on the effectiveness of continuing care likely mean that we know less than we think about how well these interventions actually work. We know that most people with alcohol or drug use disorders do not want standard substance abuse treatment, and therefore either fail to enter treatment or drop out early, long before they receive any continuing care. Of the relatively small percentage of the patients who stay in treatment long enough to be eligible for continuing care, most receive very little if any continuing care. Within this group, it does appear that continuing care treatments that have a longer planned duration of care and involve more active efforts to deliver the intervention are more likely to be effective [1, 2]. However, the evidence here is indirect – few studies have compared long vs. short forms of the same continuing care intervention – and it comes from carefully conducted research studies where investigators go to great lengths to retain participants in both the clinical interventions and the research follow-ups. Retention rates in continuing care in more typical treatment programs are likely to be lower [34].

A New Generation of Continuing Care Studies

Several relatively recent studies have examined the effectiveness of continuing care models that seek to support all patients in addiction treatment, not just those who have completed an initial phase of care. These interventions all feature active outreach efforts designed to maintain contact with patients over long periods of time so that continuing care can be delivered, even when patients have relapsed or lost motivation for recovery.

The work of Dennis, Scott, and colleagues [35, 36] addresses some of the limitations noted here in the continuing care literature. These investigators have developed and evaluated a true continuing care model, referred to as "Recovery Management Checkups," or RMC, in which all patients who enter treatment become eligible for an extended monitoring program that strives to reengage them if they relapse over the next 2–3 years. In this protocol, substance abusers who have entered treatment are followed and interviewed every 3 months. For those not currently in treatment or in a controlled environment such as jail, the need for further treatment is determined through a relatively brief assessment with very specific criteria regarding out-of-control use. Individuals who meet the criteria for need for treatment are immediately transferred to a linkage manager, who uses motivational interviewing techniques to help the participant recognize and acknowledge the problem and need for treatment, addresses any existing barriers to reentering treatment, and arranges scheduling and transportation to treatment.

The RMC protocol was first evaluated in 448 adults who were randomized to RMC or quarterly research follow-ups and followed for 24 months [35]. The results of the study indicated that the RMC intervention led to better management of the patients over time. First, patients in RMC were more likely to be readmitted to treatment (60% vs. 51%), were readmitted sooner (mean of 376 vs. 600 days), and received more treatment during the 2-year follow-up (mean of 62 vs. 40 days) than those in the control condition. Second, patients in RMC had better substance use outcomes than those in the control condition. Specifically, RMC patients were less likely to meet criteria for needing treatment in five or more quarters than patients in the control condition (23% vs. 32%) and were less likely to be in need of treatment in the final quarter of the follow-up (43% vs. 56%). These effects were generally small, but consistently favored RMC over the comparison condition.

The Chestnut Health group has conducted a second study with a new version of RMC that was modified to address the limitations observed in the first study [36]. The self-report assessment to determine need for treatment was augmented with urine testing, which increased the percentage of participants who were found to need treatment at each assessment point over the rates observed in the first study (44% vs. 30% of those interviewed). Transportation assistance was provided to increase the percentage of participants found to be in need of treatment who actually completed an intake assessment. Finally, several practices were put in place to increase retention in those participants who did complete an intake appointment at a treatment program. These practices involved closer collaboration between the research team and the treatment programs to reengage participants in treatment who drop out after intake and to prevent hasty administrative discharges.

These modifications increased the effectiveness of the intervention to a considerable degree over what was achieved in the first study [36]. A higher percentage of participants deemed in need of treatment attended the linkage meeting (99% vs. 75%), completed the assessment (42% vs. 30%), and remained in treatment for a minimum of 14 days (58% vs. 39%). Moreover, the improved RMC intervention produced significantly more days of abstinence during the 2-year follow-up (mean of 480 vs. 430, $p < 0.05$, $d = 0.29$) than the comparison condition. However, this effect, which translates into about 2 extra days of abstinence per month, was relatively small in magnitude.

Morgenstern and colleagues studied the effectiveness of an extended, intensive case management intervention in substance-dependent women receiving Temporary Assistance for Needy Families (i.e., TANF) [37]. As with the RMC intervention, participants were enrolled at the start of treatment, not after completing an initial phase of care. In this intervention, case management services were provided for 15 months. Prior to treatment entry, the case managers met with women at the local welfare office to identify barriers to treatment entry and address resistance to treatment. Plans were developed and implemented to solve childcare, transportation, and housing problems, and motivational counseling was provided as needed. Home visits and other outreach activities were also used for women who were having trouble in achieving engagement. Once the participant entered treatment, the case manager met with her weekly and continued to provide help with coordinating services. Frequency of contact was slowly titrated to twice monthly, but it could be increased up to daily during crisis periods. Small value incentives were also provided for attending treatment sessions.

The effectiveness of this intervention was compared to usual outpatient care in a sample of 302 women. Results indicated that the intensive case management intervention produced higher levels of treatment initiation, engagement, and retention, compared to usual care. Furthermore, women who received the intensive case management intervention had higher rates of abstinence throughout the follow-up, with the greatest difference obtained at 15 months (43% vs. 26% abstinent). Across the 15 month follow-up, the prevalence of abstinence within each 1 month segment was 75% higher in women who received the case management intervention (odds ratio $= 1.75, p = 0.025$). In a second study of case management, Morgenstern and colleagues have again found that participants who are provided with case management in addition to treatment as usual have better substance use outcomes than those who receive treatment as usual only [38].

Our group at Penn has also moved toward providing extended monitoring and counseling to patients who begin the protocol shortly after they enter an intensive outpatient program (IOP), rather than at graduation from IOP. The 18-month-long adaptive protocol is built around 20-min telephone contacts that consist of a brief structured assessment of risk for relapse and problem-focused counseling. The intervention includes CBT techniques such as monitoring of progress, identification of high-risk situations, and rehearsal of improved coping behaviors. The calls are scheduled at 1-week intervals early in the protocol, with the frequency decreasing over time to one call per month. When risk levels increase, participants receive stepped-up care that can include more frequent telephone sessions, several sessions of motivational interviewing [39], a course of relapse prevention, or linkage back to the IOP.

This intervention addresses most of the primary goals of the "Chronic Care Model," as described by Wagner et al. [13]. This disease management model specifies regular, extended contact between patients and service providers; interventions to increase patient confidence and skills to manage chronic conditions (e.g., goal setting, identification of barriers to reaching goals, development of plans to overcome barriers); links to patient-oriented community resources; the use of accurate and timely patient data to monitor progress and guide interventions; and provision of support to facilitate improved self-management.

The intervention was compared to two comparison conditions in a recent study. Patients who had completed 3 weeks of a 3-month long IOP were randomly assigned to continue with treatment as usual (TAU), to continue with TAU plus get the telephone monitoring and counseling condition described above (TMC), or to continue with TAU and receive brief monitoring telephone calls on the same schedule as that in the TMC intervention (TM). The calls in TM consisted of the same progress assessment used in TMC and provided very brief feedback on the results of the assessment. No counseling was provided in this condition.

The first report from this study focused on alcohol use outcomes during the 18-month period in which TMC and TM were provided [40]. With percent days alcohol use, there was a significant treatment condition × time interaction ($p = 0.03$). Planned contrast analyses indicated that TMC produced less frequent drinking than TAU at 12 months ($p < 0.02$), 15 months ($p = 0.0002$), and 18 months ($p = 0.006$), and less frequent drinking than TM at 6 months ($p = 0.2$). TM produced less frequent drinking than TAU at 12 and 15 months ($p = 0.03$). With a dichotomous outcome measure of any drinking within each 3-month segment of the follow-up, there was a significant main effect for treatment condition ($p < 0.05$). Planned contrast analyses indicated that rates of any alcohol use within each period were lower in TMC than in TAU across the follow-up ($p = .02$). TM and TAU did not differ ($p = 0.42$).

Analyses were also done to determine whether any factors moderated the main effect results in this trial. The positive effects of extended continuing care were hypothesized to be greater for patients with more severe histories of substance use problems, those with a relatively poor initial response to IOP, and those with other established risk factors for relapse as identified in the research literature (i.e., craving, low self-efficacy, low readiness for change, lack of commitment to abstinence, and negative expectancies). With TMC, the hypotheses were not confirmed. None of the 11 variables examined was a significant moderator of main effects favoring TMC over TAU, indicating that this intervention is effective for a wide range of patients. Conversely, gender and readiness to change moderated the TM effect; TM was more effective than TAU for women and for those with lower readiness to change, but not for men or for individuals higher in readiness [41].

The strong performance of TMC in this study is somewhat surprising, because about 25% of the patients who were randomized to the intervention never began it. Moreover, the patients who did begin the intervention averaged only about 10 of 36 possible continuing care contacts over the 18 months. It is possible that the intervention would produce even stronger effects if rates of participation could be raised. With that goal in mind, we are conducting another telephone continuing care study that tests the impact of low-level incentives on participation in extended telephone continuing care and outcomes. In this study, patients are randomized to receive TAU, TMC, or TMC plus incentives ($10 gift coupon for every continuing care contact completed). Initial results from this study indicate that providing these incentives increases the percentage of patients who begin the TMC protocol (82% vs. 73%) and dramatically increases the percentage of possible continuing care contacts completed (67% vs. 39%) [42].

Possible Solutions to Problems of Engagement and Retention

Reduce Patient Burden in Continuing Care Whenever Possible

Patients may be more willing to initiate and sustain participation in continuing care when the intervention is more convenient and less burdensome than standard, clinic-based group counseling. Such an approach does not need to compromise overall effectiveness. In one of our studies, for example, patients who made reasonable progress toward the goals of IOP actually had better outcomes in a low-burden, telephone-based continuing care intervention, compared to standard group counseling [20]. However, a minority of patients who did not make much progress in IOP did better if continued in regular group counseling at the clinic.

Even brief telephone monitoring and counseling continuing care sessions may be too much for some patients. However, some of these individuals may be willing to come back to the clinic occasionally for brief recovery management "checkups," which can be used to link the patient back into treatment if necessary. The work of Dennis, Scott, and colleagues, reviewed here, has demonstrated that such an intervention, delivered every 3 months for 2 years or more, results in higher rates of treatment readmission and better substance use outcomes than standard care. Although this approach may not be as effective in preventing relapses as more frequent monitoring, it clearly can interrupt relapses before the consequences become more severe. This approach is also less burdensome for patients and may be less costly to the treatment system.

When a lower intensity continuing care intervention such as telephone monitoring and counseling or recovery management checkups is provided, it is crucial that there be some provision to step up level of care when the patient's symptoms worsen or status deteriorates [1]. To facilitate this, patients should be monitored as part of these interventions, in a systematic and standardized fashion, using validated assessment tools. Algorithms should be used which specify the scores on these measures that indicate when it is time to change treatment and ideally provide guidance on which interventions to consider adding or switching too. This approach has been referred to as "adaptive treatment," or "stepped care," and it holds considerable promise as a strategy for reducing patient burden, reducing costs to the system, and improving outcomes [43]. However, in our experience, patients often are resistant to more intensive interventions when they are not doing well. Therefore, catching deterioration before it has become too severe can be very important.

Provide Incentives for Participation

There is now overwhelming evidence that providing incentives to patients leads to better attendance and higher rates of abstinence [44, 45]. These effects have been found with a wide range of patients and types of reinforcers, including low-cost gifts (canteen vouchers), chances to win prizes in drawings, cash, and gift certificates that over the course of a study can be worth up to $2,000 or more [46]. There was initially considerable resistance on the part of treatment providers to incentive-based interventions, but the results of research studies have been persuasive. The fact that incentives almost always dramatically increase treatment participation has also become seen by providers as a plus. At this point, the main barrier to wider use of incentives appears to be the cost of the incentives themselves, rather than philosophical opposition to the idea.

Rates of continuing care participation can also be increased by incentivizing the treatment providers. Shepard et al. [47] were able to increase the percentage of patients who completed at least five continuing care sessions from 33 to 59% by paying counselors a $100 bonus for each patient who reached that goal. Although five sessions may seem like a very low bar, the participants in this study were opiate-dependent patients who had been detoxified and treated in a drug-free program (i.e., no methadone). Rates of attendance in continuing care in this group have been extremely low.

Given the financial constraints virtually all addiction treatment programs operate under these days, the provision of incentives to patients in continuing care – or to the clinicians treating them – may seem impossible. However, in some studies the investigators have found creative ways to support incentives, including through the donations of goods from area business owners who see the value in reducing substance use in the community [46].

Use Leverage When Available

Positive incentives such as gift certificates and prizes are popular with patients, but they are not the only form of leverage available. In the criminal justice system, for example, patients sentenced to drug courts and other forms of mandated treatment are more likely to attend continuing care if failure to attend leads to unwanted consequences such as return to prison [48]. Patients in methadone have also been responsive to contingencies regarding ease of access to methadone that are built around attendance at counseling sessions and urine drug test results [49].

Leverage can also be provided by contracts and social reinforcement. Lash and colleagues have developed an effective intervention to increase attendance in continuing care, which includes contracts, prompts, and low-cost social reinforcements [50]. In the contracting procedures, patients are provided with information on the success rates of patients who do and do not attend continuing care, and they are asked to commit to participate in a specified amount of continuing care and other supports (e.g., AA, individual therapy). Prompts consist of letters from therapists, appointment cards, automated telephone reminders for continuing care appointments, and letters and personal telephone calls following any missed continuing care sessions. The social reinforcement consists of personal letters from counselors with congratulations for attending sessions, certificates for completion of treatment milestones (e.g., 90 days of treatment), and medallions for attending specified numbers of continuing care sessions. The certificates and medallions are typically presented in front of other patients in the therapy groups.

Combine Continuing Care with Other Services

One way to increase sustained participation in continuing care is by linking these interventions in some way to other services that patients are likely to access over time [51]. For example, continuing care can be colocated with or even provided in medical primary care practices or in community mental health centers. The effectiveness of integrated care for medical and substance use disorder problems has been demonstrated in several studies [52, 53]. There is also evidence that linking continuing care with access to housing and employment can be effective with high problem severity populations [54, 55].

Actively Link Patients to Other Recovery Supports

It may be possible to increase rates of recovery by using treatment as an opportunity to aggressively link patients to other sources of support. The most prevalent form of such support is self-help programs. However, only a minority of patients achieve sustained engagement in these programs. Timko and colleagues recently conducted a study to determine whether more intensive referral to self-help groups during outpatient treatment would promote higher and more sustained rates of participation and better outcomes than standard clinic practices [56].

The intensive referral intervention is delivered over the first three treatment sessions of outpatient addiction treatment. The content of the sessions consists of detailed lists of local self-help meetings that had been preferred by other patients, directions to the meetings, and material that describe 3 self-help meetings and addresses common questions and typical concerns about the program. The counselor also arranges a meeting between the patient and a participating member of a self-help group and provides the patient with a journal to record attendance at and reactions to the meetings. Attendance at self-help meetings is monitored over the following two outpatient sessions. For patients who had attended a self-help meeting, attempts are made to link the patient with a sponsor. For those who had not attended a meeting, the process of linking the patients with a self-help volunteer is repeated.

Results from a randomized study indicated that patients in the intensive referral condition had higher rates of overall involvement in self-help programs at 6 months than those in the standard referral condition. Interestingly, the intervention was more effective with patients who were not heavily involved with self-help in the 6 months prior to treatment. Specifically, in patients who were below the 75 percentile on prior 12-step attendance, the intensive referral intervention produced higher rates of attendance at self-help meetings than the standard referral condition (62.3 vs. 40.4 meetings during the 6-month follow-up; $p < 0.01$). With regard to substance use outcomes, the intensive referral condition produced better alcohol and drug use outcomes at 6 months, as assessed by ASI composite scores, and higher rates of total abstinence from drugs than the standard referral condition [56].

Even with a more effective intervention, there are still patients who will not attend self-help. Therefore, Litt and colleagues developed a treatment intervention designed to help patients change their larger social networks to become more supportive of abstinence [57]. Because 12-step-based self-help was the most readily available potential source of support for abstinence, the intervention still focused on participation in these programs, although making new acquaintances and engaging in enjoyable social activities at AA or other social networks were stressed, rather than other AA components like the higher power and powerlessness. For those participants who were not interested in AA, the intervention focused on increasing other forms of social support for abstinence.

This intervention, referred to as "network support," was then evaluated in a research study. Participants were randomized to a case management comparison condition (CM), network support (NS), or network support plus incentives for abstinence (NS + ContM). Data from the 1-year follow-up indicated that both network support conditions produced better alcohol use outcomes than case management, as indicated by higher percent days abstinent (about 75% vs. 63%) and higher rates of continuous abstinence in each 3-month period (as high as 40% in NS vs. 20% in CM). Moreover, NS led to greater increases in AA attendance and behavioral and attitudinal support for abstinence. The incentives did not improve outcome over network support alone [57].

Making Continuing Care More Recovery-Oriented

As was noted earlier, the Betty Ford Institute Consensus Panel [4] recently proposed that in order to be "in recovery," an individual needs to be abstinent from alcohol and drugs and also a functioning member of society. However, much of the continuing care treatment that is currently provided is focused on reducing or eliminating alcohol and drug use, not on improving functioning in other important areas such as work, parenting, and being an active and productive member of one's community. Part of the problem is that improving functioning has been seen as the purview of social workers and other professions and agencies that are outside the addiction treatment system. However, one of the best hedges against relapse is a life filled with meaningful and enjoyable activities and social connections [58, 59], and many with substance use disorders need considerable help over an extended period to achieve that kind of life. Therefore, greater focus on these goals in the continuing care phase of addiction treatment is certainly warranted, as are more active efforts to link patients to service providers and agencies where such support is available.

It is also worth considering whether the requirement for "abstinence" inhibits rather than facilitates a more recovery-oriented approach to continuing care and long-term disease management in the addictions. With other major psychiatric disorders, the concept of "recovery" is focused on the afflicted individual becoming a fully functioning member of society, despite the fact that symptoms of the disorder *are expected* to wax and wane over time [28]. No one expects a person with a psychotic or bipolar disorder to achieve the equivalent of "abstinence" from serious and significant symptoms of the disorder. Granted, for many people with serious substance use disorders, long-term abstinence is certainly the preferred outcome. However, a greater emphasis during continuing care on improving personal and social functioning, and less concern about whether the individual has remained totally abstinent, would be more consistent with a recovery focus.

Summary

- In controlled studies with treatment completers, continuing care appears to be effective, particularly if the treatment is extended and features active efforts to deliver the intervention to patients.
- However, most of these studies were done with graduates of inpatient or residential programs, which raises questions about the degree to which these findings generalize to patients in our now largely outpatient service delivery system.
- Many patients who might possibly benefit from continuing care have not been included in these studies, because they never entered treatment, dropped out of the initial phase of care too early to become eligible for continuing care, or did not successfully transition from the initial phase to the continuing care phase.
- More studies are needed that enroll patients closer to the start of treatment, rather than when they complete the initial phase of care, to test whether this approach to disease management produces stronger effects.
- Several recent studies have followed this design and have yielded positive results.
- More work is also needed to develop continuing care interventions that reduce patients' burden and increase patients' choice, include incentives for participation, make use of existing leverage when available, integrate with care for other disorders and issues, and provide more active linkage to other recovery supports in the community.

- Finally, a greater focus on nurturing strengths, skills, talents, and interests, rather than the achievement of sustained abstinence, may make continuing care both more appealing and effective and also promote stronger and more stable recoveries.

Acknowledgments This research was supported by grant P01AA016821 from the National Institute on Alcohol Abuse and Alcoholism and grant K02 DA000361 from the National Institute on Drug Abuse. Additional support was provided by the Medical Research Service of the Department of Veterans Affairs.

References

1. McKay JR. Treating substance use disorders with adaptive continuing care. Washington, DC: American Psychological Association Press; 2009.
2. McKay JR. Continuing care research: what we've learned and where we're going. J Subst Abuse Treat. 2009;36:131–45.
3. McLellan AT, Meyers K. Contemporary addiction treatment: a review of systems problems for adults and adolescents. Biol Psychiatry. 2004;56:764–70.
4. Betty Ford Institute Consensus Panel. What is recovery? A working definition from the Betty Ford Institute. J Subst Abuse Treat. 2007;33:221–8.
5. Dennis ML, Scott CK. Managing addiction as a chronic condition. Addict Sci Clin Pract. 2007;4(1):45–55.
6. McKay JR, Lynch KG, Shepard DS, Ratichek S, Morrison R, Koppenhaver J, et al. The effectiveness of telephone-based continuing care in the clinical management of alcohol and cocaine use disorders: 12 month outcomes. J Consult Clin Psychol. 2004;72:967–79.
7. Kalivas PW. Neurobiology of cocaine addiction: implications for new pharmacotherapy. Am J Addict. 2007;16:71–8.
8. Koob GF. The neurobiology of addiction: a neuroadaptational view relevant for diagnosis. Addiction. 2006;101 Suppl 1:23–30.
9. Moos RH, Finney JW, Cronkite RC. Alcoholism treatment: context, process, and outcome. New York, NY: Oxford University Press; 1990.
10. McLellan AT, Lewis DC, O'Brien CP, Kleber HD. Drug dependence, a chronic medical illness: implications for treatment, insurance, and outcomes evaluation. J Am Med Assoc. 2000;284:1689–95.
11. Hser YI, Longshore D, Anglin MD. The life course perspective on drug use: a conceptual framework for understanding drug use trajectories. Eval Rev. 2007;31:515–47.
12. Humphreys K, Tucker JA. Toward more responsive and effective intervention systems for alcohol-related problems. Addiction. 2002;97:126–32.
13. Wagner EH, Austin BT, Davis C, Hindmarsh M, Schaefer J, Bonomi A. Improving chronic illness care: translating evidence into action. Health Aff. 2001;20:64–78.
14. White WL. Recovery management and recovery-oriented systems of care: scientific rationale and promising practices. Pittsburgh, PA: Northeast Addiction Technology Center; 2008.
15. Patterson DG, MacPherson J, Brady NM. Community psychiatric nurse aftercare for alcoholics: a five-year follow-up study. Addiction. 1997;92:459–68.
16. O'Farrell TJ, Choquette KA, Cutter HSG. Couples relapse prevention sessions after behavioral marital therapy for male alcoholics: outcomes during the three years after starting treatment. J Stud Alcohol. 1998;59:357–70.
17. Bennett GA, Withers J, Thomas PW, Higgins DS, Bailey J, Parry L, et al. A randomized trial of early warning signs relapse prevention training in the treatment of alcohol dependence. Addict Behav. 2005;30:1111–24.

18. Sannibale C, Hurkett P, Van Den Bossche E, O'Connor D, Zador D, Capus C, et al. Aftercare attendance and post-treatment functioning of severely substance dependent residential treatment clients. Drug Alcohol Rev. 2003;22:181–90.
19. Horng F, Chueh K. Effectiveness of telephone follow-up and counseling in aftercare for alcoholism. J Nurs Res. 2004;12:11–9.
20. McKay JR, Lynch KG, Shepard DS, Pettinati HM. The effectiveness of telephone based continuing care for alcohol and cocaine dependence: 24 month outcomes. Arch Gen Psychiatry. 2005;62:199–207.
21. Brown BS, O'Grady K, Battjes RJ, Farrell EV. Factors associated with treatment outcomes in an aftercare population. Am J Addict. 2004;13:447–60.
22. Godley MD, Godley SH, Dennis ML, Funk RR, Passetti LL. The effect of assertive continuing care on continuing care linkage, adherence, and abstinence following residential treatment for adolescents with substance use disorders. Addiction. 2006;102:81–93.
23. American Society of Addiction Medicine. ASAM PPC-2R- ASAM patient placement criteria for the treatment of substance-related disorders. 2nd ed. Chevy Chase, MD: American Society of Addiction Medicine; 2001. Revised.
24. Substance Abuse and Mental Health Services Administration, Office of Applied Studies. Treatment Episode Data Set (TEDS): 2005. Discharges from Substance Abuse Treatment Services, DASIS Series: S-41, DHHS Publication No. (SMA) 08-4314. Rockville, MD: Substance Abuse and Mental Health Services Administration, Office of Applied Studies; 2008.
25. Rosenman MB, Holmes AM, Ackermann R, et al. The Indiana chronic disease management program. Milbank Q. 2006;84:135–63.
26. Project Match Research Group. Matching alcoholism treatments to client heterogeneity: Project MATCH posttreatment drinking outcomes. J Stud Alcohol. 1997;58:7–29.
27. Carroll KM. A cognitive-behavioral approach: treating cocaine addiction. Rockville, MD: National Institute on Drug Abuse; 1998. NIH publication 98-4308.
28. Davidson L, O'Connell MJ, Tondora J, Lawless M, Evans AC. Recovery in serious mental illness: a new wine or just a new bottle? Prof Psychol Res Pract. 2005;36:480–7.
29. Monti PM, Abrams DB, Kadden RM, Cooney NL. Treating alcohol dependence: a coping skills training guide. New York, NY: Guilford Press; 1989.
30. Rothman AJ. Toward a theory-based analysis of behavioral maintenance. Health Psychol. 2000;19 Suppl 1:64–9.
31. Institute of Medicine. Crossing the quality chasm: a new health system for the twenty-first century. Washington, DC: National Academy Press; 2001.
32. Institute of Medicine. Improving the quality of health care for mental and substance-use conditions: Quality Chasm series. Washington, DC: National Academies Press; 2006.
33. Harris AHS, McKellar JD, Moos RH, Schaefer JA, Cronkite RC. Predictors of engagement in continuing care following residential substance use disorder treatment. Drug Alcohol Depend. 2006;84:93–101.
34. McKay JR, Foltz C, Leahy P, Stephens R, Orwin R, Crowley E. Step down continuing care in the treatment of substance abuse: correlates of participation and outcome effects. Eval Program Plann. 2004;27:321–31.
35. Dennis ML, Scott CK, Funk R. An experimental evaluation of recovery management checkups (RMC) for people with chronic substance use disorders. Eval Program Plann. 2003;26:339–52.
36. Scott CK, Dennis ML. Results from two randomized clinical trials evaluating the impact of quarterly recovery management checkups with adult chronic substance users. Addiction. 2009;104:959–71.
37. Morgenstern J, Blanchard KA, McCrady BS, McVeigh KH, Morgan TJ, Pandina RJ. Effectiveness of intensive case management for substance-dependent women receiving temporary assistance for needy families. Am J Public Health. 2006;96:2016–23.
38. Morgenstern J, Hogue A, Dauber S, Dasaro C, McKay JR. A practical clinical trial of care management to treat substance use disorders among public assistance beneficiaries. J Consult Clin Psychol. 2009;77:257–69.

39. Miller WR, Rollnick S. Motivational Interviewing: preparing people for change addictive behavior. 2nd ed. New York, NY: Guilford Press; 2002.
40. McKay JR, Van Horn D, Oslin D, Lynch KG, Ivey M, Ward K, Drapkin M, Becher JR, Coviello D. A randomized trial of extended telephone-based continuing care for alcohol dependence: within treatment substance use outcomes. Journal of Consulting and Clinical Psychology, in press.
41. Lynch KG, Van Horn D, Drapkin M, Ivey M, Coviello D, McKay JR. Moderators of response to extended telephone continuing care for alcoholism. Am J Health Behav. 2010;34 (6):788–800.
42. Van Horn D, Ivey M, Drapkin M, Thomas T, Domis S, Abdalla O, Herd D, McKay JR. Impact of low level incentives on participation in an extended continuing care intervention. Drug and Alcohol Dependence, in press.
43. Murphy SA, Lynch KG, McKay JR, Oslin DW, Ten Have TR. Developing adaptive treatment strategies in substance abuse research. Drug Alcohol Depend. 2007;88:S24–30.
44. Lussier JP, Heil SH, Mongeon JA, Badger GJ, Higgins ST. A meta-analysis of voucher-based reinforcement therapy for substance use disorders. Addiction. 2006;101:192–203.
45. Prendergast M, Podus D, Finney J, Greenwell L, Roll J. Contingency management for treatment of substance use disorders: a meta-analysis. Addiction. 2006;101:1546–650.
46. Petry NM. A comprehensive guide to the application of contingency management procedures in clinical settings. Drug Alcohol Depend. 2000;58:9–26.
47. Shepard DS, Calabro JAB, Love CT, McKay JR, Tetreault J, Yeom HS. Counselor incentives to improve client retention in an outpatient substance abuse aftercare program. Adm Policy Ment Health. 2006;33:629–35.
48. Marlowe DB, Festinger DS, Arabia PL, Dugosh KL, Benasutti KM, Croft JR, et al. Adaptive interventions in drug court: a pilot experiment. Crim Justice Rev. 2008;33:343–60.
49. Brooner RK, Kidorf MS, King VL, Stoller KB, Peirce JM, Bigelow GE, et al. Behavioral contingencies improve counseling attendance in an adaptive treatment model. J Subst Abuse Treat. 2004;27:223–32.
50. Lash SJ, Burden JL, Fearer SA. Contracting, prompting, and reinforcing substance abuse treatment aftercare adherence. J Drug Addict Educ Erad. 2007;2:455–90.
51. Miller WR, Weisner C. Integrated care. In: Miller WR, Weisner CM, editors. Changing substance abuse through health and social systems. New York, NY: Kluwer Academic/ Plenum; 2002. p. 243–53.
52. Willenbring ML, Olson DH. A randomized trial of integrated outpatient treatment for medically ill alcoholic men. Arch Intern Med. 1999;159:1946–52.
53. Weisner C, Mertens J, Parthasarathy S, Moore C, Lu Y. Integrating primary medical care with addictions treatment: a randomized controlled trial. J Am Med Assoc. 2001;286:1715–23.
54. Milby JB, Schumacher JE, Wallace D, Frison J, McNamara C, Usdan S, et al. Day treatment with contingency management for cocaine abuse in homeless persons: 12-month follow-up. J Consult Clin Psychol. 2003;71:619–21.
55. Silverman K, Svikis D, Wong CJ, Hampton J, Stitzer ML, Bigelow GE. A reinforcement-based therapeutic workplace for the treatment of drug abuse: three-year abstinence outcomes. Exp Clin Psychopharmacol. 2002;10:228–40.
56. Timko C, DeBenedetti A, Billow R. Intensive referral to 12-step self-help groups and 6-month substance use disorder outcomes. Addiction. 2006;101:678–88.
57. Litt MD, Kadden RM, Kabela-Cormier E, Petry N. Changing network support for drinking: initial findings from the network support project. J Consult Clin Psychol. 2007;75:542–55.
58. Moos RH, Moos BS. Treated and untreated alcohol-use disorders: course and predictors of remission and relapse. Eval Rev. 2007;31:564–84.
59. Vaillant GE. A 60-year follow-up of alcoholic men. Addiction. 2003;98:1043–51.

Part III
Recovery Management in Practice

Chapter 11
Recovery-Focused Behavioral Health System Transformation: A Framework for Change and Lessons Learned from Philadelphia

Ijeoma Achara-Abrahams, Arthur C. Evans, and Joan Kenerson King

Abstract The concept of recovery is fast becoming the prevailing paradigm in behavioral health policy arenas. Consequently, behavioral health care systems are trying to align their services with a recovery-oriented approach. To date, no blueprint exists to guide systems and communities through the complex process of transformational change. The vision of "what" a recovery-oriented system looks like is becoming increasingly clear, but the process for "how" systems transform and align themselves with this vision remains obscure. This chapter draws upon work in the City of Philadelphia to propose a framework for the recovery-focused transformation of behavioral health systems. Concrete examples of change strategies and lessons learned are discussed.

Keywords Addiction recovery management · Recovery-oriented systems of care · Holistic services

Introduction

A new paradigm in behavioral health care is emerging. At its core, this movement represents a shift away from crisis-oriented, deficit-focused, and professionally directed models of care to a vision of care that is directed by people in recovery, emphasizes the reality and hope of long-term recovery, and recognizes the many pathways to healing for people with addiction and mental health challenges. As a result, sweeping changes are being called for in behavioral health systems [1–5].

These changes are nothing short of revolutionary. They entail far reaching policy, practice, fiscal and regulatory realignments, and fundamentally alter the

I. Achara-Abrahams (✉)
Department of Behavioral Health and Mental Retardation Services, 1101 Market St.,
7th Floor, Philadelphia, PA 19107, USA
e-mail: ijeoma.achara@yahoo.com

J.F. Kelly and W.L White (eds.), *Addiction Recovery Management: Theory, Research and Practice*, Current Clinical Psychiatry, DOI 10.1007/978-1-60327-960-4_11,
© Springer Science+Business Media, LLC 2011

relationships between service providers and service recipients and between local service providers and federal, state, and local administrative authorities. As systems grapple with the complexity of transformational change, those leading these efforts can be overwhelmed with the sheer immensity of the challenges involved. Without informed, visionary, and skilled leadership, the transformation process can easily stagnate, further demoralizing system stakeholders. Despite these challenges, recovery transformation is possible and is happening at national, state, and local levels [6–9].

This chapter is written for system administrators, local treatment program managers, and directors of recovery community organizations who are playing leadership roles within a recovery transformation process. The chapter reviews the conceptual framework that is being used in the City of Philadelphia to guide such a process and uses this experience to suggest a road map for facilitating systems transformation.

The History of Recovery-Focused Transformation in Philadelphia

The impetus to transform Philadelphia's behavioral health system came from the convergence of several distinct yet interrelated national trends [1]. These include the proliferation of diverse recovery mutual aid societies, and the rise of new independent recovery community organizations, coupled with the explosive growth in the recovery advocacy arena and emerging research highlighting the limitations of prevailing acute and palliative care treatment models [1, 10–16].

At the local level, several milestones paved the way for Philadelphia's current transformation efforts. The closing of the Philadelphia State Hospital in 1990 was a critical shift from an institutional to a community-based model of behavioral health care. Philadelphia's visionary leadership continued with the development of Community Behavioral Health (CBH) in 1997, which brought the formerly separate funding streams for mental health and addiction treatment together under one plan and set the stage for the integration of all behavioral health services in Philadelphia. These initiatives laid a strong foundation for the development of a service system responsive to and driven by the needs of people being served.

The progression toward a transformed service system in Philadelphia was taken to the next level when Dr. Arthur Evans was recruited in 2004 to lead the newly created Department of Behavioral Health and Mental Retardation Services. Dr. Evans initiated the current recovery transformation process in 2005 with the vision of a radically transformed service system that would better meet the needs of people seeking long-term recovery. The transformation was intended to shift the emphasis of treatment from bio-psychosocial stabilization to the goal of equipping people with the services, supports, and opportunities to sustain long-term recovery and achieve full lives in their communities.

The Case for a Guiding Framework

Shifting service delivery paradigms, increasingly diverse communities, shrinking resources, and public demands for greater accountability all place the task of managing change at the center of the work life of behavioral health care managers. Despite this reality, few system and organizational leaders in the public sector have formal training in change management. Consequently, many people find themselves ill-equipped to lead a major change effort, particularly in the midst of an economic downturn, when people mistakenly assume that substantive systems change can only occur with an influx of additional resources.

Models of Approaching Systems Transformation

The authors have observed three basic approaches to behavioral health systems transformation: *additive*, *selective*, and *transformative*. Each of these takes a different approach to the development of a recovery-oriented system of care.

The Additive Approach

In the *additive approach,* the development of a ROSC is thought to be achieved by adding "recovery services" to the existing treatment system. This approach is based on the view that treatment is effective in initiating change, but that recovery support services are needed to sustain these changes. In this approach, existing treatment practices remain unchanged, but are supplemented by adding such support services as peer run recovery support groups, recovery houses, peer-based telephonic aftercare, family support groups, or a community-based recovery center.

The hallmark of additive thinking is the belief that a ROSC is achieved through the "addition" of nonclinical recovery support services and the belief that such supports cannot be added without "new dollars." In this approach, a rigid boundary often exists between formal treatment providers and informal recovery supports either within the treatment organization or between the treatment organization and a recovery community organization providing recovery support services. In addition, important treatment variables such as service planning, the nature of service relationships, and the focus of services remain unchanged [1].

While the additive approach to the development of a ROSC is still an improvement over nonrecovery-focused systems, the approach falls short of making the policy and practice changes that would fully align the system with recovery principles. Furthermore, it does not change or challenge assumptions that are inconsistent with a recovery framework, such as deficit-based treatment services. The overall conceptual alignment necessary for complete system transformation is lacking in this approach.

The Selective Approach

Another emerging approach to the development of a ROSC is the *selective approach*. In this approach, there is recognition that treatment practices must be changed and better aligned with recovery principles. This may be achieved through a combination of strategies including adding new recovery-oriented treatment services, modifying existing treatment services, and incorporating recovery support services into the system. The emphasis is on changing the practices of select programs or levels of care and ensuring that recovery-oriented supports are available within select parts of the system.

What distinguishes the selective approach is that certain portions of the treatment system are chosen strategically and targeted for changes related to recovery transformation while other elements of the system remain virtually unchanged. For example, systems that take this approach might choose to change an existing intensive outpatient system to one focused more on recovery-oriented practices and might change the funding mechanism to allow for the integration of peer support services. These select services may experience powerful change and the infusion of hope and energy that accompanies recovery transformation. These specific service changes do not, however, for the most part, impact other parts of the treatment system. This creates confusion for people receiving services in the system as they receive conflicting messages from different parts of the system.

The Transformative Approach

In the *transformative approach* to developing a recovery-oriented system, the entire treatment system including the context in which it operates is aligned with recovery principles. This includes treatment services, support services, as well as the policy, community, and social context of the system. The nature of treatment itself radically changes to align itself with the values and principles of recovery-oriented care. Peer and community-based recovery supports are developed and integrated into treatment settings and community contexts. Funding and regulatory policies are examined and modified through the lens of recovery-oriented care. In the transformative approach, the entire system is aligned to support long-term recovery for individuals and families and to promote community health. Peer and community-based recovery supports and treatment services are regarded as not only equal in importance, but also indispensable in promoting sustained recovery, and they are provided in a seamless, integrated manner. Peer and community-based recovery supports and services inform the treatment system and support the continued transformation of staff attitudes and practices.

Philadelphia's vision of a ROSC is based on the transformative approach. This approach moves beyond change at the margins of the system to assuring that every aspect of the system is aligned to support the goal of long-term recovery for individuals and families and community wellness. That means that every aspect of how individuals and families experience the system must be evaluated in light of recovery principles and aligned to support this long-term recovery process. This requires an aggressive and wide-ranging set of change activities; from the language that is used to services that are available, to reimbursement policies, to the availability of indigenous helpers, to community education, and to specific treatment practices such as recovery planning. The treatment system itself must be fundamentally changed. In fact, all domains in the system including, but not limited to, its design, leadership, management, quality improvement, fiscal and administrative policy, cross-systems collaboration, community relations, training, and all service delivery functions are realigned.

The Philadelphia model moves beyond the historical focus on pathology and disease processes to an emphasis on building individual, family and community recovery capital strength and capacity with the goal being to increase resilience and support recovery. In this approach, the community is not solely seen as something into which individuals with behavioral health challenges are "integrated," but also as a resource for healing. Consequently, the community itself becomes a target for intervention. It is integral in the overall strategy to ensure that individuals are able to sustain their recovery and that the community itself can act as a resource for prevention, early intervention, and sustained recovery support.

We will now describe the strategies that were employed by system administrators, providers, and the recovery community in Philadelphia to align concepts, practices, and context with this vision of a recovery-oriented system of care.

Overview of the Change Framework

The change strategy employed to transform Philadelphia's behavioral health system has three components – conceptual alignment (core values and principles), practice alignment, and contextual alignment (regulations, funding, relationships, and community context) – all directed toward supporting the long-term recovery of individuals and families and promoting community health.

Conceptual alignment targets the promotion of conceptual and philosophical clarity regarding the system's collective vision of recovery transformation. During this process, the core values, principles, and ideas upon which a recovery-oriented system of care will be built are defined through an inclusive process. Change leaders facilitate activities and opportunities that help stakeholders understand and create their vision of what a recovery-oriented system of care looks like in their unique community.

Practice alignment is focused on changing behaviors and processes across the system so that they are consistent with the stated vision of recovery. Change leaders are focused on developing mechanisms to translate the theoretical concepts of recovery into concrete practices across various levels and within diverse parts of the system.

Finally, contextual alignment consists of activities that are designed to sustain and support the transformation over time. While practice changes are a necessary part of the process, these changes cannot be implemented in a vacuum. To be sustained over time, they must be simultaneously accompanied by contextual changes that will facilitate their long-term success and will impact the very culture of organizations and the larger systems within which they are embedded. Many of these changes in context include policy and fiscal changes, political advocacy, activities that increase community support for people in recovery, as well as efforts that address stigma and enhance recovery capital within the communities in which people live.

Kotter [17], a leading expert in change management, presents a change strategy that is consistent with these three components. He contends that in a successful change strategy, the first stages in the transformation process help "defrost the hardened status quo" (conceptual alignment). The next stages introduce changes in behaviors (practice alignment), and the final stages help embed the new behaviors into the culture and "make them stick" (contextual alignment). In Philadelphia, the conceptual alignment phase of the transformation process set the stage for change, the practice alignment phase focused on implementing change, and the contextual alignment phase is ensuring that the new changes are sustainable within an environment that promotes continuous innovation. Each strategy informs the other in a continuous feedback loop.

While the three change strategies do not take place in a linear fashion, they are time sensitive. At various phases in the change process, one component may play a more central role than the others. Practice changes, for instance, should not be made before the conceptual foundation is laid, and the values, principles, and overall vision for the system are clarified. This critical work of conceptual alignment helps guide the practice changes and direct their ongoing development. It provides the philosophical foundation and the "north star" directional system for innovation. Similarly, effective contextual alignment, which includes fiscal and policy alignment, is most effective after obtaining a clear understanding of the types of practice and behavioral changes that are desired and the systemic barriers that stand in the way of their implementation.

Strategies that Advance Conceptual Alignment

Establish a Sense of Urgency

One of the first and most critical tasks in leading any transformational change effort is establishing a sense of urgency. Without it, obtaining the cooperation and buy-in needed to move things forward is an arduous, if not impossible, process. Urgency is needed to overcome the generalized complacency that often exists in many organizations and systems [17].

In Philadelphia, system administrators utilized system assessments, community meetings, and conferences with all stakeholders to establish and communicate a sense of urgency. In addition to collecting local data, national data was used to outline many of the gaps in behavioral health treatment systems around the country. Stakeholder meetings were held to explore the impact these gaps were having on people with behavioral health needs and to generate consensus that the status quo was no longer acceptable. Framing the transformation within the national context not only increased credibility for moving in this direction, but also reduced defensiveness on the part of local stakeholders as systems change was no longer a Philadelphia issue, but a national imperative – and one in which Philadelphia could play a leadership role.

Form Powerful Guiding Coalitions to Assist with Developing a Vision

It is imperative in making practice changes in a system or organization to first develop a guiding vision of how the system/organization should look in the future. In the absence of a clear and compelling vision of a future desired state, change processes are often motivated only by problems severe enough to generate a call to action. As a result, they inevitably run out of steam as soon as the problems driving the change are perceived as less pressing [17,18]. One of the first strategies employed in Philadelphia's system transformation efforts was developing a strong coalition to assist with refining the emerging vision for the future and leading the change process. The Recovery Advisory Committee (RAC) was the first coalition established, and it was charged with the responsibility of overseeing and guiding the transformation process. Among the initial tasks were the development of a recovery definition for the system and a set of values/guiding principles for the system.

Going through this process with the RAC underscored the importance of allowing stakeholders the time needed to develop a shared vision of a transformed system. At the inception of the RAC, several definitions of recovery and guiding principles for a ROSC already existed in the field. Consequently, it was assumed that coming to consensus regarding a recovery definition would be a relatively quick task, as it would require only minor modifications to the existing concepts. Instead, however, committee members did not want to merely adopt the definitions of others. They needed to personally struggle with the concept of recovery. In doing so, attitudes and beliefs linked to the prevailing models surfaced and were challenged, and stakeholders were able to consequently develop a new and dramatically different vision for the system.

The process of developing a recovery definition and a set of guiding principles took approximately 6 months. The group emerged with a vision that went far beyond rhetoric or words on a page. It reflected a shared sense of hope and a deep commitment to change. The resulting values became the compass for the system transformation effort.

Connect the Vision to Other Initiatives and Over Communicate it Times Ten

One of the primary functions of the emerging vision was to establish an overarching framework that could help to align and coordinate all the activities that were occurring in the system. The vision of a recovery-oriented system of care helped connect the dots between different initiatives so that the change process did not appear fragmented. In the absence of this, any transformation effort would be quickly reduced to a number of well-intentioned, but disparate projects unlinked to any common goal. Having this comprehensive vision and stating and restating it, is critical to the ongoing evolution of an effective change process [17].

Change leaders need to be able to clearly and succinctly communicate how the various efforts within the system are a part of the developing ROSC. In Philadelphia, leaders communicated that all the transformation initiatives converged around the holistic needs of individuals. They repeatedly stated that in traditional systems of care, services are shaped primarily by historical practice and the demands of funding and regulatory bureaucracies. In recovery-oriented systems, services and supports are viewed from the perspective of the person and/or family receiving them. What do they need in order to build a meaningful life in the community? They need effective treatment (such as evidence-based practices and trauma informed care) that integrates essential components of their identity (gender and culture) and facilitates access to supports and opportunities (housing, education, employment, spiritual, and social support) that are critical to having a life in the community.

In an effort to advance each of these areas and align them with the vision of a recovery-oriented system of care, additional workgroups and initiatives were formed, such as the Trauma Taskforce, the Evidence Based Practices Workgroup, the Faith Based Initiative, and the Person First Initiative.

Ensure that Stakeholders Understand the Nature of Transformational Change

One cautionary note is necessary before stakeholders embark on the transformation journey. Transformational change is different than the staged or top down change normally facilitated by organizations and systems. It is marked by a radical reorientation of the way everything within a system is done. Early on in Philadelphia's transformation process, leaders sought to shape stakeholders' expectations by communicating that transformational change is unique in three critical ways.

First, the future is unknown and only through forging ahead it is discovered. It requires entering a process without a clearly defined outcome, guided by values and the evidence that currently exists. The very nature of a recovery-oriented transformation process requires that leaders resist the urge to be prescriptive (telling stakeholders what to do). Instead, leaders of transformational change set a direction and facilitate a process that engages everyone in the development and pursuit of a shared vision.

Second, in transformational change, the future state is so different from the traditional state that a shift in mindset is required to invent it [19]. With regard to recovery-focused transformation, practice changes that are not accompanied by profound changes in how people think are unsustainable and represent only superficial compliance. For example, recovery-oriented care cannot be implemented simply by replacing treatment planning with recovery planning. Recovery planning is not about a change in language, the forms utilized, or the final product. It is about the process, the shift in power dynamics, a change in focus, and moving from an expert orientation to one of collaboration so that people can be supported in developing plans that work for their lives [20]. The process cannot be effectively implemented without attitudinal changes on the part of service providers.

Finally, because transformational change does require changes in organizational culture and mindset, the process and the human dynamics are much more complex [19]. Feelings of chaos are characteristic of the process and have to be normalized for all stakeholders. In some ways, the chaos supports the process because it causes old assumptions to be called into question and reorganized. Without understanding chaos as part of the process, the tendency to revert to a "central office" clarifying the vision and communicating new mandates will be great. Transformational change requires a new style of leadership [21].

Utilize a Transparent and Participatory Approach at All Times

Perhaps the single most important guiding principle is the recognition that the transformation process involves a form of recovery for everyone. Multiple stakeholder groups feel demoralized and discouraged regarding the state of behavioral health systems. People in recovery and their families are often angry at providers whom they believe are not meeting their needs and not allowing them to have a meaningful voice in directing their own care. Providers are often frustrated with regulatory agencies that they feel are impeding their ability to provide effective care, and the regulatory agencies are frequently annoyed with providers for not providing what they deem to be high-quality services. Rather than explore the issues behind these feelings, systems become locked in battles of blame, control, and maneuvering for resources [22].

While traditional change efforts rely heavily on authoritarianism and micro-management [17], in Philadelphia there was recognition that due to the nature of transformational change and the generalized discontent among stakeholders, these strategies were unlikely to create lasting change. To transition from recovery concepts to practices, systems transformation had to unfold as a shared vision of change. Thus, stakeholders had to have more than a voice. They needed opportunities to shape and direct the process rather than simply react to it. Consequently, one of the initial steps in the transformation process was developing mechanisms to ensure that the entire process was transparent and promoted participation, healing, and reconciliation at all levels.

During the process, there were times when DBHMRS made critical decisions that were not transparent – actions that were later conceptualized as organizational relapse. These instances threatened to erode trust among stakeholders and initially resulted in lost credibility. What became most important was utilizing these opportunities to reestablish that recovery transformation is a process and that all stakeholders including DBHMRS itself would grow, but occasionally relapse along the way. What is critical is that leadership acknowledges the missteps, takes corrective action to address them, and uses them to increase communication and renewed commitment to the shared vision.

Create Forums for Knowledge Sharing and Exploration of New Ideas

While visionary leadership is a critical component of any successful change process, ideas and energy also have to naturally emerge from other parts of the system. Provider learning collaboratives, cross-system workgroups, recovery luncheons, and training approaches and venues that include all stakeholders provide an opportunity for people in recovery, family members, providers, staff of DBH/MRS along with the members of the broader community to come together and discuss promising practices that are emerging as the system transforms.

Address Perceived Loss and Facilitate Engagement

Change of any kind can precipitate anxiety. Large-scale transformational change can trigger a myriad of fears and concerns. People are concerned about what the change will mean for them. Will the new vision require the development of new skills and/or will their expertise be viewed as irrelevant? What about their status within the organization or system? Bridges, a leading change management expert, contends that stakeholders in a change process cannot grasp the new thing until they have let go of the old thing [23]. It is the process of loss that people resist rather than the change itself.

> ..many of these losses aren't concrete. They are part of the inner complex of attitudes and assumptions and expectations that we all carry around in our heads. These inner elements of "the way things are" are what make us feel at home in our world. When they disappear, we've lost something very important [23].

In response to this sense of loss, people often tend to dig in and protect their turf, role, function, and way of doing things. In Philadelphia's transformation process, it was critical that these concerns and anxieties were appreciated. Dismissing them as "resistance" generated division between those charged with leading the change efforts and those continuing to manage day-to-day operations. Instead, those leading the transformation effort needed to learn to accept the importance of subjective loss and openly acknowledge it [23].

It was also critical to provide staff within DBHMRS with opportunities to develop meaningful roles that advanced the transformation process. In contrast to the "no pain, no gain" mantra, Bridges contends that change efforts frequently fail because the stakeholders only experience the pain [23]. Instead they need opportunities and roles to help them build new, meaningful identities. To assist with this, an interest assessment was created, which identified many skills, interests, and knowledge domains that would be needed during the initial stages of transformation. DBH/MRS staff interested in assisting with the transformation process completed the interest inventory and was then assigned to a particular workgroup or task. This served to energize and motivate many individuals within the Department and provided an opportunity to identify emerging leaders.

Mobilize the Early Adopters and Recovery Champions

In his book, *The Tipping Point*, Malcolm Gladwell describes an epidemiological model of social change [24]. He contends that ideas proliferate like diseases and that change occurs when dissemination becomes an epidemic. He offers three rules to explain the nature of epidemics. One of these he terms, "The Law of the Few." The basic premise of this law is that a small group of people with a particular perspective and unique social abilities can effect enormous change. He describes these individuals as "mavens," "connectors," and "persuaders." They are knowledgeable, passionate, and have significant influence with people. Gladwell maintains that just a few of these people can have a profound and lasting impact.

Early in Philadelphia's recovery transformation process, individuals within the Department and system were identified as those who not only shared the same philosophical perspective of recovery, but also possessed the unique ability to connect with and influence people within their social network. These individuals varied with regard to their role and formal status within the organizations. Some of them were support staff within the Department while others were executive directors of treatment organizations. Regardless of their roles, what they shared was a commitment to spreading the message that this recovery transformation was vital. While the Department had formal mechanisms to communicate key messages, such as newsletters, memos, presentations, etc., this informal network began to generate the excitement, energy, and hope that were essential to the early success of the transformation process.

Strategies that Advance Practice Alignment

Establish Priorities

While obtaining conceptual clarity and creating a shared vision is critical in the initial stages of transforming a system, aligning practices and processes with that vision becomes increasingly important as the transformation progresses. As such, the next change strategy, aligning practices, is focused on translating the conceptual information into concrete practice changes throughout the system. In Philadelphia, one of the concerns increasingly voiced as the transformation process progressed was, "Recovery-oriented care sounds great, but what does it look like in practice?" In an effort to answer this question, DBH/MRS identified initial system transformation priorities, which were derived from the feedback from stakeholders. The initial priorities were: holistic care, community integration, peer culture, support and leadership, family partnership and leadership, partnership, sustained recovery supports, and quality of care.

These priorities provided direction and focus in the midst of ambiguity and massive change. Rather than asking the broad question, "What does recovery-oriented care look like?," stakeholders began to explore how to promote community integration or how to develop a culture of peer support and leadership. These priorities had implications for all stakeholders at all levels of the system. The question for everyone became, "How does this particular priority impact my day-to-day functioning?" and "What helps to advance it and what impedes it?" The priorities also provided a way to align administrative functions, plan for and direct training efforts, and gave policy and fiscal decisions a point of reference.

Identify Practice Changes Associated with the Priorities

Stakeholders at all levels of the behavioral health field have witnessed the rise and fall of many new initiatives and service philosophies, most of which have failed to have any lasting impact on clinical practices [1]. With a values-driven transformation process, even when a common agenda emerges, the concepts being described can sound abstract and ethereal, leaving individuals to wonder about the practical implications. Based on the system transformation process to date in Philadelphia, clinical practices are in the midst of changing in the following ways (Table 11.1).

In addition to outlining the above practice changes [25], the Department also developed a *tools for transformation series* to identify the types of practice changes that coincide with each priority area. Each priority area, such as community integration, has a resource packet that is composed of a white paper, a list of relevant resources, and checklists for providers, people in recovery, and staff members of DBHMRS to assist them in evaluating their own practices relative to the particular priority (see http://www.dbhmrs.org/technical-papers-on-recovery-transformation/).

Table 11.1 Desired practice changes in Philadelphia's ROSC

Service engagement: Greater focus on early engagement via outreach and community education. Emphasis on removing personal and environmental obstacles to recovery through meeting basic needs; responsibility for motivation to change shifts from client to service providers; inclusive admission criteria rather than emphasis on *exclusionary* criteria

Assessment: Greater use of holistic, culturally relevant, strengths-based assessment procedures and interview protocols; shift from assessment as an intake activity to assessment as a continuing activity focused on the developmental stage of recovery

Retention: Enhance the rates of service retention and reduce the rates of service disengagement and administrative discharge by utilizing outreach workers, enhancing peer-based recovery support services in the treatment context, providing culturally competent services, providing a menu of service options so that care is individualized, and incorporating family members and other important allies as desired

Service access: Assure rapid access to treatment with minimal wait times. During unavoidable wait times, clients are engaged through peer-based supports within treatment. Ensure that there are no limitations to accessing treatment based on past utilization and/or treatment outcomes

Role of client: Shift toward philosophy of choice rather than prescription of pathways and styles of recovery, greater client authority, and decision making within the service relationship, emphasis on empowering clients to self-manage their own recoveries, and identify their personal life and treatment goals

Service relationship: Shift the primary service relationship from a hierarchical expert/patient model to a partnership/consultant model. The helping stance changes from "This is what you must do" to "How can I help you?"

Clinical care: Provide clinical services that are recovery-focused, evidence-based, developmentally appropriate, gender-sensitive, culturally competent, trauma informed, and integrated with a broad spectrum of nonclinical recovery support services. Clinical care also extends to strengthening the family and community contexts so that individuals have increased access to long-term recovery supports. Focus of treatment is expanded to include the development of recovery maintenance skills rather than limited to recovery initiation

Service delivery sites: Increase the delivery of community integrated, neighborhood-, and home-based services and expand recovery support services in high-need areas. Utilize and link clients to existing community-based resources rather than duplicating efforts and recreating resources within segregated, institutional environments. Assist clients in developing a network of natural recovery supports in order to increase their recovery capital

Peer-based recovery support services: Expand the availability of nonclinical, formal (paid), and informal (nonpaid) peer-based recovery support services and integrate them with professional and peer-based services

Dose/duration of services: Provide doses of services across levels of care that are associated with positive recovery outcomes. Facilitate continuity of contact in a primary recovery support relationship over time and across levels of care

Posttreatment checkups and support: Shift the focus of service interventions from acute stabilization to sustained recovery management via posttreatment recovery checkups, stage appropriate recovery education, and, when needed, early reintervention. Shift from passive aftercare to assertive approaches to continuing care

Attitude toward readmission: Returning clients are welcomed, not shamed

Relationship to community: Collaborate with indigenous recovery support organizations (e.g., faith community); assertively link clients to local communities of recovery; participate in local recovery education/celebration events in the larger community and advocate on issues that effect long-term recovery in the community (e.g., issues of stigma and discrimination)

Develop Mechanisms for Attitudinal Change and Skill Building

When trying to transform a complex service system, a multidimensional approach to skill building is required. In recent years, a call to action has emerged regarding the "substantial, if not fundamental, change in the education and training of the behavioral health workforce" [26, p. 320]. Graduate and continuing education programs have not kept pace with the dramatic changes that have been occurring in the field in recent years [27, 28]. As a result, there are grave concerns that current educational approaches are not sufficient to equip professionals to function within a rapidly evolving healthcare system [28].

Given this reality, in order for sustainable changes to take root in the system, concerted attention is being devoted to the issue of workforce development. The recovery foundations training (RFT) series was the first of its kind in the system to include people in recovery, family members, multiple levels of provider staff (from those that provide direct services to executive level staff), and staff of DBHMRS all in the same training. The training provided an opportunity for participants to discuss these issues together and become exposed to the experiences and perspectives of other stakeholders in the system in a nonthreatening environment. In addition to participating in the training itself, people in recovery with relevant life experiences were trained and paired with professional staff to facilitate the trainings and serve on panels.

This training was followed by the development of the advanced recovery training series and several other strategies to further develop the workforce. These include activities such as:

- Web-based and distance learning techniques
- Partnerships with area universities to support graduate training
- Unit recovery planning processes to examine how each DBHMRS unit would align practices and/or processes to support the recovery transformation effort
- Development of practice guidelines in partnership with people in recovery and providers.

Empower All Stakeholders

Given the disenchantment and cynicism that is rampant in behavioral health systems, strategies that empower stakeholders are among the most important and potent in transformation processes. Some of the activities that helped to empower people in recovery and their family members included:

Story telling training that prepared more than 600 recovering people and their families to share their recovery story in multiple community venues; trainees were subsequently hired as trainers, consultants, and employees throughout the behavioral health system.

A peer specialist initiative that equipped more than 140 individuals with the skills necessary to be hired to provide recovery supports within Philadelphia's behavioral health system.

A peer leadership academy (26-week training program) that prepared more than 60 individuals and family members to assume leadership roles in Philadelphia's recovery-focused systems transformation process.

A peer group facilitation training that equipped people in recovery with the knowledge and skills to develop and facilitate recovery support groups.

Strategies used to empower DBH/MRS staff and local services providers included:

Creating a quality of life committee composed of DBHMRS staff drawn from all levels (including administrative support staff and executive staff) whose charge was to align the organizational culture with a recovery orientation.

Changing the composition of planning and decision-making committees to include staff from all levels of the organization rather than restricting membership to senior management.

Creating new planning groups with significant provider representation to ensure that providers were partnering with city administrators and people in recovery to design a new service system.

Create Short-Term Wins

Transformational change does not occur overnight, but rather unfolds with time, usually over a long period of time. In the absence of any demonstrable successes, cynicism and doubt festers and motivation wanes. Kotter [17] warns that change agents can become so focused on the vision that they neglect to effectively manage the current reality. Consequently, when asked for evidence that the investment of resources has actually made a difference, there is little to substantiate and validate the new direction. To prevent this scenario from occurring, well-timed and carefully planned short-term wins are essential.

Given that transformation was taking place within the context of a complex system of care, Philadelphia developed a multitiered approach to demonstrating short-term wins. The antagonistic relationship that existed between stakeholder groups permitted early wins to be defined in the form of developing processes and mechanisms that facilitated a truly collaborative approach. As time progressed, however, there was an increased need to demonstrate wins that were less process oriented and more outcome oriented. The wins needed to be visible, unambiguous, and clearly connected to the transformation. The question that preoccupied everyone was: "How was this paradigm shift making a difference in the lives of people in recovery?" Short-term wins that lent early credibility to Philadelphia's change process include:

- Populations with serious behavioral health conditions were experiencing improved quality of life.
- Men and women with serious mental illness and/or co-occurring disorders who had become dependent on the system and whose lives revolved around attending partial hospitalization programs were participating in the community at increased levels and utilizing emergency care at significantly lower levels.
- Cost efficiencies were demonstrated as a result of the provision of recovery-oriented care. For instance, provider agencies implementing integrated peer- and professionally based services experienced increases in retention rates from 50% to over 75%.

Celebrate the Successes

Generating the types of successes noted above is necessary for building and sustaining momentum, but it is not sufficient. Celebrating the successes acknowledges the hard work and dedication of stakeholders, renews motivation, and disseminates new knowledge so that innovations proliferate [17]. One of the most visible ways Philadelphia celebrated early successes of transformation was by hosting a recovery conference for providers, people in recovery, family members, members of the broader community, and staff of DBHMRS. Representatives from all stakeholder groups highlighted transformation successes within their respective areas of influence and shared lessons learned. At the program level, many agencies have instituted their own annual recovery celebrations, graduation ceremonies, and other events geared to highlighting individual, staff, and program successes.

Strategies that Advance Contextual Alignment

In a ROSC, the administrative components of the system are aligned with the recovery vision. The temptation must be avoided to create a network of model programs or pilot projects rather than to take on the more difficult task of transforming the fundamental philosophy, infrastructure, mission, and methods of the whole system. Aligning the context means that all administrative functions, including policies and financing strategies, are examined through the lens of recovery and modified to facilitate rather than impede the provision of recovery-oriented care. In addition, the context in which services are embedded includes the community at large. If the ultimate goal of recovery-oriented systems of care is to provide people with the services and supports to assist them in developing a meaningful life in the community, then it follows that the system also has a role in developing recovery capital in the community. The following are some principles and strategies that guided and continue to guide Philadelphia's efforts to align the context and ensure that all of the changes being created as a result of the recovery transformation will be sustainable.

Align Organizational Structure

One of first strategies Dr. Evans employed to create the organizational structure necessary to support transformation was to establish a dedicated transformation team. He hired a Director of Strategic Planning, who was charged with planning and implementing the recovery transformation and reassigned existing staff to ensure that she had the necessary support to carry out the work. Over time the strategic planning unit grew to include people in recovery and family members who are now playing key roles in leading the redesign of the service system. Currently, key functions within the organization such as provider credentialing, monitoring, and system evaluation strategies are being aligned with the vision of recovery.

Address Policy and Fiscal Issues for Long-Term Sustainability

While many providers in Philadelphia's behavioral health system expressed great hope and tremendous excitement about the changes unfolding through system transformation, there were others who experienced anxiety regarding how recovery-oriented care would be provided within the existing reimbursement and regulatory structure. Current funding mechanisms in behavioral health systems evolved in tandem with the reigning treatment paradigms of isolated, episodic treatment that focuses on symptom reduction and/or stabilization. Over the years, funding in the public sector has shifted from a program funding model (via grants) to the fee-for-service model characteristic of private health care. This shift contributed to a narrowing of services to only those approved for reimbursement and billing in the current fee-for-service system. This created a system poorly designed to support the broad range of services and supports needed by many people to sustain long-term recovery and build a healthy and meaningful life in the community [1].

The creation of recovery-oriented systems of care is even more vital in an economically strained environment in which treatment providers are forced to become more vigilant about reimbursement. Examples of the types of policy and fiscal changes that have occurred in Philadelphia to support the provision of recovery-oriented care include:

- Alternative payment arrangements so that more flexible menus of service can be developed to meet individuals' changing needs over time.
- Changing reimbursement policies that require on-site service delivery so that services can be delivered in the community rather than only within traditional treatment settings.
- Incentivized performance-based contracting to support recovery outcomes.

- Rate negotiations to include recovery support services. One of the misconceptions encountered during system transformation is the belief on the part of providers and system administrators that recovery-oriented services cannot be created without the influx of additional resources to support new programming. While there is undoubtedly a need for fiscal alignment, there are also many cost neutral practice changes that can be implemented even prior to any changes in funding. Examples include:
- Mobilizing the community of people in recovery to provide informal peer-based support such as outreach and continued care,
- Expanding leadership opportunities for people in recovery within treatment settings,
- Conducting holistic, strengths-based assessments,
- Shifting from treatment planning to recovery planning,
- Developing reciprocal community partnerships,
- Shifting the service approach from an expert to a consultation approach,
- Assertively including family members and other important allies in recovery planning and service delivery as desired, and
- Developing a menu of supports and services for people to develop their own individualized recovery plan, rather than providing a one-size-fits-all program.

Strengthen the Community and Build Indigenous Recovery Capital

Within a recovery-oriented system of care, the institutional focus on getting people into treatment programs shifts to exploring how we connect the process of recovery to the individual or families' natural environment, the community [1]. Toward this end, recovery-oriented systems of care focus on decreasing stigma and environmental obstacles to recovery while simultaneously strengthening recovery support resources within the community. These efforts often encompass prevention services, which serve to make the community healthier for everyone. Philadelphia's transformation process has involved building community recovery capital through the development of several key projects. Examples include:

- The opening of Philadelphia's first recovery community center which served more than 2,300 individuals in its first 7 months of operation.
- The Faith Based Initiative which was designed to assist the faith community in providing community-based supports to those individuals and families impacted by behavioral health challenges.
- The distribution of mini-grants to grassroots community organizations to seed new or enhance existing recovery support services in the community.
- The creation of seven coalitions composed of community-based organizations, faith-based organizations, and treatment providers to strengthen neighborhood-based recovery supports through the prevention or early intervention services within Philadelphia.

Another strategy for increasing community recovery capital was participation in Philadelphia's mural arts initiative through the creation of three murals that focus on recovery. This process brought together artists, community members, providers, and people in recovery and their families to create beautiful murals that address stigma and increase awareness that recovery is possible. Both the process of creating the murals, and the murals themselves, were instrumental in dispelling myths regarding people in recovery and making recovery more visible within the City of Philadelphia.

Move Beyond the Choir – Link It to Other Political Agendas

At any given point in time, different issues rise and recede within the hierarchy of community concerns. This hierarchy has the power to determine the resources available to social institutions and consequently influences the fate of the people they serve. Historically, the focus of behavioral health systems has been so insular that minimal attention has been given to building political capital to support long-term recovery support resources. Recovery-oriented systems of care deliberately link the agenda of recovery to prominent community concerns to engender broad-based support. Without this, systems are not well-positioned to survive in an economic crisis that forces policy makers to decide among roads, schools, day care, and behavioral health treatment and recovery support resources [1].

Philadelphia's DBHMRS has made a concerted effort to build allies within the City's political arena by applying the principles of recovery-oriented care to some of the most challenging social issues confronting the community. The issue of homelessness is one of these concerns. DBHMRS transformed some of its existing residential addiction treatment programs into recovery-oriented programs for chronically homeless men and women. Men and women who previously had difficulty with the rigidity, that is, characteristic of traditional residential substance abuse treatment facilities, were able to not only initiate recovery, but also transition to living independently in their own apartments in the community. Successes such as these are helping to build the political capital necessary to embed the recovery transformation into the culture of the City.

Summary

The framework detailed in this paper provides organizational and system leaders with a set of principles to guide the development of a recovery-oriented system of care that is responsive to the unique needs of the communities they serve. While transformation is a long-term and complex process, it is one that holds tremendous opportunity and hope for people and communities.

The experiences in the City of Philadelphia have revealed that:

- Recovery transformation is not about developing new programming or tweaking what currently exists. Recovery transformation revolves around developing more holistic services that are consistent with what people in recovery and science tells us works. The focus of these services is not just on managing symptoms, but on helping individuals to fulfill their highest potential and find meaningful roles in their communities. This vision requires that systems undergo revolutionary changes at all levels and that they assertively promote changes in the surrounding community.
- Of paramount importance is the recognition that this new paradigm of recovery-oriented care is not a model to be superimposed on any community regardless of its unique variables. Such indiscriminate replication would be antithetical to the philosophical underpinnings of recovery-oriented care. While the elements of recovery-oriented systems of care are consistent across cultures, geographic locations, and time, they should manifest themselves differently in different contexts to match the unique needs of the people and communities being served.
- Three change strategies have been helpful in promoting systems transformation in Philadelphia: aligning concepts, practices, and contexts.
- Three approaches to developing a ROSC have emerged in the field. The additive, selective, and transformative approaches all have significant practice and policy implications for the system.
- The critical role of informed leadership cannot be overstated. Leaders must understand the nature of transformational change processes, be willing to empower formal and informal leaders around them, and facilitate participatory, transparent processes.

References

1. White W. Recovery management and recovery-oriented systems of care: scientific rationale and promising practices. Chicago, IL: Northeast Addiction Technology Transfer Center, the Great Lakes Addiction Technology Transfer Center, and the Philadelphia Department of Behavioral Health and Mental Retardation Services; 2008.
2. Davidson L, Tondora J, Lawless MS, O'Connell M, Rowe M. A practical guide to recovery oriented practice. New York: Oxford University Press; 2009.
3. Davidson L, Harding C, Spaniol L. Recovery from severe mental illness: research evidence and implications for practice. Boston, MA: Center for Psychiatric Rehabilitation; 2005.
4. Anthony WA. A recovery-oriented service system: setting some system level standards. In: Davidson L, Harding C, Spaniol L, editors. Recovery from severe mental illness: research evidence and implications for practice. Boston, MA: Center for Psychiatric Rehabilitation; 2005.
5. Jacobson N, Curtis N. Recovery as policy in mental health services: strategies emerging from the states. In: Davidson L, Harding C, Spaniol L, editors. Recovery from severe mental illness: research evidence and implications for practice. Boston, MA: Center for Psychiatric Rehabilitation; 2005.

6. White W. Peer-based addiction recovery support: history, theory, practice, and scientific evaluation. Chicago, IL: Great Lakes Addiction Technology Transfer Center; and the Philadelphia Department of Behavioral Health and Mental Retardation Services; 2009.

7. Clark W. Recovery as an organizing concept. In: White W. *Perspectives on Systems Transformation: How Visionary Leaders are Shifting Addiction Treatment Toward a Recovery-Oriented System of Care.* (Interviews with H. Westley Clark, Thomas A. Kirk, Jr., Arthur C. Evans, Michael Boyle, Phillip Valentine and Lonnetta Albright). Chicago, IL: Great Lakes Addiction Technology Transfer Center; 2008.

8. Kirk T. *Creating a recovery-oriented system of care.* In: White W. *Perspectives on Systems Transformation: How Visionary Leaders are Shifting Addiction Treatment Toward a Recovery-Oriented System of Care.* (Interviews with H. Westley Clark, Thomas A. Kirk, Jr., Arthur C. Evans, Michael Boyle, Phillip Valentine and Lonnetta Albright). Chicago, IL: Great Lakes Addiction Technology Transfer Center; 2008.

9. Evans A. The recovery-focused transformation of an urban behavioral health care system. In: White W. *Perspectives on Systems Transformation: How Visionary Leaders are Shifting Addiction Treatment Toward a Recovery-Oriented System of Care.* (Interviews with H. Westley Clark, Thomas A. Kirk, Jr., Arthur C. Evans, Michael Boyle, Phillip Valentine and Lonnetta Albright). Chicago, IL: Great Lakes Addiction Technology Transfer Center; 2008.

10. Gottheil E, Sterling RC, Weinstein SP. Pretreatment dropouts: Characteristics and outcomes. *Journal of Addictive Diseases.* 1997;16:1–14.

11. Substance Abuse Mental Health Services Administration, Office of Applied Studies. Treatment Episode Data Set (TEDS): 2004 Treatment Discharges. Available at: http://www.oas.samhsa.gov/TEDSdischarges/2k4/TEDSsk4chp2.htm. Accessed January 30, 2008.

12. Shearer J. Psychosocial approaches to psychostimulant dependence: A systematic review. *Journal of Substance Abuse Treatment.* 2007;32:41–52.

13. Stevens A, Radcliffe P, Sanders M, Hunt N. Early exit: Estimating and explaining early exit from drug treatment. *Harm Reduction Journal.* 2008;5:13.

14. Anglin MD, Hser YI, Grella CE. Drug addiction and treatment careers among clients in the Drug Abuse Treatment Outcome Study (DATOS). *Psychology of Addictive Behaviors.* 1997;11(4):308–323.

15. Wilbourne P, Miller W. Treatment of alcoholism: Older and wiser? In: McGovern T, White W, eds. *Alcohol Problems in the United States: Twenty Years of Treatment Perspective.* New York: Haworth Press; 2002:41–59.

16. Hubbard RL, Flynn PM, Craddock G, Fletcher B. Relapse after drug abuse treatment. In: Tims F, Leukfield C, Platt J, eds. *Relapse and recovery in addictions.* New Haven, Conn: Yale University Press; 2001:109–121.

17. Kotter JP. *Leading Change.* Boston, MA: Harvard Business School Press; 1996.

18. Senge P. *The fifth discipline: The art and practice of the learning organization.* New York: Doubleday; 2006.

19. Ackerman L. Development, transition, or transformation: The question of change in organizations. In: Van Eynde D, Hoy J, Van Eynde E, eds. *Organization Development Classics.* San Francisco: Jossey Bass; 1997.

20. Borkman, T. (1998). Is recovery planning any different from treatment planning? *Journal of Substance Abuse Treatment,* 15(1):37–42.

21. Anderson D, Ackerman-Anderson L. *Beyond change management: Advanced strategies for today's transformational leaders.* San Francisco: Jossey Bass; 2001.

22. Lamb, R., Evans, A.C, & White, W. (2009). The role of partnership in recovery-oriented systems of care: The Philadelphia experience. Accessed October 29, 2009 at www.facesand-voicesofrecovery.org

23. Bridges W. *Managing transitions: Making the most of change.* Cambridge, MA: Perseus Publishing; 2003.

24. Gladwell M. *The tipping point.* NY, NY: Back Bay Books; 2002.

25. White W. A recovery revolution in Philadelphia. *Counselor.* 2007;8(5):34–38.

26. Adams N, Daniels AS. Sometimes a great notion . . . a common agenda for change. *Administration and Policy in Mental Health*. 2002;29(4/5):319–333.

27. Hoge MA, Selby J, Belitsky R, Migdole S. Graduate education and training for contemporary behavioral health practice. *Administration and Policy in Mental Health*. 2002;29(4/5):335–358.

28. Daniels AS, Walter DA. Current issues in continuing education for contemporary behavioral health practice. *Administration and Policy in Mental Health*. 2002;29(4/5):359–376.

Chapter 12
Connecticut's Journey to a Statewide Recovery-Oriented Health-care System: Strategies, Successes, and Challenges

Thomas A. Kirk

Abstract Approaches to the treatment of addiction at state level have typically been fragmented, costly, and inefficient. This chapter describes Connecticut's journey in designing and implementing a transformation of its entire public/private behavioral health-care system, treating 90,000 adults annually, to a recovery-oriented model driven by quality improvement, continuity of care vs. an acute service emphasis, and supported by innovative resource development strategies and service delivery infrastructures. With broad stakeholder collaboration and based on Recovery Core Values created by recovery communities, a Commissioner's Recovery Policy set the initial tone and direction. The chosen approach addressed interventions for facilitating sustained change at the practitioner/client, program, and overall system levels. The tools for change, such as baseline system assessments, recovery-oriented practice guidelines inclusive of those for co-occurring disorders and gender, trauma and culturally responsive care, all tied to the IOM quality domains, centers of excellence, and state agency linkages with child welfare, criminal justice, and social service systems, are detailed. Critical is a model for innovation, reinvestment, and enhanced outcomes.

Different large databases reveal improvements on traditional and new dimensions — 62% decrease in use of acute care and 78% increase in ambulatory care, with 14% lower cost even after adding extensive recovery-support services such as housing and transportation, 40% increase in first time admissions, and 24% decrease in average annual cost per client, especially for high service utilizers. In tough fiscal times, these findings support the value of a recovery-oriented behavioral health-care system and the use of health-care business plans for state systems even more.

Keywords Addiction recovery management · Health-care systems · Recovery core values · Recovery-oriented system of care

T.A. Kirk (✉)
Department of Mental Health and Addiction Services, 100 Sorghum Mill Drive, Cheshire, CT 06410, USA
e-mail: ta129kirk@aol.com

J.F. Kelly and W.L. White (eds.), *Addiction Recovery Management: Theory, Research and Practice*, Current Clinical Psychiatry, DOI 10.1007/978-1-60327-960-4_12,
© Springer Science+Business Media, LLC 2011

Introduction

This chapter describes the journey of the Connecticut Department of Mental Health and Addiction Services (DMHAS) [1], a state operated private/public partnership treating 90,000 adults annually, including 900 inpatient beds for persons with forensic issues, drug dependence, and/or mental illness, in designing and implementing a recovery-oriented system of care (ROSC) notable for its continuing care, long-term "health-care" management focus, and its commitment to quality as the defining characteristic of an ROSC. What is unique in this effort is the fact that its aim has been to create a full statewide transformation of its existing service system for persons with mental illness and/or substance use disorders rather than being a project or limited initiative.

What are some of the challenges that justify a statewide transformation?

- *The language perpetuates stigma and* reinforces the dim view that some have about addiction and mental health treatment (Fig. 12.1) (Table 12.1).
- *It conveys a weak message to funders and policy makers*: Who would be optimistic about investing funding in such a system? Do these terms offer a tone of hope to individuals and families in need of care?

Table 12.1 The Power of Language

What message are we conveying?
"Addicts"
"A chronic, relapsing disease"
"Severe, persistent mental illness"
Doesn't anybody ever get better?

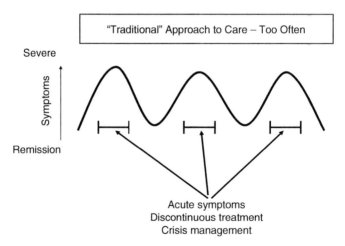

Fig. 12.1 Cyclical and Recurrent

- *Use of acute care service and funding model*: The Cyclical and Recurrent graphic reflects the costly and ineffective service response for persons with substance use and/or mental health disorders that leads policy makers and funders to question the quality of the behavioral health-care system and its relevance to easing other public sector challenges, e.g., criminal justice, child welfare, public safety, and health. Who would be optimistic about investing funding in such a system?
- *Customers vote with their feet*: Dropout rates tend to be high. Is this the message from persons and families who use the system?
- *Less than meaningful outcome measures*: Focusing on numbers of persons out-reached or in care is less relevant than reporting how many get "better."

New Collaboration Sets the Stage for the Recovery Movement

Given the challenges of a statewide transformation, where does one start? This effort involved a progression of eras beginning in the late 1990s. The initial driver was the Governor's Blue Ribbon Task Force on Substance Abuse [2] and the subsequent formation of the Connecticut Alcohol and Drug Policy Council (ADPC), cochaired by the then Deputy Commissioner, Thomas Kirk, and the Governor's Legislative Director. The ADPC *served to crystallize the collective energy and collaborative force of Connecticut's legislative, judicial, and executive branches*. It formulated the most significant and sustained thematic end result of the ADPC era: addiction issues are essential parts of a progressive, informed, and solution-oriented approach for policies, practices, and costs of the criminal justice, child welfare, and public health and safety systems in Connecticut [3]. The right players and "systems" were now at the same table and have been ever since.

The initial systemic approach that DMHAS selected and implemented beginning in late 1999 had three key phases: (1) determine direction, (2) initiate and implement change and system integration, and (3) increase depth and complexity, and preparedness for future phase. It is important to note that the development of a statewide ROSC is not a linear process but rather one of simultaneous and inter-acting operational and strategic tracks, which gradually begin to emerge into one integrated cohesive system.

Phase I: Determine Direction

Core Values and Premises

The first phase in addressing the problems and challenges facing Connecticut was to determine what the "ideal" system would look like and map out how to get there. In 1999, DMHAS charged the recovery community (advocates and persons in recovery from mental illness and substance use) to be the major source for developing *core values and premises of a recovery system*. The initial "oil and water" process of two historically very different advocacy groups succeeded, over several months of spirited, thoughtful, and progressively productive meetings, to produce the DMHAS Recovery Core Values that articulated four major premises and 24 Recovery Core Values, grouped into four categories: Participation, Programming, Direction, and Funding – Operations.

The premises were:

- All individuals are unique and have specific needs, goals, health attitudes and behaviors, and expectations for recovery.
- Persons in recovery with mental illness, alcohol or drug addiction, or both, share some similarities. However, management of their own lives and mastery of their future will, at times, require different pathways.
- All persons shall be offered equal access to treatment and have the opportunity to design their own recovery process.
- DMHAS shall support a ROSC that requires funded and/or operated treatment programs to treat individuals in accordance with recovery-based core values (Fig. 12.2).

The product was a cornerstone in Connecticut's movement into the recovery era in 2000 and remains so in 2009.

Another important contextual component leading to the recovery movement was the creation of the Connecticut DMHAS in July 1995. As commissioner of this newly created state agency, the late Dr. Albert Solnit was clear that this was not a merger of the mental health field over that for addiction or vice versa. Rather, the history, values, and practices of each field would yield something new and greater

Programming
- Individually tailored care
- Culturally competent care
- Staff know resources

Direction
- Equal opportunity for wellness
- Recovery encompasses all phases of care
- Entire systems to support recovery
- Input at every level
- Recovery-based outcome measures
- New nomenclature
- System wide training
- Culturally diverse, relevant and competent services
- Consumers review funding

Participation
- No wrong door
- Entry at any time
- Choice is respected
- Right to participate
- Person defines goals

Funding-Operations
- Funding and Operations
- No outcomes, no income
- Person selects provider
- Protection from undue influence
- Providers don't oversee themselves
- Providers compete for business

Fig. 12.2 Recovery Core Values

than the sum of its parts. The Recovery Core Values and Premises is a solid example of Dr. Solnit's mantra.

Define Recovery and Establish Policy

Armed with the Recovery Core Values and Premises, in early 2000, the process of formally defining what we mean by "recovery" began. Very ably led by the then Deputy Commissioner, Arthur Evans, it took well over 18 months to reach a consensus. An extraordinarily heavy emphasis was placed on developing consensus and was accomplished through hosting retreats and focus groups for state-operated and private nonprofit CEOs, consumers, persons self-described as being "in recovery," medical directors, trade associations, and generally the broadest network of possible stakeholders one could gather.

Commissioner's Policy #83: Promoting a Recovery-Oriented Service System, (available at: www.ct.gov/dmhas/recovery), the first of its kind in the nation, was completed after a long journey with signing in September 2002. The definitions were:

> We endorse a broad vision of recovery that involves a process of restoring or developing a positive and meaningful sense of identity, apart from one's condition, and a meaningful sense of belonging while rebuilding a life despite or within the limitations imposed by that condition.

> A ROSC identifies and builds on each individual's assets, strengths, and areas of health and competence to support the achievement of a sense of mastery over his or her condition while regaining a meaningful, constructive sense of membership in the broader community.

Inherent in the policy was the unequivocal message that *recovery* would be *the guiding principle and operational framework* of the DMHAS system and that recovery:

- Is a process and not an event
- Encourages hope and emphasizes respect
- Involves addressing needs over time and across levels of disability
- Requires identifying and building on one's strengths and areas of hope

Of particular importance were these action words in the policy: We must "embed the language, spirit, and culture of recovery throughout the system of services, in our interactions with one another and with those persons and families who entrust their care to us." These words convey that the recovery movement is not owned by any one leader or person and will survive after "leaders" move on to other tasks and interests. The sense of empowerment, energy, self-esteem, and new ideas is so ingrained in the culture that the system is highly unlikely to regress to its past.

The final piece of Dr. Solnit's great legacy at DMHAS was leading, as chair of the Governor's 2000 Blue Ribbon Commission on Mental Health (BRCMH), the Commission in its recommendations (July 2000) [4] to formally add "recovery" into the mental health lexicon in Connecticut. Further, the recommendations of the BRCMH and the ADPC were very much in the same direction – increased access, quality of care and improved outcomes, recovery and health promotion.

Identify DMHAS as a Health-care Service Agency

As the early work on recovery evolved, a new strategic action plan was developed. The Department's plan, released in January 2000 and entitled *"Partnership for Healthy Communities – The DMHAS Strategic Action Plan,"* established the theme that mental illness and addiction are health issues and that DMHAS as a health-care service agency has a twofold mission: (1) to promote wellness through prevention and intervention services, and (2) to support recovery and sustained overall health – physical, mental, social, economic, and community – through treatment and recovery support services (RSSs).

Besides helping to offset the stigma that envelops substance use and mental illness, the health-care theme also would communicate that any individual accessing services from DMHAS should hope and expect to get *better* from the care. Yes, mental illness and substance use disorders are chronic health-care conditions for many. But those who need and seek care, and all policy and funding stakeholders would be better served by a descriptor such as "Continued Care Disorder" rather than "chronic" and these disorders can be best stabilized and improved with "Long-Term Recovery Management Services" over one's lifetime.

In sum, the concepts of health and recovery were gradually threaded into the strategic and operational fabric of this new state agency called DMHAS.

Establish a Strategic Action Plan

The January 2000 Strategic Action Plan identified four major goals that would serve as additional pillars of Connecticut's recovery movement and system transformation.They were, in their most succinct form:

1. Quality care
2. Services for people with challenging needs
3. Effective DMHAS management
4. Resource base to support goals

When the author assumed his role as Commissioner in May 2000, an overarching goal was added to the DMHAS Strategic Action Plan to reinforce the evolving recovery focus: *Create a Value-Driven, Recovery-Oriented Health-care System. Value-driven?* This means the quality and the cost of a service are assessed to ensure highest quality at the most efficient cost. These goals reinforced and directly supported Connecticut's recovery direction, serving as policy and operational drivers for the journey to an ROSC.

Goal One – Quality: DMHAS' view from the outset has been that *Recovery is not a stand-alone discrete initiative. It is the overarching theme for everything we do in our system of services.* Connecticut's approach embeds the recovery focus into the core of *all* parts of the system, whether it is a traditional level of care or a RSS such as transportation or temporary housing support before, during, or after formal treatment. Goal One, thus, served to link quality and recovery together. That said, one key tool of the recovery transformation path can be noted as: *Quality – The Driving Force in Creating a Recovery-Oriented System of Services* [5].

Goal Two – Services for People with Challenging Needs addressed the repeated use of acute-care services for persons with seemingly complicated continuing care conditions. Data from 1997 through 2001 demonstrated that heroin was an increasingly frequent part of the substance use profile of persons presenting for care into the more costly settings, e.g., residential detoxification, 42% in 1996 and 64% in 2002. During the same period, the percentages for marijuana, cocaine, and alcohol all decreased. The second theme was that the rate of readmissions of persons into these costly levels of care was high, resulting in their using up a disproportionate amount of our resources and with little sustained benefit. Effectively addressing these findings would improve care and could yield better allocation of resources.

One by-product of Goal Two and the overarching goal to create a ROSC was a new term, *Recovery Zone* – a state of sustained periods of stability with the opportunity to rebuild an improved and fullest possible quality of life in support of the goals a person may have. Thus, a key direction of the DMHAS' ROSC is to provide the tools that one can choose from to enter and have a sustained stay in their *Recovery Zone* (Fig. 12.3).

Goal Three – Effective DMHAS Management: One impetus for this action goal involved the extraordinarily important decision that DMHAS would train existing state staff and recruit others from the private provider and managed care fields into state service to help the agency adapt itself to using quality-driven and fiscally sound managed care techniques, but always based on public sector values and with not a penny to be made by denying care.

Given the variability of public funding and the over arching goal of completely transforming the DMHAS system into a ROSC, it was essential that we included the

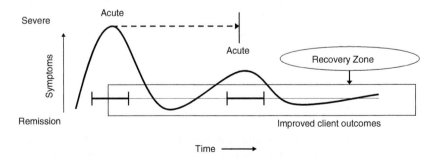

Fig. 12.3 Goal: Help People Move Into Recovery Zone

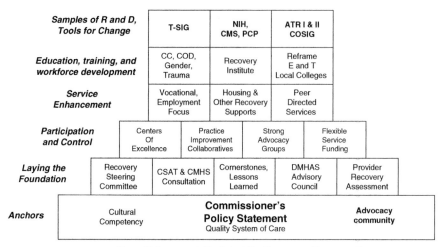

Fig. 12.4 Connecticut Implementation Process

goal of a strong resource development strategy within Phase 1. This strategy would support the testing of new ideas and the addition of innovative services resulting from pilot work (Fig. 12.4).

Phase II: Initiate and Implement Change in System Integration

The intensive and extensive process of arriving at a Recovery Policy in September 2002, given all the groups involved, resulted in an initial buy-in which would need to be continually reinforced. Additional critically important stakeholders had to be engaged and informed if a large state agency was to be transformed into one based on a recovery paradigm. Those included the Governor's Office and staff, his/her budget agency, and state legislators and their staffs – all being the ultimate approval authority for funding and policy. Other state agency leadership with whom DMHAS would interact, directors of DMHAS-funded private agencies, the thousands of administrative and direct line staff who are part of the system, family members, and the major media outlets who influence opinion about government needed to be brought on board.

Spread the Word

A multifaceted and sustained communication strategy was designed and implemented in 2000 to spread the word and create awareness. The initial components included:

Interviews with the editorial boards of newspapers, individual local reporters, and similar regional sessions with service providers and their boards of directors.

"Messages from the Office of the Commissioner" – One page commentaries written by the commissioner, senior managers, and others explain the meaning of recovery and the purpose of changes as they occurred. They address the critics, and publicly congratulate staff, providers, and others for their work. Beginning in October 2000 and continuing through September 2009, over 175 Messages were distributed electronically to an estimated 5,000 recipients once or twice a month. Quick perusal of the titles of the *Messages* (all available at www.ct.gov/dmhas/oocmessages) reflects a steady stream of recovery-focused themes. Consider just a few: *Promoting a ROSC* (1/11/01), *Join the Voice of Recovery: A Call to Action* (9/5/02), *The Changing Culture of Recovery* (2/10/05), *Myths and Facts About Work and Recovery* (4/24/08), and *Have Some Fun and Be Renewed* (9/25/09).

Quality Improvement and Collaboration

Given the premise that quality is the driver of an ROSC, four areas were initially selected for improving quality: *gender, cultural competence, trauma* [6], and *co-occurring substance use and mental health disorders* [7, 8]. The figures below are evidence of some early findings in support of the rationale for selecting these choices. The first figure, *Aggregate Data*, reflects that continuity of care (i.e., timely linkage from the time of discharge from one level of care to entrance – not simply referral into the next level) over a 3-year period for Black and Latino clients in the DMHAS service system was far lower than for Whites or the overall population, thus indicating the importance of addressing race and culture as components of quality (Fig. 12.5).

The following co-occurring figure, based upon a sample of 2,086 admissions for residential detoxification services, shows that the greater number of admissions an individual had into residential detoxification in a 1-year period, the more likely the presence of a co-occurring mental health disorder (Fig. 12.6).

DMHAS operational staff working in the four service areas (gender, culture, trauma, and CODs) led focus groups throughout the state to elicit the views of

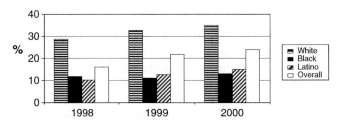

Fig. 12.5 Aggregate data masks important differences among groups. Continuity of Care Rates from Acute Substance Detoxification to Rehabilitation

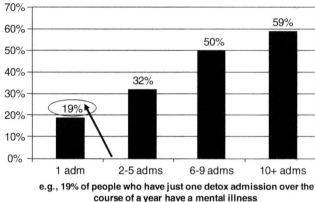

Fig. 12.6 Persons with co-occuring disorders are more likely to be multiple detox users

individuals/family members/advocates who directly or indirectly experienced the services. Findings were used to design and implement an Agency Self-Assessment Tool. Practice or Quality Improvement Collaboratives (QIC) comprised of state and invited private provider staff were then created, and 1 year of federally funded technical assistance consultation services was provided. These initial QICs engendered significant buy-in from participants and eventually resulted in a body of new policies, practice guidelines, identification of training needs, program performance, and suggested outcome indices in each of these areas. The products were, and continue to be, incrementally integrated into the operations of the DMHAS service system and serve as visible evidence for all stakeholders of how improved outreach, competencies, and service innovation yield better access and engagement, maximum use of the existing system capacity, and positive recovery orientations for those persons. Additional collaboratives created are on preferred practices, health disparities, and enhancement of employment and educational opportunities for clients. Details and products can be accessed at www.ct.gov/dmhas; visit and then click on "Programs and Services."

Change and full transformation must occur at three different levels: system, program, and practitioner. The policy development and participatory decision making of the care providers and persons in recovery who are or were part of the QICs are examples to support system-level change. The improvement collaborative process and technical assistance reinforce program level change while more formal training activities, addressed in greater detail below in *Identify and Apply Tools of Change,* are examples of practitioner-level change agents.

Examples of actual QIC data and implementation can be accessed as follows: gender, *Women's Services Practice Improvement Collaborative,* 5/24/07; trauma, *Meeting the Needs of Trauma Survivors,* 11/8/07, both available at www.ct.gov/ dmhas/infobriefs. Additional material regarding trauma can be accessed at www.ct. gov/dmhas/trauma. Linkages for cultural competence and for CODs are www.ct.gov/

dmhas/oma and www.ct.gov/dmhas/cosig, respectively. Findings from one highly successful example of an employment joint venture between the Connecticut Community for Addiction Recovery, Inc. and an addiction service agency is described in *Recovery is Working*, 11/7/08, available at www.ct.gov/dmhas/infobriefs.

Identify and Apply Tools for Change

Formally defining recovery and publishing the Recovery Policy created a sense of urgency and interest among administrators, care providers and advocates to "get on with it." How do we go about creating an ROSC? How will we know when we have one?

Assessment Instruments – One interesting tool was the *Recovery Self-Assessment (RSA)*, developed by DMHAS colleagues at Yale's Program for Recovery and Community Health. It is a 36-item assessment scale that was completed by a total of 974 persons (CEOs, care staff, consumers, persons in recovery, family members/significant others) associated with 82 service agencies. Participants rated their degree of agreement to statements such as:

People in recovery work along side agency staff on the development and provision of new programs and services

At this agency, participants who are doing well get as much attention as those who are having difficulties

Staff use a language of recovery (i.e., hope, high expectations, respect) in everyday conversations.

Scores for each type of respondent group were determined on five factors:

- Diversity of treatment outcomes
- Consumer involvement and recovery education (lowest rated)
- Life goals and symptom management
- Rights and respect (highest rated)
- Individually tailored services

An expanded recovery assessment instrument, *RSA-Revised* [9] set a strong guidance path due in part to its format of a lead line to questions as follows: Person in Recovery Group – *To me recovery means...* Direct Service Provider Group – *I can support people in recovery by...* Manager/Administrator Group – *I can lead an organization that supports recovery by...* The scale also includes a "Recovery Marker" section that has the lead line – *We will know that we are working together toward recovery when...*

Benefits of the *RSA-R* tool for change? Each agency funded by DMHAS could now use such an instrument to assess their recovery strengths and weaknesses and implement a plan for improvements. DMHAS subsequently modified its service provider contract to require such an assessment and the submission of an Annual Recovery Plan for critique and approval. Another overall benefit was to highlight areas of training, skills building, and competency enhancement that DMHAS

should address in its education and training offerings, and differentiated by participant group.

The Recovery Marker aspect of RSA-R set the framework for two major Practice
Guideline documents. The first edition of *Practice Guidelines for Recovery-Oriented
Care for Mental Health and Substance Use Conditions* was developed in 2006 by
the Yale PRCH group in concert with DMHAS and a second edition released
December 2008. An extraordinary tool for change, the Guidelines use a "how to"
format, and the 2008 edition integrated the Institute of Medicine (2001) [10] quality
measures as well as the standards and guidelines developed in the four quality areas
described above – gender, culture, trauma, and CODs. The Guidelines hold great
potential for performance and outcome measures at system, program, and practitioner
levels. Both editions are available on the DMHAS website at www.ct.gov/dmhas/
recovery and hard copies by request to DMHAS or to PRCH.

The *"Recovery Institute,"* a tool for change on both the system and practitioner levels, began in 2003 to provide a group of innovative recovery-oriented
course offerings. Essentially a Recovery Education and Training Institute, it became
part of the DMHAS Education and Training (E&T) Division with decisions regarding
courses made by forums heavily inclusive of persons in recovery. Persons in recovery
are key members of the "faculty." In addition to the usual menu of clinical classes are
newer areas such as *Faith, Spirituality, and Recovery; Nine Passages into the Journey
of Recovery; Collaborative Treatment Planning in an ROSC*; and an especially strong
group of offerings on person centered and individualized recovery planning
supporting the 2008 Commissioner's Policy #33: *Individualized Recovery Planning.
The DMHAS Recovery Institute 2006* (5/25/06, available at www.ct.gov/dmhas/
infobriefs), describes how practice enhancements for *Illness Management and
Recovery*, the *Telephone Recovery Support Program* and *Peer to Peer Support*
(paid and volunteer) were among the highlights for FY06. The number of Recovery
Institute classes has more than doubled since FY03. Thousands of staff, consumers,
and persons in recovery annually are "students" in these classes where there is also a
significant focus on cultural competence, faith-based services, CODs, trauma, and
gender-responsive practices in support of the quality areas described above. Onsite
and video conferencing supervision and fidelity to model processes must be part of
these efforts and are thus increasingly supported.

Centers of excellence (COE) – First introduced in 2005, specific types of service
activities were selected to increase the skill sets of the DMHAS system as a whole
and the staff providing the services. A total of 16 COEs were initiated and among
them were Outreach, Engagement, and Motivation-Based Treatment; Case Management and Recovery Guides; Training and Supervising Peer Staff; Person-
Centered Planning and Self-Determination; Providing Peer Support; Core Clinical
Skills/Recovery Guiding; Supportive Community Living and Community Collaboratives; Development of Self-Help Peer-Run Programs; and Cultural and Developmental Competence.

The COE format provides consultation and training to develop exemplary
programs, with Centers then serving as models for other care providers who are
focusing on recovery-oriented services. Agencies or programs had to apply on a

competitive basis to become a COE. While DMHAS leadership went to some length to publicly recognize and celebrate the COE agencies with awards and other nonfund ceremonies, the motivational driver of the agencies seemed to be the learning of new skills, the provision of better care, and the desire to be perceived as a step above others – an effective tool for system change similar to the quality/ practice improvement collaboratives.

Annual Consumer Satisfaction Survey (CSS) – Required by provider contract, the CSS taps the degree of satisfaction of persons receiving services in seven domains: *General Satisfaction, Access, Quality and Appropriateness of Care, Outcomes, Participation in Treatment, Respect, and Recovery*. The 2008 and 2009 survey included the 26-item World Health Organization Quality-of-Life instrument (WHOQOL) which addresses four domains: Physical, Psychological, Social Relationships, and Environment. The number of respondents reached over 25,000 in 2009. The areas assessed are very indicative of the degree of satisfaction and fullness of one's life.

The Annual Consumer Survey Report for each year is posted on the DMHAS website www.ct.gov/dmhas/site. An example of a General Satisfaction item is: *If I had other choices, I would still get services from this agency*. Outcome items elicit responses as to whether an agency's services are helping the person to deal more effectively with daily problems, control his or her life, deal better with stress, get along well with family and others, and asks about relief of symptoms. Five recovery questions inquire about involvement in community life and control of one's treatment. As a tool for change, the CSS has appreciable system and program benefit. Agency directors receive individual program results that offer insights about strengths and weaknesses, and these are used to identify quality improvement initiatives for the upcoming year. An incentive award, a recognition ceremony at the State Capitol, was held for agencies that were tops in individual categories or had impressive results over three consecutive years. A sense of pride was evident for all attendees, especially for members of the agencies' boards.

Cross-State Agency Collaboration is an interesting tool for change on a system level in particular. Special legislative or governor-established commissions have addressed issues such as prisoner-reentry, jail diversion, emergency room overcrowding, workforce issues, poverty, homelessness, and prevention. It is expected that Commissioners or senior designees attend and actively participate in these forums resulting in highly innovative policy and service initiatives. As occurred with the ADPC, they have reinforced that attention to addiction/mental health issues is part of the solution to challenges of these other state systems. Also, because most DMHAS-funded private agencies receive funding from other state agencies (Social Services – Medicaid, Child Welfare or one of the Criminal Justice entities), participating agencies often collaborate on funding proposals, thus affirming shared views on policies, practice guidelines, and other dimensions of care. For example, DMHAS entered into a Cooperative Purchasing Agreement, whereby the Judicial Branch agreed to purchase residential services through DMHAS at rates and similar contract terms.

Statewide Conferences – With support from SAMHSA, DMHAS has either jointly or solely hosted large state conferences on three topical areas in recent years. A 2004 Faith Conference highlighted the emergence of faith-based recovery in Connecticut. Two major Recovery Conferences (2001 and 2006) and a recent CODs Conference were held for 2 days each and included plenary and workshop sessions tailored to the needs of each state-agency cosponsor. Nationally recognized keynote speakers, and workshops designed with strong participation of persons in recovery were featured. Persons in recovery participated in planning and as presenters. Over 400 persons attended each day with others on wait list or turned away. The collective substance and spirit of the conferences was a powerful force in energizing stakeholders throughout the state to raise the journey of creating an ROSC to a whole new level.

Have a "Recovery Plan" to Protect the Overall Strategic Goal

In 2002 and extending into 2003, Connecticut had an estimated $650 million to $1.5 billion state budget deficit. Every aspect of the DMHAS budget was under intense scrutiny. Approximately 450 individuals (15% of total staff) were laid off or took an early retirement. The overarching goal of creating a *ROSC was at risk of crumbling or at least being stopped in its tracks.* Views were resurfacing that recovery was an add-on to the system and should be jettisoned. Other stakeholders were realistically concerned about the stability of care for those in the current system due to the time, energy, and resources required for the ROSC focus. Overtime ballooned in our state-operated hospitals and community centers as units still needed staffing for clients/patients.

DMHAS initiated a "recovery plan" that included implementing a host of administrative and clinical stabilization actions and identifying our cornerstones for success and lessons learned to date. DMHAS leadership reinforced its commitment to creating and maintaining an ROSC, detailed their view of the benefits accomplished, and emphasized that our shared responsibility was to find a path to provide the best services possible to people with psychiatric and/or substance use conditions as these disorders did not simply abate because of a stressed budget. Five cornerstones of DMHAS' success to date were identified: (1) *Skilled and Dedicated People Make it Work,* (2) *Continued Focus on Quality,* (3) *Recovery Orientation,* (4) *Effective Advocacy,* and (5) *Its Reputation for Achievement and Success.* The collective residual effect was strengthening staff morale and highlighting successful work such as results from implementing recovery-oriented approaches in the Greater Hartford area (DMHAS, *Substance Abuse Treatment Enhancement Project – SATEP,* 10/25/02. Available at www.ct.gov/dmhas/info-briefs). SATEP results included a 26% increase in residential rehab admissions with no increase in bed capacity, a 24% decrease in readmission for detox services, a 60% increase in female admissions as well as the addition of a 24/7 access call line and transportation service staffed by persons in recovery. These and other lessons were touted to affirm the care benefits of a recovery-oriented approach and the rate of growth and cost controls that DMHAS could contribute to the state's fiscal crisis. In so doing, DMHAS was fostering positive brand recognition to the major policy and fiscal bodies in state government. The "recovery plan" helped the leadership to stabilize the system though the fiscal pressures lasted into 2004; yet on the whole, DMHAS was able to stay on the course set in 2000. The challenges arising from the "fiscal tsunami" of 2009/2010 are addressed in Phase III below.

Complete a Lessons Learned Initiative

The transformation journey is one of repeated reviews, and refining and sharpening of the road map. This is especially necessary when resources are under siege. Such reviews can lead to an impression, especially for long-term staff, that their hard work and dedication were not worth much. Given these periodic and sustained fiscal constraints, what should one reinforce in services and costs in building an ROSC? In 2004, DMHAS completed a Lessons Learned Initiative [11]. The LL effort evaluated findings that had yet to reach evidence-based status, yet were clearly worth weighing for inclusion in an ROSC based upon reasonable, well-defined criteria. With quality as the driver, DMHAS wanted to meet the highest standards, yet was willing to consider and include services that met the defined criteria of other forms of evidence. The LL process involved systematically gathering knowledge by reviewing all DMHAS programs, and selecting those programs, services, or strategies that increased quality of care, utilized resources better, and/or positively influenced service characteristics (Table 12.3).

The LL products not only served as a bridge to acknowledge "the shoulders we all stood on" as we continued our journey but also helped to set and refine the next steps. They affirmed past tools for change and led to new ones in the content, infrastructure, and other aspects of the evolving ROSC such as the need to increase the emphasis on housing and employment/education as part of a life in the community, to reinforce our linkages with the recovery community, and to emphasize the value of data analyses.

Expand the Resource Base Beyond State Funding

Aggressive pursuit of federal and other grants supported Connecticut's recovery vision and the contents of an ROSC. From 1997 through to 2008, over $154 million of new nonstate funding was awarded to DMHAS (*Expanding a Resource Base for CT's Behavioral Health-care System*, 10/6/05. Available at: http://www.ct.gov/dmhas/infobriefs). Grants provided flexible funding to test and refine new approaches and offered major research and development opportunities as tools for change. Findings were used to redefine our purchasing strategies in terms of content and/or financing mechanisms (Table 12.2).

Table 12.2 Sampling of Connecticut Federal and Foundation Grant Awards

Access to Recovery I and II	Women's jail diversion programs (gender and trauma responsive)
Co-occurring State Incentive Grant	Strategic Prevention Framework
Mental Health Transformation	Project Nueva Vida (culturally responsive)
RWJ Recovery Purchasing Project	Community Reentry Program
Recovery Community Support Program	Treatment Needs Assessment I and II
Treatment Outcomes/Performance Pilots	CT Community for Addiction Recovery
Hartford Engagement and Recovery Program (culturally and gender responsive)	Promoting adoption of evidence-based practices in addiction treatment

Table 12.3 Systems change and what works: six lessons learned

Emphasize and focus on community life and natural supports

Recognize that people in recovery have valuable and useful contributions to make at all levels and throughout all components of care

Use multiple forms of "evidence" to guide policy, not just evidence-based but also evidence-supported, informed or suggested

Use a combination of approaches to address cultural needs and to eliminate health disparities

Establish clear service expectations for providers and for monitoring

Use Practice Management Tools adapted from the private sector

Phase III: Increase Depth, Complexity, and Preparedness for Future Phase

Access to Recovery

The 2004 *Access to Recovery (ATR I)* grant, valued at $22.8 million over 3 years, had considerable impact and very promising system transformation value. It:

- Required that clients have choice for where they would receive services.
- Encouraged new services to support recovery at every input level.
- Led DMHAS to request proposals for "regional or local networks" of current providers and vendors not usually part of the service system, e.g., housing, transportation, child care, supermarkets and clothing stores for basic needs, and educational and employment agencies.
- Resulted in operational skill set development to meet new infrastructure needs, e.g., certification/credentialing processes and fraud-protection claim audits.

The progress made in Connecticut's ROSC transformation efforts during and after ATR I represent the most significant gains in implementation of the ROSC in the entire period to date (DMHAS. *ATR: A Good Return on Investment*, 7/26/07. Available at: www.ct.gov/dmhas/infobriefs). ATR I also offered the opportunity for DMHAS to build on strengths including:

- Adapting the Connecticut Client Placement Criteria based on the American Society of Addiction Medicine (ASAM) criteria, for tracking use of levels of care.
- Cultivating partnerships with care providers, the recovery community and other state agencies to facilitate ATR I start-up.
- Supporting an Administrative Service Organization, Advanced Behavioral Health (ABH), Inc. to apply criteria for service authorization and continued stay reviews, link authorizations with claims for quality analyses, and function effectively on a fee for service (FFS) payment basis for new levels of care and RSSs.
- Establishing a contract linkage since 1997 with a faith-based leader and hosting a Faith-Based Conference in 2004 to support training and the emergence of religious leaders for effective outreach and referral of persons into care.
- Implementing a pilot "Basic Needs Program (BNP)" in 1998 that provided a person-centered approach through recovery supports and personal care items to people in treatment. Subsequent analyses in 2007 *Getting Down to Basics* and 2008, *The General Assistance Recovery Supports Program* (both available at www.ct.gov/dmhas/infobriefs) demonstrated that the connect to care rate for those leaving inpatient status with BNP support was 68% vs. 38% for those without and, for persons transitioning from outpatient 50% vs. 40% without BNP support. Of added importance, the dropout rate from follow-up care after inpatient care for persons with BNP was 11% vs. 25% without the support.

One of the most significant benefits resulting from ATR I was improved capability for data and quality analysis. DMHAS had reasonably good data analysis staff, but only a fair data system that was compromised by less than desired accuracy or cleanliness, fragmentation, and limited linkage to the claims, thereby sharply curtailing quality and cost-containment studies. The Comprehensive Data Analysis section in (a) below documents the depth of findings resulting from the increased volume and new outcomes from better data. Also detailed below are selected categories of highlights of Connecticut's ATR I which led to national recognition.

ATR I Increased Access, First-Time Admissions, Diversity, and Points of Access – It served 18,000 individuals, over 40% being first-time admissions to the DMHAS system. The diversity was 41% African American, 40% Caucasian, and 17% Hispanic; 60% male and 40% female. The majority of individuals reached entered through the Judicial Branch probation and reentry units, the Departments of Correction, Children and Families and Social Services, and from the faith community.

Five regional networks of treatment and recovery support providers – comprised of 32 clinical substance abuse treatment and 86 recovery support providers established to provide a full continuum of clinical and RSSs.

Grant resources – predominately for new or current nonclinical RSSs (67%) including temporary housing (defined durations/amounts), peer-operated transportation services, faith- and peer-based mentoring/coaching, vocational and educational activities, basic needs (food, clothing, utilities, etc.), and recovery-oriented case management provided by trained peers or Recovery Guides/Coaches.

New or expanded capacity of clinical services – Introduced Brief Treatment and Cocaine/Methamphetamine Intensive Outpatient (IOP), and supported increased capacity for Ambulatory Detox, Methadone Maintenance, and IOP services.

Congregate sober housing or independent housing – Provided for 6,000 persons, through expansion of Recovery House sites and Alternative Living Centers and helped with security deposits.

Connecticut's ATR II $14.9 million award, covering September 2007–2010, concentrates on housing, transportation, employment, and peer- and faith-based support. It also supports new clinical services, e.g., Buprenorphine, clinical recovery check-ups, and specialized IOP care for persons with COD provided by agencies who have met credentialing standards for enhanced COD capability. An incentivized reimbursement rate (25% higher than for traditional IOP) rewarded improved quality and resulting cost-containment benefits.

It has become increasingly apparent that RSSs complement treatment, outreach, engagement, and other strategies used to assist people in establishing an environment supportive of recovery and in gaining skills and resources to initiate and maintain them in the "Recovery Zone." They help to remove personal and environmental obstacles (e.g., transportation or child care) and promote identification and participation in the recovery community. Further, they expand the individual's "recovery capital" [12] by assisting people with their basic needs, employment, education, and sober relationships. Are there also intangible benefits recipients talk about? Yes. An improved sense of hope for recovery, time spent in self-selected prosocial community-based activities, and interest in areas such as educational advancement and work searches are achieved.

It is important to emphasize that the collective federal discretionary funds awarded to Connecticut were a crucial part of its resource development strategy for designing, implementing, and improving our ROSC. Because the applications submitted by DMHAS reflected its clear vision and identified points of opportunity and linkages (criminal justice, child welfare, employment) that would help to advance a full ROSC.

Finance and Quality Models

Conduct comprehensive data analyses of innovative financing/quality enhancement models: Health-care financing is a tool within a health-care system that can stimulate enhancements with respect to access and quantity of care and create the ability to improve outcomes, while containing or reducing cost. The result is improved value, i.e., better bang for the buck. DMHAS, in accord with Lesson Learned 6 described above in Phase II, (Use "Practice Management Tools") increased its focus on experiences from the operations of its ASO since its inception in the late 1990s and pooled those with its ATR I lessons. DMHAS was now

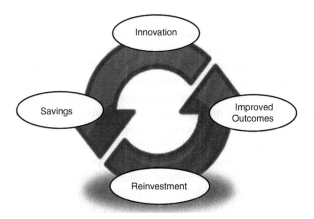

Fig. 12.7 Reinvestment System Enhancement Cycle

positioned to formalize an innovative model of financing/quality enhancement and assess the benefits based on large pools of accumulated data. The examples below demonstrate the efficacy of the approach, now labeled the *Reinvestment, System Enhancement Cycle Model* (Fig. 12.7).

This approach creates an environment in which recovery support and clinical service innovations are implemented resulting in cost savings. Some of these savings are reinvested in the system creating a continuous cycle of improvement, while others serve to demonstrate the impact of a ROSC in controlling the rate of growth of costs. Examples that follow demonstrate this approach from the DMHAS General Assistance Behavioral Health Program's (GABHP) Intensive Case Management (GA-ICM) initiative, the Opioid Agonist Treatment Protocol (OATP), and the total overall GABHP results.

Connecticut's GA Intensive Case Management (GA-ICM) program was designed to assist individuals with multiple acute care admissions within very short intervals. GA-ICM initiatives have been added and refined since its inception in 2001/2002. They include a focus on *High Service Utilizers* of inpatient or residential-based detox services and brief inpatient mental health care due to presenting at Emergency Departments with expressed suicidal threats (*Out of the Emergency Department and into Treatment*, 1/25/08. Available at: www.ct.gov/dmhas/infobriefs).

The OATP, introduced in April 2001, included interventions for those with a primary diagnosis of opioid dependence and who had four or more admissions into inpatient or residential detox within a 6-month period. The eligibility was expanded in May 2007 to include persons with three detox admissions in 90 days or two within 30 days. The final component, the *Acute Care Initiative*, took effect in April 2004 and expanded the criteria for GAICM to include those with three admissions to brief inpatient mental health care (5–7 days) within 90 days.

Originally, DMHAS created Behavioral Health Units (BHUs) placed at different provider locations whose staff operated the GA-ICM. This decentralized delivery methodology cost the state approximately $5 million per year. After a thorough quality analysis, a less costly, more effective approach was taken. By applying the Reinvestment, System Enhancement Cycle Model, DMHAS eliminated the BHUs and reinvested $2.5 million in a centralized version administered by the ASO. The ASO hired Recovery Specialists/Managers who were trained and well versed in performing in vivo case management with active client participation. By centralizing operations at the ASO, care management (clinical utilization management) could be directly integrated with case management. The remaining $2.5 million was used for targeted interventions designed to connect people to treatment and RSSs that help sustain recovery and develop a stable lifestyle, thus interrupting the futile cycle of their serial readmissions to acute care. Among the supports these resources purchased were Recovery Houses – a new form of residential recovery support (DMHAS. *Recovery House*, 7/1/04. Available at: www.ct.gov/dmhas/infobriefs.)

Findings for a recent (2008) large group of 2,185 GA-ICM clients vividly demonstrate the favorable care and fiscal benefits of the intervention. Comparisons of cost and types of services, used 12 months pre- and post-participation in the intensive case management (ICM) intervention, show that there was an *overall 62% decrease (2,441 vs. 6,365) in the use of acute service (inpatient and residential detox, brief inpatient mental health stays)* and a *78% increase (3,568 vs. 1,999) in the use of IOP, methadone maintenance, and standard outpatient services.* The corresponding *total treatment costs* were *14% lower* ($15.2 vs. $17.7 million) and, even after factoring in the GA-ICM case management operational and administrative costs, $725,699 was saved [13].

The OATP is another outstanding example of the Reinvestment, System Enhancement Cycle Model. OATP is a mix of motivational interviewing, access to opioid agonist treatment, education/information, service coordination, and culturally competent services (significant Hispanic cohort). It led to the average annual number of admissions per OATP person into detox dropping from 4.3 to 0.7. The cost of treating this group, as evident below in *Better Care, Resource Management*, declined from a high of $3.7 million in 2003 to less than $1 million in 2008. The decline in residential detoxification bed use by the OATP group also offered opportunity for increased access by others or for potential conversion of the beds to alternative purposes (Fig. 12.8) [14].

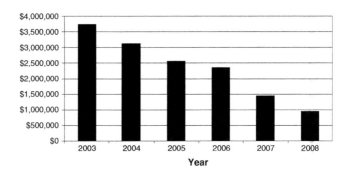

Fig. 12.8 Better Care, Resource Management Acute Care Claims Expenses for OATP Clients

Overall GABHP Results: Service fragmentation, disproportionate allocations in cost, and inefficiency are too often evident in state or public systems for treatment of substance use disorders. The following description of the overall operations of the recovery-oriented, innovative, and clinically effective DMHAS GABHP offers an alternative. The total effort creates greater value for every health-care dollar that is invested. A *46% increase* was achieved in the number of *people served* from 2003 to 2008 (15,324 vs. 22,428), with a *24% decrease* ($2,489 in 2003 v. $1,913 in 2008) in *average cost per person*. Outcomes have improved, dropout rates have decreased and recovery supports have been made available for more individuals. This was achieved through a variety of innovative strategies including ICM, creating enhanced access to care, increased housing and employment, medication-assisted therapy, and basic needs and recovery supports. It is projected that without these innovative strategies, GABHP costs, using a baseline of 2003, would have been $65.5 million more from 2004 through 2008 (DMHAS. *Quality Health care: A Good Investment*, 2/25/09. Available at: www.ct.gov/dmhas/infobriefs).

Connect the Dots

Connect the dots – QIC, practice guidelines, quality measures. Creating a ROSC and transforming an existing behavioral health system has not been a linear process. Rather, there have been multiple tracks such as defining Recovery and establishing the Recovery Policy and, at the same time, a host of work on the original four QIC (Gender, Culture, Trauma and CODs), with Health Disparities, Preferred Practices, Health Promotion and Wellness, and Employment/Education further along the way. While the DMHAS leadership position has been that the multiple tracks are related given that quality is the driver of a ROSC, all of these activities periodically led to concerns by staff about too many agendas and too much to do. Although there was appreciable buy-in and implementation of recovery activities, there is need to answer new questions, e.g., what are the quality indices?

To help connect the dots Dr. Larry Davidson and his staff from Yale's PRCH in concert with DMHAS staff created the first edition of *Practice Guidelines for Recovery-Oriented Care for Mental Health and Substance Use Conditions* in 2006 [15]. It identified and proposed eight domains of recovery-oriented care ranging from Promoting Access and Engagement to Identifying and Addressing Barriers to Recovery. The document clearly showed the utility of Practice Guidelines as a blueprint for change.

A second edition was released December 2008 that identified domains in a format that accomplished at least three aims: (1) It linked domains from the first edition to domains included in the Institute of Medicine Crossing the Quality Chasm Report (2001). Why the tie? The IOM measures are generally accepted as the "gold standard." Recovery-oriented measures, on the other hand, are new and do not have the instant credibility that to read IOM's have. Consistent with the DMHAS policy that it is a health-care organization wherein one should expect to get better from continuing care conditions such as substance use and/or mental illness, it would be an appropriate linkage to make. Six practice domains were identified in this new linkage. Recovery-oriented Care for mental health and substance use conditions is

Consumer and family driven	Timely and responsive
Effective, equitable and efficient	Person-centered
Maximizes use of natural supports and settings	Safe and trustworthy

Second, the new edition integrated guidelines and related products from the four initial QICs and was reviewed by the key DMHAS leader/manager in each area for congruence with the QIC emphases. Third, as a "how-to" document, it includes domain self-assessment checklists, examples of strength-based conceptualizations and source documents from DMHAS initiatives. In so doing it lends itself to offering performance and outcome measures at the system/agency and practitioner/person in recovery levels. Its format offers extraordinary potential as a tool for change due to its "how to" format [16].

When designing and implementing an ROSC, one should consider traditional as well as new performance and outcome measures that are important from the perspectives of persons in recovery, clinical managers, and system funders. *Persons in recovery* want a respectful, welcoming, accessible setting, staffed by highly qualified persons who listen to, and work with the person; offer hope and an expectation that s(he) can get "better," and has tools that can be used to manage their own recovery and be renewed rather than having to repeatedly come in and out of the system. *System clinical managers* focus on access, retention, and dropout indices; percent of first-time admissions out of the total population of persons served; qualitative ratings on identified indicators; rates of dropout, readmission, and connect to lower levels of care. *System funders* want satisfied customers and good "brand recognition," to know the degree of maximization of the existing system, overall rate of growth of costs, percent of persons in the different levels of care and the costs associated with each, costs pre- and posttreatment and RSS interventions, actual adjusted fee-for-service rate after factoring in repeated admissions within 30, 60, or 90 day intervals into the higher cost levels of care, and cost indices of any new definitions of bundled services and rate in a "continuing care, long-term recovery management service system." Many of the above have been referenced with examples at earlier points in this chapter. Others are in the developmental pilot stage.

Organizational Structure and Business Plan

Align organizational structure and health-care "Business Plan" communication strategy, identify new cornerstones, integrate operations and strategic planning. The DMHAS vision was modified in early 2008 after review of accomplishments since 2000 and other considerations. The new vision – *Healthy People, Healthy Communities. Let's Make It Happen!* – is intended to convey the pursuit of an even more expansive environment of recovery, the fullest level of economic, educational, physical health, social inclusion, and community integration.

As the benefits and positive "brand recognition" of the continually evolving ROSC were more known and touted within Connecticut, it seemed wise to employ the concept of a "Health-care Business Plan" to communicate the needs and qualities of the system in submissions to the Governor's Budget Office. The template for budget submissions in late 2008 was titled "Health-care Business Plan for Systematic Budget Cost Containment and Service Innovations." The schematic reflected continually increasing state agency collaborations and thus increased populations for DMHAS vs. the traditional and limited DMHAS core population. Four levels of action strategies, labeled *Innovative, Quality Improvement, Cost-Containment Strategies; Growth Control, Containing Cost Strategies; Management Infrastructure Strategies;* and *Revenue Enhancement and Discretionary Grant Strategies* were noted. The overall effect was to emphasize care-, cost-, and revenue-*enhancement* approaches developed in creating an ROSC, while also noting organizational management and staffing *reductions* and traditional "downsizing" approaches. The business plan keyed in on varied actions to be accelerated and new ones to be introduced in the midst of the "economic tsunami" that hit in the last part of calendar 2008. The plan recognized that, as a state agency, reductions had to be made but that DMHAS knew how to do so better than the usual "batten down the hatches" approach. On the whole, the budgets proposed by the Governor and later integrated with that from the Legislature were not bad. As the crisis has continued, the final bottom line has yet to be set. However, the ROSC approach remains embedded.

The new fiscal times required a leaner organizational structure and a faster, action-oriented decision making process. A senior-level Commissioner's Strategic Analysis and Implementation Group (CSAIG) was established in 2008 to capitalize on the extraordinary talents of senior DMHAS leadership and staff by meshing their operational and strategic planning skills. An anticipated outcome of this group is a new strategic action plan to prepare for DMHAS' future phases.

Other organizational units evolved or were reinforced. A very key one is a small *Health-care Finance Group,* which tests potential new finance models such as partial conversion of grants to fee-for-service, rates for bundles of recovery support, and/or clinical services and funding tied to "episodes of care/recovery." Also created was a redefined *Evaluation and Quality Management Information Unit* that focuses on better data quality, analyses of quality improvement initiatives and the annual CSS, and helping with two new information systems coming online in 2009 and 2010.

The importance of identifying a new set of cornerstones that support DMHAS is heightened and timely now just as were the cornerstones set in 2003 with the previous fiscal crisis. They help to renew the spirit of staff and anchor strategies to the strengths of organization. The proposed new *DMHAS Cornerstones* are: *Professional, Knowledgeable Workforce; Service Infrastructure; Informed, Involved Respected Service Users; and Community Health Focus.*

Closing Note: Based on the Connecticut experience, it is suggested that rather than speaking about discrete evidence-based services, it is better to think in terms of an ROSC that is comprised of components for a continued care, long-term *Recovery Management System*. Ten key components of such a system are as follows:

- Expanded care continuum
- Person and family centered
- Data-driven decision making
- Finance reinvestment strategies
- Local/regional service collaboratives
- Dynamic service/innovation approaches
- Strong recovery community relationships
- Strong multifaceted communication strategy
- Best practices tied to "episode of care" model
- Many recovery support and peer-directed services

Key Points:

- Set a clear vision – *"Healthy People, Healthy Communities...Let's Make It Happen!"* – tweak it occasionally and only to raise the bar. Link it to a two-minute "stump speech" that can be adjusted to different audiences.
- Transformation toward recovery-orientation for large health-care systems must be quality-driven, requires changes at the system, program, and practitioner levels as well as redefinition and innovation in the service content, delivery/infrastructures, finance mechanisms and outcomes. Combinations of the latter, described as the Reinvestment, System Enhancement Cycle Model, are highly effective in maximizing resource allocations to reach more clients and more effectively.
- Broaden "the choir" as much as possible, address your critics. Successful initiatives have many fathers and mothers. Failed initiatives are orphans.
- Recognize and build on lessons learned from your predecessors, add your own, and build on both. We all stand on the shoulders of those who came before us.
- Reduce actions to incremental steps with observable products lest the movement is seen as too risky and complicated. Celebrate small accomplishments and people along the way.
- Form collaborative partnerships to demonstrate that substance use and mental health issues, though not *"the agenda,"* are part of many agendas.
- Develop positive "brand recognition" for products and services and create a "health-care business plan" to emphasize control over the rate of growth of cost, especially in tough fiscal times.
- Refine the system along the way as lessons are learned and research and practical experiences bring new knowledge.
- Expect periodic plateaus and get used to redesigning the plane while in mid-flight, helping stakeholders to stay calm and confident.

Acknowledgment This chapter reflects the work of many people who believed in the vision of a recovery-oriented system of care in the late 1990's and whose skill, creativity and passion helped to bring it to fruition thereafter. Especially noteworthy to the author are the late Jerry Croog, Paul DiLeo, Arthur Evans, Sue Tanner, Sabrina Trocchi, Doreen DelBianco and Irene Williams as well as David Crompton, Wayne Dailey, Steve Fry, Barbara Geller, Julienne Giard, Tom Gugliotti, Dianne Harnad, Karen Kangas, Ken Marcus, Pat Rehmer, Peter Rockholz, Yvette Sangster, Bob Savage, Phil Valentine, and Larry Davidson and his colleagues at the Yale Program for Recovery and Community Health. Many other staff in DMHAS and its private affiliate agencies also paved the way. To all of them a hearty Thank You! Their legacy is improved lives for thousands who learned that recovery is possible and to be expected, and who had the courage to begin the journey into recovery. I will forever be in awe of them and thankful for what they taught me over the last 15 years.

References

1. Connecticut Department of Mental Health and Addiction Services (DMHAS). Partnership for healthy communities: the DMHAS strategic action plan. Hartford, CT: DMHAS; 2000.
2. State of Connecticut Office of the Governor. The Governor's Blue Ribbon Task Force on Substance Abuse. Hartford, CT: State of Connecticut; 1996.
3. Kirk TA, Croog G. The reality of substance abuse in Connecticut. An overview. What will be our response? First meeting of Connecticut Alcohol and Drug Policy Council. September 11, 1996. Hartford, CT.
4. State of Connecticut Office of the Governor. The Governor's Blue Ribbon Commission on Mental Health. Hartford, CT: State of Connecticut; 2000.
5. Kirk TA. Quality – the driving force in creating a recovery-oriented system of services. Center for Substance Abuse Treatment. East Coast Regional Conference. August 20, 2003. Nashville, TN.
6. Najavits L, Weiss R, Shaw S, Muenz L. Seeking safety: outcome of a new cognitive-behavioral psychotherapy for women with post-traumatic stress disorder and substance dependence. J Trauma Stress. 1998;66:61–70.
7. Kirk TA. A new systems framework for approaching the problem of co-occurring disorders. Annual meeting of National Association of State Alcohol and Drug Abuse Directors. June 9, 1999. St. Pete Beach, FL
8. Sachs S. Co-occurring mental health and substance use disorders: promising approaches and research issues. Subst Use Misuse. 2000;35(2–14):2061–93.
9. O'Connell M, Tondora J, Evans AC, Croog G, Davidson L. From rhetoric to routine: assessing recovery-oriented practices in a state mental health and addiction system. Psychiatr Rehabil J. 2005;28(4):378–86.
10. Institute of Medicine. Crossing the quality chasm: a new health system for the 21st century. Washington, DC: National Academies Press; 2001.
11. Kirk TA, Evans AC, Dailey W. The Connecticut lessons learned initiative: How one state found evidence in its own background. NASMHPD Research Institute Annual Conference on State Mental Health Agency Services Research, Program Evaluation and Policy. February 9, 2004. Arlington, VA.
12. Granfield R, Cloud W. Coming clean: overcoming addiction without treatment. New York: New York University Press; 1999.
13. DiLeo PJ. Facilitating addiction recovery using healthcare financing and program innovation. Federal Center for Substance Abuse Treatment. July 18, 2008. Rockville, MD. Webcast
14. Kirk TA. Continuing care, long term recovery management service SYSTEM? What will the evidence look like? National Institute on Drug Abuse Blending Conference. June 2, 2008. Cincinnati, OH.

15. Connecticut Department of Mental Health and Addiction Services (DMHAS). Practice guidelines for recovery-oriented care for mental health and substance use conditions. Hartford, CT: DMHAS; 2006.
16. Connecticut Department of Mental Health and Addiction Services (DMHAS). Practice Guidelines for recovery-oriented care for mental health and substance use conditions:2008 (Prepared by the Yale University Program for Recovery and Community Health.

Chapter 13
Implementing Recovery Management in a Treatment Organization

Michael Boyle, David Loveland, and Susan George

Abstract This chapter will provide an overview of how a large behavioral health provider has implemented the principles of recovery management for treating individuals with a substance use disorder over the past 10 years. The story begins with the launching of the Behavioral Health Recovery Management (BHRM) project in 1999 and the subsequent funding of the grant project from the Illinois Division of Alcohol and Substance Abuse. We will briefly review the differences between recovery management and the broader disease management model. The BHRM project was the catalyst and incubator for implementing many of the principles outlined in this book. We will review the trials launched, successes achieved, barriers encountered, mistakes made, and lessons learned while incorporating the principles of recovery management within the existing, publicly funded addiction and mental health treatment system in Illinois. We will highlight the challenges involved in translating recovery principles into the existing medical or professional model of treatment. In particular, we will discuss the philosophical challenges involved in altering the views and values of staff, limitations with the Federal and State funding streams, and structural barriers associated with publicly funded organizations. The chapter will close with a discussion of how to translate the lessons learned to other organizations, future applications of the BHRM principles in an emerging concept of integrative care, and expanding the model to include emerging technologies.

Keywords Addiction recovery management · Principles of recovery management · Behavioral health recovery management · Acute care model · Evidence-based treatment

M. Boyle (✉)
Fayette Companies, 600 Fayette Street, Peoria, IL 61603, USA
e-mail: mboyle@fayettecompanies.org

J.F. Kelly and W.L. White (eds.), *Addiction Recovery Management: Theory, Research and Practice*, Current Clinical Psychiatry, DOI 10.1007/978-1-60327-960-4_13,
© Springer Science+Business Media, LLC 2011

Introduction

The goal of this chapter is to provide the reader with an overview of one organization's ongoing process of implementing the principles of recovery management. The chapter begins with an overview of the Behavioral Health Recovery Management (BHRM) project and how it was used as a platform to implement the principles of recovery management at Fayette Companies. We review the successes and barriers encountered in the process of moving toward this model of care within a large, urban, not-for-profit behavioral health organization. The chapter also includes an example of the implementation process using recovery coach services, which were a product of the BHRM project. The chapter concludes with a discussion of lessons learned and future directions of the recovery management model in the not-for-profit behavioral health-care field.

BHRM Project

The first author, Michael Boyle with assistance from a local state representative, wrote legislation in the spring of 1999 mandating our organization to develop a disease management approach to serious mental illness and addiction. The legislation passed the Illinois House and Senate and was signed into law by the Governor. During this process, the Secretary of the Illinois Department of Human Services stated that he had become intrigued with the concept and pledged $1,000,000 over a 3-year period to support development of the project.

M.B. became the Project Director and recruited Bill White [1] from Chestnut Health Systems to be Associate Director for addictions and David Loveland, the second author of this chapter, to be Associate Director for mental health. Pat Corrigan [2–4], Director of the Center for Psychiatric Rehabilitation at the University of Chicago subsequently joined the project.

The project began with a mission to resolve the paradox between the theoretical formulation of serious mental illness and addiction, which views these diseases as chronic conditions, similar to diabetes or hypertension, and the applied behavioral health treatment system, which treats these diseases with an acute care model [5]. Addiction, for example, is described as a chronic, relapsing disease; however, most addiction treatment interventions are delivered in acute, discrete episodes of care [6, 7].

Researchers in the medical field developed a chronic disease model to address conditions, such as diabetes or hypertension, for which there is no cure, but can be treated and managed over an individual's lifespan [8]. The model is often referred to as *disease management* because of its focus on helping individuals learn how to manage their chronic medical conditions over time through the integration of effective medical care, ongoing support, and self efficacy.

The chronic care model, as articulated by Wagner et al. [9], served as the framework for developing a behavioral health treatment model for chronic conditions of mental illness or addiction. Bill White proposed the term "recovery management" rather than disease management for the BHRM project to emphasize the realistic possibility of recovery from either addiction or serious mental illness (or both). This model of care included consumers as partners in the process and utilized community resources while focusing on a long-term orientation to recovery. When initially challenged that disease management was a known treatment process while no one has heard of recovery management, Bill replied "they will in 3 years." With this inspiration, the BHRM project was launched.

The BHRM team outlined an action plan for the project along with the initial principles of recovery management. An agreement was reached on an overarching purpose: to change the world of addiction and mental health treatment. One of the significant differences between disease management and recovery management was the inclusion of the community as a significant resource for recovery support. Charles Rapp [10], in his work on a strength-based approach for the treatment of serious mental illnesses, characterized the community as "an oasis of resources" that could be used to help individuals achieve their goals in life. This view of the community was adopted as a major BHRM principle.

The first task of the project was to outline the essential principles of recovery management. We established 11 guiding principles of recovery management over the course of 4 years. These principles include the following:

1. Maintaining a recovery focus
2. Promoting consumer empowerment and self-management
3. Supporting the de-stigmatization of experience
4. Adopting evidence-based practices
5. Developing and applying clinical algorithms
6. Utilizing emerging technologies
7. Integrating addiction, mental health, and primary health-care services
8. Establishing recovery partnerships
9. Incorporating the ecology of recovery
10. Providing ongoing monitoring and support
11. Promoting the continual evaluation of the model

A description of these principles can be accessed on the project web site at http://www.bhrm.org.

The next task was the dissemination of the recovery management principles and concepts through peer-reviewed journals and trade journals [5, 11–15]. The third task was promoting the application of evidence-based treatment approaches, which is a key component of the disease management model. A notable problem in the dissemination of evidence-based behavioral health practices is the significant lag in time between the development of effective practices within research settings and the eventual application of these interventions in applied settings [16]. This lag in time can exceed 17 years, on average, from development to application [17]. In contrast, new medications and medical technologies are rapidly adopted in both primary and specialty medical treatments. One explanation is that private corporations with a profit motive develop most medications and technologies in medical care. Significant resources are spent in marketing and sales staff to convince practitioners to use new medications and medical instruments. In contrast, research in behavioral health lacks "detailers" who go into clinical settings to promote and train on new clinical technologies.

The BHRM project identified and contracted with researchers and clinicians to write guidelines that were posted on the project's web site. The authors were asked to write materials that could be utilized by clinical staff and supervisors, including

- A brief review of the research establishing the effectiveness of the practice.
- An overview of how the components and how the approach is utilized.
- A section that identifies manuals, books, videos, CDs, and other resources that can be used to learn and implement the practice.

Implementing BHRM Principles at Fayette Companies

Fayette became the beta site for piloting the BHRM principles. Using Fayette as a pilot site was a natural choice considering that the primary architect of the BHRM, M.B., was and still is the president of the organization and could provide internal leadership. Moreover, the organization had already launched several initiatives around the same time period that reflected and informed the BHRM principles. These overlapping initiatives included

- The integration of mental health and addiction treatment services for those with co-occurring conditions
- Integrating behavioral health and primary care services for all clients
- Training staff on evidence-based practices, such as Motivational Interviewing and the Community Reinforcement Approach.

Despite the advantages of piloting recovery management principles at Fayette, the BHRM team encountered multiple barriers in the process of implementing evidenced-based practices. The first challenge was to create an infrastructure to support evidence-based practices. Initially, we assumed that the first step in the implementation process was to train staff on evidence-based practices. Most counselors at HSC, including those with advanced degrees, had received minimal or no training on evidence-based practices. It became clear, however, that Fayette lacked the capacity to support these interventions. For example, the organization had sponsored multiple trainings by national experts on various evidence-based practices to a large portion of clinicians at HSC. Nonetheless, it became apparent that providing training was insufficient without follow-up. Notable barriers identified, included

- Supervisors would support some but not all aspects of an evidence-based practice (i.e., poor fidelity to the model).

- Staff would continue to use outdated modes of service delivery, such as confrontational techniques, along with aspects of motivational interviewing or strength-based case management.
- Counselors received minimal structured supervision. Most counselors received hallway supervision (i.e., random communications based on crisis rather than proactive training) or weekly meetings that focused on process issues (e.g., reviewing cases for billing or paperwork, but not for outcomes) rather than improving the skills of the clinicians.

These barriers highlighted the differences between academic settings and not-for-profit behavioral health operations in the implementation of EBPs. We were able to translate the technologies associated with the EBPs, but not the oversight, feedback and ongoing supervision that support the development of these interventions within academic environments. In other words, EBPs don't exist in a vacuum; they require an environment that supports and nurtures data collection, fidelity, quality improvement procedures, and an outcome-based vision of treatment. While some researchers have noted that community-based organizations lack the resources to conduct the quality training and supervision utilized in research [18], it became apparent that this was exactly what was needed to change clinical behaviors.

We shifted resources from expensive trainings to developing an organizational structure to support EBPs based on the results of the initial round of training. Fayette Companies created the position of Vice President of Clinical Services to oversee the development of an organizational infrastructure and subsequent guidelines for implementing and sustaining EBPs. The third author of this chapter, Susan George (S.G.), was hired into the position in 2006.

S.G. initiated a supervision-training protocol that was adopted across the agency. The process involved multiple steps, including

- Establishing a monthly meeting for all supervisors and program directors (this included over 30 employees) to develop action plans, providing training, and disseminate practices.
- Establishing requirements for training for all supervisors that would be subsequently applied to all counselors.
- Initiating the training with a basic skill set for all supervisors and counselors, i.e., active listening, as well as identifying ineffective techniques that can undermine active listening, such as arguing, confronting, or dictating treatment solutions without understanding the client's stage of change or personal goals.
- Developing competency standards for supervisors, followed by counselors, which included an internal certification program.
- Requiring all supervisors to audiotape individual sessions with clients and submitting the tapes to S.G. for review and feedback.
- Training supervisors to audiotape counselors to evaluate their performance and to provide constructive, informative feedback (as well as learning how to rate the fidelity of the counselor's performance).

Changing Organizational and Administrative Structures

Each staff-level change required a parallel change at the administrative-level of the organization. For example, the administration had to commit time and resources to modifying the supervision structure. Moreover, many changes were required within the electronic medical records to support the changes in clinical approaches. The process was and still is time consuming; therefore, administrators had to adopt a long-term view that required dedication and vigilance against drifting away from the process of change.

Integrating Treatment for Addiction, Mental Health, and Physical Conditions

An important principle of the recovery management model is using a holistic view of individuals. The concept implies that we treat individuals not diseases or diagnostic categories. The principle is intuitive, but again, creates a challenge in the behavioral health field that was structured to treat specific, nonoverlapping diseases. Individuals who need behavioral health services are more likely to have co-occurring conditions, particularly medical complications related to extensive alcohol or drug use or neglect as a result of an ongoing SMI [19–25]. As an example, 25% of women entering our residential programs test positive for Hepatitis C. Yet, only four out of ten women who test positive are aware that they have the virus.

The Comprehensive, Continuous, Integrated Systems of Care approach developed by Minkoff [26] was chosen as a guideline to integrate behavioral health services for individuals with both mental illness and substance use disorders. A multidisciplinary quality improvement committee of addiction and mental health professionals was organized to oversee planning and implementing changes in policies and procedures at the program level. In addition, clinical staff were trained to address both conditions. Some of the changes included

- Implementing a single access point for all services using an integrated assessment for substance abuse, mental health disorders, and physical health disorders.
- Developing a policy that an individual receiving services anywhere in the organization had priority for all services provided.
- Providing easy access to psychiatric assessments and medications for persons receiving addiction treatment.
- Assisting all clients in completing medication scholarships for those who don't have access to insurance or resources to purchase medications.
- Requiring mental health counselors to participate in ongoing treatment planning sessions with their clients while they are enrolled in a residential addiction treatment program.

- Providing specialized groups for persons with co-occurring conditions at the mental health outpatient facility with effective addiction treatment interventions.

Counselors are also required to connect all clients with a medical care provider. Most clients are referred to the local Federally Qualified Health Center (FQHC). FQHCs receive enhanced Medicaid and Medicare rates for persons without insurance, which allows these centers to serve our primary population. The FQHC in Peoria also assumed operations of a primary care clinic within the Fayette mental health facility. The satellite clinic allows integration of primary care and psychiatry and utilizes a shared medical record. The clinic provides medical services to many of our clients who have co-occurring conditions. In the Winter of 2009, Fayette and the FQHC will open a crisis center to divert persons with behavioral health problems from unnecessary use of hospital emergency departments or arrest as a result of a police encounter (for nonviolent offenses that could be diverted from arrest or booking).

We also developed a set of guidelines for establishing a relationship with an existing or new primary care provider [27]. The guidelines include sample referral forms and letters for physicians that can be used integrate medical care and ongoing recovery management from an addiction (or mental illness). Primary care providers can play a supportive role in implementing the BHRM principle of ongoing monitoring and support.

Addressing Culture

Another challenge was addressing the institutional norms that existed within all programs across the agency, such as the beliefs and values of counselors which had been passed down from generation to generation of behavioral health-care providers. This process can be compared to societies where the elders pass down stories and wisdom to the youth of the tribe around the campfires. These beliefs and values exist, even if they are not documented.

We introduced a series of "fire starter" meetings with staff to see if we could uncover some of these latent values that could undermine the recovery management model. Staff members from different service areas were brought together to discuss a list of statements that were meant to evoke passion and start fires in the discussions. Examples included are as follows:

- "Medications can be an effective strategy in the treatment of both substance use and mental health disorders"
- "It is more important to convey caring and concern than to avoid being manipulated or conned – even at the cost of "enabling" "
- "All persons should be retained in service and treated with great respect in spite of nonadherence with treatment plan recommendations, including not taking prescribed psychiatric medications or a return to use of the drug of choice."

Discussion among staff in these facilitated groups assisted people in examining their beliefs by hearing opposing views and real-life stories. For example, a person who believed an individual could not be in recovery if taking methadone was able to hear from a staff member working in a methadone program about clients who, for years, are employed, supporting a family, and not using illegal drugs. The need to address staff beliefs and values is a continual challenge.

During implementation of BHRM, the organization has needed to address the following cultural and philosophical issues (Table 13.1).

Reimbursement and Regulatory Challenges

Another significant issue to consider when implementing principles of recovery management is the identification of viable funding sources. There are many regulatory and financing challenges to implementing BHRM that vary significantly from State to State. Further, most of these funding mechanisms for behavioral health are based on an acute care model and office-based services. For example,

Table 13.1 Contrasting professional-driven and recovery management practices

Practice	Professional-driven model of care vs. recovery management model of care	
Path to recovery ➡	One path to recovery, as designed by the professional staff, for all persons	Multiple paths to recovery and all can be valued based on the needs and motivation of individuals
Clinical practice ➡	Clinical approaches based on firmly held folklore, eclectic mix, or personal experiences	The application of evidence-based treatments based on manual-driven protocols and measures of fidelity
Dealing with relapse ➡	Zero tolerance for any alcohol or drug use are mandatory	Harm reduction approach and the use of multiple, stepped interventions to keep individuals engaged
Treatment philosophy ➡	Use of the professional expert or paternalistic approach	A collaborative and strengths-based model
Treatment plans ➡	Development of staff-driven treatment plans	Working with persons to develop their personally owned recovery plans
Focus of treatment ➡	Utilization of an office-based "they come to us" treatments	Working with persons in the community and working with the community to support recovery
Family involvement ➡	Isolating individuals in residential treatment to focus on his or her addiction, minimal family involvement	Emphasize ongoing connections with the community and involvement of family and friends as a crucial treatment component

- Treatment reimbursement may be restricted to services that occur after an individual has been classified as eligible (i.e., meets target population) following a full assessment process. Services needed to engage individuals in the community may not be reimbursed under an office-based model that assumes that all individuals who need services are capable and ready to enter the program.
- Posttreatment monitoring and support services may not be reimbursed by a State's funding mechanism, particularly for clients who have completed a formal phase of treatment.

A couple options may be used to address these administrative issues. First, providers can collaborate with state agencies to make changes to licensing, certification, and funding rules to facilitate change in delivery systems that may enhance effectiveness. The Substance Abuse and Mental Health Services Administration's Strengthening Treatment Access and Recovery – State Initiative (STAR_SI) and the Robert Wood Johnson Foundation's Advancing Recovery provided funding to states to implement provider–state partnerships. For example, Fayette and the Illinois Division of Alcohol and Substance Abuse worked together through a STAR-SI collaborative to identify funding options for preenrollment services to help engage individuals in treatment.

The second option is for a provider to request an exemption to current rules from their state authorities. Fayette initially used this approach by requesting exemptions to allow billing of recovery support services for 9 months following active treatment without requiring periodic treatment plans updates and to allow use of a personal recovery plan rather than a professionally developed discharge plan. This exception significantly facilitated the development and implementation of recovery coaching (reviewed next).

The Recovery Coach Model

All the changes that occurred within our organization that have been reviewed in this chapter set the stage for implementing recovery management interventions. The recovery coach program is one of our longest standing innovations resulting from these changes and provides an example of how we translated the theory of recovery management to a real-world application. The recovery coach model is based on the BHRM principles (noted in this chapter and Bill White's review of recovery management [1]) and the concept of recovery capital [28]. The model is implemented through a community-based case management program developed in addiction treatment research. All three concepts are reviewed next.

Recovery Capital

Research with general samples of substance users has shown that as many as 50% of all individuals who have achieved full or partial recovery from their SUD, did so without the help of a professional-based intervention [29–33]. Individuals who require professional interventions to overcome their SUD:

- Experience more alcohol and drug related problems
- Have a more intensive pattern of drug or alcohol use
- Have limited or no social support
- Are in lower paying jobs or unemployed
- Have higher rates of mental illness
- Their SUD had an earlier onset than those who are able to achieve recovery without a formal intervention [28, 31, 32, 34]
- Cloud and Granfield [35] used the term "recovery capital" to refer to resources that support peoples' recovery from an SUD. The authors found that people who achieved recovery without treatment had substantial recovery capital, such as a strong social support network of sober friends and family members, well-paying jobs, education, and a range of coping skills [28, 35]. The authors postulated that people who require formal addiction treatment services have less recovery capital and that the goal of treatment should be to increase these recovery-supporting assets.

We used the recovery capital concept as well as White's [36] elements of recovery management as a framework for constructing an intervention for those who are less likely to achieve recovery on their own. Specifically, we postulated that

- Capacity for recovery from a substance use disorder exists on a continuum of skills.
- The goal of addiction treatment is to teach individuals how to achieve their own recovery.
- Full recovery is not essential at completion of treatment as long as individuals leave with the capacity to eventually achieve recovery without additional treatment interventions.
- All individuals are capable of achieving sufficient recovery capital if given the skills or access to the resources.
- Addiction treatment is one of multiple resources used to help individuals achieve a sustainable recovery from alcohol and other drugs.

Research on Case Management

A community-based case management model was selected as the vehicle for delivering recovery coach services. Case management interventions have received extensive attention in addiction treatment research [37]. Individuals assigned to a case management condition (with or without standard addiction treatment services) were more likely to engage and remain in treatment, report lower rates of drug and alcohol use, be linked to needed ancillary services, and report better outcomes in other problem areas, such as employment, housing, and involvement in the criminal justice system compared to individuals who received only standard addiction treatment services [38, 39, 40, 41, 42, 43].

The research of Siegal and colleagues [44, 42, 45] was particularly informative of the potential for case management in addiction treatment. The researchers combined case management services with a standard continuum of addiction treatment services for veterans with a SUD. Individuals who received the enhanced condition, which included a strengths-based case management component, stayed in treatment longer, and had lower reported drug and alcohol use [41]; had better outcomes on multiple indicators of criminality [45]; and, for those who wanted to work, had better employment outcomes compared to a randomized group of individuals who received the same addiction treatment services without the case management component [44]. The authors also found that approximately a third of the individuals assigned to the enhanced treatment condition dropped out of the addiction treatment services, but stayed engaged with the case management component [42]. This subgroup within the enhanced condition had similar outcomes to those individuals that remained engaged in treatment. Siegal et al.'s research as well as others highlighted the potential of using a community-based model that could simultaneously augment treatment or function as the primary intervention for individuals with a SUD. Case management is useful because:

- It provides a direct link to the community.
- Can be used to engage individuals entering any point of the addiction treatment continuum, such as at detoxification or at assessment for services [32].
- Can be coordinated with office- or residential-based programs.
- Case managers can use a harms-reduction approach to relapse, even when the office-based or residential programs may not [38].
- Case management services are fairly low cost compared to office-based program.
- Effective case management models:
- Are community based (office-based models are less effective; [46, 47]).
- Maintain small caseloads of below 25 individuals [48, 37].
- Train case managers in evidence-based techniques, including motivational interviewing and behavioral-skills training [38, 49, 48].

Recovery Coach Program at Fayette

Translating both White's [36] and Cloud and Granfield's [35] concepts into a model of case management, the goal of treatment is to improve peoples' resources and tools so that they can sustain their recovery after the formal treatment program has been completed [50]. An essential function of a case manager in the addiction treatment field, therefore, is to help people build their recovery capital.

The recovery coach model was constructed as a pilot test of the BHRM principles [51] and based on the established protocols for case management in addiction treatment. The integration of these elements included

- A community-based case management program that coordinated services with the continuum of addiction treatment services offered at Fayette, including detoxification, residential treatment, intensive outpatient, outpatient, and medication-assisted programs.
- Case managers who were also in recovery from a SUD, i.e., peers who were trained as case managers.
- A strength-based model of service delivery.
- A continuum of care based on the treatment needs and goals of consumers.

The recovery coach program was initiated in Fall 2004 with two female recovery coaches serving women leaving residential treatment (we made the assumption that recovery coaches would be more effective if they were matched on gender).

A training manual was developed that outlined the principles of the recovery coach model as well as the skills needed to be a recovery coach [52]. The training protocol included effective practices of case managers and evidence-based practices in addiction treatment. Specifically, we adapted training protocols from Motivational Interviewing [53], the Community Reinforcement Approach (CRA; [54]), and the assertive continuing care model for adolescents [55].

The second author (D.L.) provided most of the training and supervision of recovery coaches. The training protocol included weekly supervision and individual training sessions with consumers. An interactive training format was used and involved working with recovery coaches and consumers in the learning sessions.

The recovery coaches were initially assigned to a supervisor within the existing addiction treatment programs at HSC, while receiving weekly clinical training from D.L. This split management model proved to be ineffective, particularly when it became clear that the recovery coaches were receiving conflicting messages on how to work with clients. The approach was modified to have D.L. train and supervise the recovery coaches. This modification in training and supervision reduced the risk of recovery coaches drifting toward the institutional, office-based treatment model within these programs. Further, we implemented a clinical team structure similar to the one developed by Bond and colleagues [56, 57] for their supported employment program. Bond and colleagues [56] designed a community-based model that promoted fidelity of supported employment though a cohesive team unit, while simultaneously promoting continuity by assigning employment specialists to work with specific mental health teams. Employment specialists work and train as a team under one supervisor but also meet weekly with mental health teams to receive referrals and integrate treatment planning.

Recovery coaches are trained and supervised as a team but are also assigned to specific programs at Fayette. Coaches meet weekly with counselors to receive referrals or coordinate services with clients. All clients who live or plan to reside in the Tri-County area of Peoria are eligible for recovery coach services.

Counselors refer clients who show an interest in receiving recovery coach services. Specific elements of the program include

- *Voluntary services*: Recovery coach services are always voluntary and based on the clients' willingness to meet with coaches, regardless of their needs, involvement in the criminal justice system, or recommendations of counselors.
- *Time-unlimited service*: Recovery coach services are time-unlimited, although most clients require <3 months of recovery coach services.
- *Community based*: Recovery coach services are provided in the community, but coaches will meet with clients on site at a residential facility to establish an engaging relationship, develop an initial personal recovery plan or provide support.
- *Open-ended policy*: Clients have the option of working with recovery coaches after they complete or if they withdraw from treatment.
- *Harms-reduction approach*: Recovery coaches continue working with clients who have relapsed or returned to active use of alcohol or other drugs. One goal of recovery coaching is to encourage individuals to stay engaged in treatment or consider returning to treatment after a relapse, if needed. A recovery coach can also assist a person in working through a brief relapse without returning to treatment.
- *The Vegas Rule (confidentiality of information)*: What is said with recovery coaches remains with recovery coaches, regardless of the clients' involvement in treatment or the criminal justice system. Recovery coaches encourage clients to maintain open communication with their counselors or probation officers about their addiction but won't share information without the clients' approval, including relapse.

Research on the Recovery Coach Model

As of June 30, 2009, 503 women (398) and men (105) have been enrolled in the recovery coach program. Table 13.2 provides a summary of the individuals who have been engaged in the program. Individuals are considered enrolled if they received at least three contacts from a recovery coach (a combination of phone and face-to-face contacts). Approximately 30% of men and women who are referred to a recovery coach decline the service or cannot be reached after the referral has been made. More men and women accept referrals in the residential programs, whereas nearly half decline the offer in the outpatient programs or cannot be reached. Individuals with more need are also more likely to accept a referral.

Table 13.2 provides information comparing treatment continuation of 84 women who received RC services compared to 84 women who completed the same residential program during the same time period but did not receive RC services (Discharged between July 30, 2005 and February 24, 2009). Women in the matched group were

Table 13.2 Demographics of RC clients

	Total	Female	Male
Number opened	503	398	105
Ethnicity			
Minority (95% African American) (%)	32	26	53
White (%)	68	74	47
Legal involvement (%)	53	50	66
Martial status			
Single (%)	58	58	60
Married (%)	13	13	12
Divorced/separated (%)	24	26	17
Widowed (%)	2	3	0
Unknown (%)	3	1	10
Child welfare involvement (women only)	23	23	n/a
Has a co-occurring mental illness			
Yes (%)	42	50	11
No (%)	58	50	89
Education level			
Some college (%)	27	33	12
HS/GED (%)	41	41	41
Less than HS (%)	27	25	34
Unknown (%)	5	3	12

included if they lived in the local area and were referred to one of the organization's intensive outpatient program after leaving the residential program. We reviewed 90 days of treatment records for all women after discharge from the residential program. All women were referred to HSC's outpatient programs (women who did not complete the residential program, moved out of the county or were not referred to outpatient services were excluded from these analyses). The groups were similar in age and race (diagnostic information was not compared) (Table 13.3).

Women who received RC services were significantly more likely to engage in outpatient services after leaving the residential program and stay longer in treatment compared to women who did not connect with a recovery coach. Of course, it is also possible that women who voluntarily agreed to work with a recovery coach were more motivated to stay engaged in treatment. The results are encouraging but require research using a randomized design (i.e., eliminate the possible confound of motivation for treatment) to further evaluate the effectiveness of the model.

Preliminary results indicate that recovery coaches have been successful at helping women obtain employment, improve their housing, and acquire essential resources in the community.

The initial success of the recovery coach program led to several expansions through grant projects. The first adaptation of the model occurred through a US Department of Justice grant to expand treatment services for a drug court program. The grant project allowed us to provide recovery coach services to men involved in the criminal justice system. We recently developed an outreach program with two recovery coaches – one male and one female – who are receiving referrals directly

Table 13.3 Treatment continuation for women receiving RC services

	Connected with IOP	Average no. of IOP – groups	Average no. of groups for those who connected
Recovery coach (n = 84)	78 (93%)*	22 (SD = 13)*	24 (SD = 12)*
No recovery coach (n = 84)	61 (73%)	13 (SD = 14)	18 (SD = 13)

* Significant at 0.05

from the County's probation program. The outreach program was a product of our ongoing research with the drug court program.

We acquired a grant in 2009 through the Illinois Department of Healthcare and Family Services to develop a 24-h crisis center that can divert individuals from either an emergency room or jail. The program will focus on individuals who are in crisis due to a psychiatric condition or substance use disorder and can be treated in an outpatient setting. Recovery coaches will help engage individuals who are diverted to the program as well as assist in triaging them to treatment or other needed resources in the community.

A third grant project will use the recovery coach model with adolescents enrolled in a US Department of Labor's Youth Build Vocational Training Program (2009). One recovery coach will work with young adults who have an SUD and are enrolled in the vocational and educational program. The grant project was awarded to a workforce program in Peoria and is slated to begin in January 2010.

Challenges and Modifications of the Recovery Coach Model

The recovery coach program continues to evolve at Fayette. Limited research at HSC provides initial support for the model, although more research is needed to thoroughly evaluate the intervention. Below is list of challenges and barriers that have been encountered over the course of 5 years of the recovery coach program.

Adapting a Consumer-Driven Model to a Professional-Driven Treatment Program

Combining a consumer-driven model with an established, professional-driven addiction treatment system was the first challenge encountered in the implementation process. Many of the counselors working in the Fayette programs in 2004 tended to use a hierarchical, i.e., paternalistic, model of care that viewed the clinician as the expert and the client as the patient needing care and guidance. Recovery coaches, on the other hand, are trained to use a collaborative model that views the consumer as the expert of their own recovery and the coach as a consultant. These divergent philosophies of care led to conflicting strategies, such as

- Counselors wanted recovery coaches to become community extensions of the treatment plan as developed by the clinical team; whereas recovery coaches tended to provide services based on the goals of clients.
- Counselors wanted recovery coaches to monitor and report back client activities in the community, whereas recovery coaches allow clients to control the flow of information that is delivered back to the counselors.
- Counselors would discontinue treatment to clients who continued to relapse, whereas recovery coaches continued to work with clients, regardless of their relapse.
- Counselors would discourage clients from acquiring a job or returning to the community before achieving particular treatment plan objectives, whereas coaches would encourage clients to acquire a job or other activities the clients wanted.
- Counselors would discourage clients from accessing family and friends in the early stages of residential treatment, whereas recovery coaches would facilitate these connections upon clients' request.

These philosophical or ideological conflicts will likely be amplified if the two interventions are provided by independent agencies.

As noted previously, the solution at Fayette was to change the treatment approaches of counselors and the overall institutional culture to make it consistent with the philosophy and approach of the recovery coach program and recovery management model.

Maintaining Fidelity of the Recovery Coach Program

Maintaining the fidelity and mission of recovery coaching is another ongoing challenge of the program. Recovery coaching is designed to help individuals' access resources (internal coping skills and external resources) that will help individuals achieve recovery, based on the principles of recovery capital. The overall mission of the recovery coach program was articulated to treatment staff, but we neglected to outline services that were not considered within the framework of the model. For instance, the majority of our treatment population lives at or below the poverty level. Most of our clients need assistance with housing, transportation, clothing, childcare, food, and other necessities of basic living; however, many of these needs are not related directly to abstaining from alcohol and other drugs. Counselors often confused recovery coaching with services to address poverty. For example, recovery coaches were frequently viewed as cab drivers who could provide clients with transportation services, regardless of how these trips were related, if at all, to the overall goal of recovery. Moreover, many of the clients struggled to differentiate their own goals for recovery from other objectives. To maintain fidelity of the recovery coach model, our recovery coaches have been trained to

- Provide transportation services to clients who have a clear, recovery-based objective; otherwise, clients are encouraged or trained to ride the bus or acquire other forms of transportation (e.g., purchasing a bicycle).
- Engage family and friends in the treatment planning process to help clients address both recovery- and non-recovery-based activities.
- Coordinate services with counselors and assign responsibility for achieving specific objectives.
- Provide in-service training to counselors about the goal of recovery coaching.
- Provide pamphlets to counselors, clients, and family members on the services provided and not provided by recovery coaches.

Next Steps in Fayette Companies' Transformation

We continue to encounter practices and institutional policies that require modifications as we integrate principles of recovery management. Three additional challenges encountered in the process of transformation are (1) sustaining a viable workforce, (2) modifying residential treatment for individuals with a SUD, and (3) providing alternative treatment interventions for individuals in the early stages of a substance use illness (i.e., those who require brief interventions in nonconventional settings). The following discussions highlight three recent developments in the recovery management process to address these challenges.

Development and Utilization of New Technologies

The addiction treatment field is extremely labor intensive with salary and benefit costs comprising an average of 76% of total costs. Overall, salaries are low resulting in both high turnover and challenges in recruiting highly qualified counselors [58]. Dave Gustafson determined early in his work as Director of NIATx that the addiction treatment field was not sustainable due to the factors discussed above. He organized an international group of experts in various technology fields, such as genetics, bio-informatics, and nanotechnology, to identify or develop technological interventions that could overcome the deficiencies in the behavioral health workforce. This think-tank of experts identified numerous technological innovations that were already available and could be used to augment addiction treatment interventions. Gustafson and colleagues used the information from this think-tank to launch the Innovations for Recovery project (http://www.innovationsforrecovery.org) within the Department of Industrial Engineering at the University of Wisconsin.

Fayette has partnered with Dr. Gustafson and his staff to develop and implement technological innovations for addiction treatment services. A product of this partnership was the acquisition of a 5-year National Institute of Alcoholism and Alcohol Abuse (NIAAA) grant to develop and evaluate the use of smart phones to provide recovery support for persons with an alcohol use disorder. Persons leaving residential treatment programs at Fayette will be randomly assigned to the study beginning in November 2009. The web-connected smart phones will have a variety of recovery support features ranging from 24 h immediate access to a counselor if in a high risk or crisis situation to reminders of upcoming rewarding social and recreational activities based on individual interests. The phones will have a variety of recovery support features, such as a GPS function that can provide individuals with a warning when they near high-risk relapse zones (e.g., a previously frequented local bar), relapse prevention reminders, and easy access to social support networks.

Restructuring Residential Treatment

Residential addiction treatment presented a unique set of barriers in the process of implementing principles of recovery management. Most short- and long-term residential treatment programs, as designed, create a safe treatment milieu for clients. The inpatient environment can be used effectively as both respite and treatment for individuals who are living in chaotic situations and are unable to abstain from alcohol or other drugs. Unfortunately, the sterile sanctuary of residential care can also lead to isolation from the community, which poses a direct conflict to the principles of recovery management. The longer an individual resides in a residential treatment setting, the more difficult it becomes for them to integrate back in to the community where they will eventually live (this is an unavoidable outcome associated with any institutional program). In fact, it is common that we hear clients say that "I can *do* residential but I cannot make it in the outside." When the BHRM project began in 1999, our residential programs had "black-out" periods where people could not make phone calls or have visitors during their first few weeks of treatment. The folklore rational was that people would become lonesome or be influenced by individuals in their social system resulting in their leaving treatment. We eliminated the black-out policies in our three residential programs, which led to a significant *decrease* in early withdrawals (i.e., AMAs) from treatment. More recently, we altered the admission policy so that clients could keep their cell phones and laptops in treatment (if they had them).

It became apparent that we had to redesign residential treatment. Some people need this level of care as to achieve a break in their addiction and to regain basic health through nutrition, rest, and lifestyle modification. Nonetheless, individuals who need residential treatment are, by default, the ones who need more recovery capital, i.e., access to community resources, such as housing, medical, or mental health care, employment, problem solving skills, and social support. The challenge for our agency was to create a residential treatment intervention that could effectively treat an individual's severe addiction to alcohol or other drugs while simultaneously helping the person rebuild or develop a recovery support system in the community. Our goal was to help individuals increase their recovery capital before they leave residential treatment.

We instituted several low-cost modifications that promoted access to recovery capital while men and women were in the residential program. These modifications included

- Constructing computer labs that clients could use to learn basic computer skills, study for a GED, improve typing, develop a resume, taking online course or to email friends and family members (emails reduced the cost of communication for clients compared to cell phone minutes or pay phones).
- A pilot program was developed that allowed residents to acquire and maintain employment in the community in the evenings and on weekends.
- A second pilot that evolved out of the first allowed women to continue to reside in one of the residential programs while they establish a savings account from their income, complete an initial phase of school, or acquire stable housing. Women could decrease their involvement in clinical groups while they increased their support in the community through work, school, and social outlets.

A major barrier to assisting people to start employment, a GED program or course at the local community college was the State of Illinois licensing requirement that persons in residential treatment receive a minimum of 25 h of treatment weekly. This requirement also limited the time counselors had available for individual and family counseling. The primary mode of treatment within a residential program is group therapy. Thus, we were faced with a conflict between wanting to change the service delivery system to a model that we believed would be more effective and the need to earn revenues to support operations.

The breakthrough came when the Manager of Clinical Records and State Reporting challenged the funding box we were living within. Residential services were paid on an all inclusion per diem rate. She calculated that we could unbundle the services, while earning the same dollars. This unbundled model includes billing a residential rate for recovery home services while billing a mix of individual, group, and case management services at their rates for each service. As a result, we can now decrease the number of group therapy hours while increasing services that can help individuals increase their recovery capital, such as family sessions, couples therapy, supported employment services, and recovery coaching (e.g., access to medical care, housing, or education). Having more time for individual and family sessions will allow greater use of evidence-based practices such as the Community Reinforcement Approach [54] and Behavioral Couples Therapy [59]. An evaluation will be conducted to measure the impact of these changes on retention in treatment, employment, involvement in educational activities, and living conditions at discharge.

Outpatient Buprenorphine-Assisted Program

Clients with an addiction to opiates can now receive buprenorphine treatment combined with individualized outpatient services. The program was developed in response to the long waiting list of clients who had entered the detoxification program and were successfully stabilized on buprenorphine. Fayette adopted the use of buprenorphine for opiates in the medical detoxification program in 2004. The usual length of detoxification for opiates was 5–7 days. With buprenorphine, most individuals could be medically stabilized within 24 h. As a result, most individuals were no longer in need of inpatient care after 1 or 2 days. Unfortunately, there was often a waiting list for residential or intensive outpatient services; thus, individuals in detoxification had to wait for a treatment slot or leave the unit without being transferred to a treatment program. An outpatient buprenorphine service was implemented in 2007 to reduce the stay in the inpatient setting, allow a longer period of detoxification at home and provide ongoing outpatient services.

We initially established a 13-day in–outpatient detoxification program based on a NIDA study [60]. We combined the detoxification program with a four-night weekly IOP. A focus group was held with participants after a few weeks of implementation to see if the program was meeting their needs. Participants wanted two significant changes to the medication-assisted program. First, most did not want a short detoxification. Instead most clients wanted to continue the medication-assisted treatment. Second, nearly all participants wanted a reduction in group time during the week from four to two nights but an increase in individual counseling. The program immediately was modified to meet these requests and participation and retention has remained high. Several clients tapered to a low maintenance dose while others chose to finish the detoxification process. The key word is this process was and still is the consumer choice.

True-North Solutions Outpatient Program

Over 87% of those who may benefit from substance abuse treatment do not seek these services [61]. Perhaps one reason is that they don't feel they need or want what is being offered. Addiction treatment consists mostly of residential and intensive outpatient interventions. Both models of treatment are very intrusive to an individual's life. Some people may desire a more individual and private approach. Based on this assumption, Fayette developed an alternative addiction treatment intervention for people who desire an individualized model of care.

Individuals with a SUD who are willing to pay privately or have access to private insurance can now enroll in an alternative treatment program, True North Solutions. Clients in this program are provided with a menu of choices including individual and family-couples counseling, pharmacological treatments to augment therapy (e.g., naltrexone or buprenorphine), and psychiatric care. Counselors also provide the Community Reinforcement Approach Family Training (CRAFT; [62]) for concerned others who wish to assist their loved ones in entering addiction treatment. The services package has a lower cost than traditional private pay treatment programs. Based on experience, an episodic rate may be offered. It is hoped that the demonstration of this model may influence the public sector to reconsider their payment system.

Lessons Learned

Albert Einstein was correct when he noted that insanity is doing the same thing over and over again and expecting different results [63]. Repeatedly admitting someone to the residential or intensive outpatient services, providing the same treatment within these settings and thinking maybe this time will be successful is wasting health-care resources. The BHRM team was aware that change was needed. The challenge, of course, is transcending a behavioral health system that was built and funded on an acute care model. Below is listing of lessons learned in the process of transitioning from an acute care model to a recovery management model.

1. Implementing evidence-based treatment approaches is really, really hard. Ongoing intensive supervision including observation or review of taped sessions and use of fidelity tools is an absolute necessity.
2. Integrating addiction, mental health, and physical health care is essential to wellness.
3. Empowering is not enabling. Our job is to listen to an individual's goals, provide a menu of treatment choices for their selection, provide them with the skills and resources needed, support and celebrate their successes, and assist them to learn from setbacks.
4. Listen to those we serve and involve them in both the design and evaluation of services. Provide the services they need and want when they need and want them.
5. Align written treatment plans with EBPs. Our service model before the BHRM project consisted of treatment plans reflecting a counselor-driven perspective that was influenced more by the requirements of our funding sources than by specific needs and goals of our clients. Recovery management plans require collaboration between clients and counselors, need to be written in behavioral terms (rather than in clinical jargon), include specific EBPs focused on measurable outcomes (rather than on the quantity or frequency of services provided), are tailored to the specific capacities and level of motivation of the client and include the integration of client objectives and needs into the plan.
6. Partner with state organizations who fund and regulate addiction, mental, and physical health services to facilitate needed changes to funding, licensure/ certification or other regulations to promote changes that may facilitate application of recovery management principles.

The 10-year journey to implement Behavioral Health Recovery Management at Fayette Companies resulted in significant learning and changes that were never anticipated. We have many more miles to go.

References

1. White W. and Kelly JF. The Theory science and practice of recovery management. In Kelly JF and White W. (eds.), Addiction Recovery Management: Theory, Research and Practice, *Current Clinical Psychiatry*, DOI 10.1007/978-1-60327-960-4_14, © Springer Science+ Business Media, LLC 2011.
2. Corrigan PW, Steiner L, McCraken, SG, Blaser B, Barr M. Strategies for disseminating evidence-based practices to staff who treat people with serious mental illness. *Psychiatr Serv.* 2001; 52(12):1598–1606.
3. Corrigan PW. Place-then-train: an alternative service paradigm for persons with psychiatric disabilities. *Clin Psychol: Science & Practice.* 2001; 8(3):334–339.
4. Corrigan PW, Phelan SM. Social support and recovery in people with serious mental illness. *Community Ment Health J.* 2004; 40(6):513–523.
5. White WL, Boyle MG, Loveland DL. Alcoholism/Addiction as a chronic disease: from rhetoric to clinical reality. *Alcohol Treat Q.* 2002; 20(3/4):107–130.
6. McClellan AT, Lewis DC, O'Brien CP, Kleber HD. Drug dependence, a chronic medical illness: implications for treatment, insurance and outcomes evaluation. *J Am Med Ass.* 2000; 284:1689–1695.
7. O'Brien CP, McClellan, AT. Myths about the treatment of addiction. *Lancet.* 1996; 347:237–240.
8. Wagner EH, Austin BT, Davis C, Hindmarsh M, Schaelfer J, Bonomi A. Improving chronic illness care: translating evidence into action. *Health Aff.* 2001; 20(6):64–78.
9. Wagner EH, Austin BT, VonKorff M. Organizing care for patients with chronic illness. *Milbank Q.* 1996; 74(4):511–544.
10. Rapp CA. *The Strengths Model: Case Management with People Suffering from Severe and Persistent Mental Illness.* New York: Oxford University Press; 1998.
11. White WL, Boyle MG, Loveland DL. A model to transcend the limitations of addiction treatment. *Behav Health Manage.* 2003; 23(3):38–43.
12. White WL, Boyle MG, Loveland DL. Recovery from addiction and recovery from mental illness. In Ralph R, Corrigan P, eds. *Consumer Visions and Research Paradigms.* Washington DC: American Psychological Association; 2005:233–258.
13. Loveland DL, Weaver- Randall K, Corrigan PW. Research methods for exploring and assessing recovery. In Ralph R, Corrigan P, eds. *Consumer Visions and Research Paradigms.* Washington DC: American Psychological Association; 2005:19–60.
14. Corrigan PW, Boyle MG. Mental health system change: evolution or revolution? *Adm Policy Ment Health.* 2003; 30(5):379–395.
15. Corrigan PW, Larson JE, Watson AC, Boyle MG, Barr L. Solutions to discrimination in work and housing identified by people with mental illness. *J Nerv Ment Dis.* 2006; 194(9):716–718.
16. Miller WR, Sorenson JL, Selzer JA, Brigham GS. Disseminating evidence based practices in substance abuse treatment: a review with suggestions. *J Subst Abuse Treat.* 2006; 31:25–39.
17. Institute of Medicine's Committee on Quality Health Care in America. *Crossing the Quality Chasm: A New Health System for the 21st Century.* Washington DC: Institute of Medicine; 2001.
18. McClellan AT, Chalk, M, Bartlett J. Outcomes, performance and quality: what's the difference? *J Subst Abuse Treat.* 2007; 32:331–340.
19. Stein MD, Friedmann P. Need for medical and psychosocial services among injection drug users: a comparative study of needle exchange and methadone maintenance. *Am J Addict.* 2002; 11:262–270.

20. Crandall LA, Metsch LR, McCoy CB, Chitwood DD, Tobias H. Chronic drug use and reproductive health among low income women in Miami Florida: a comparative study of access, need and utilization. *J Behav Health Serv Res.* 2003; 30(3):321–331.
21. Hser Y, Polinsky ML, Maglione M, Austin MD. Matching client's needs with drug treatment services. *J Subst Abuse Treat.* 1999; 16(4):299–305.
22. Marsh JC, D'Aunno TA, Smith BD. Increasing access and providing social services to improve drug abuse treatment for women with children. *Addiction.* 2000; 95(8):1237–1247.
23. McClellan AT, Arndt IO, Metzger DS, Woody GE, O'Brien CP. The effects of psychosocial services in substance abuse treatment. *J Am Med Ass.* 1993; 269:1953–1959.
24. McClellan AT, Hagan AT, Levine M, et al. Supplemental social services improve outcomes in public addiction treatment. *Addiction.* 1998; 93:1489–1499.
25. Vaughn-Sarrazin MS, Hall JA, Rick GS. Impact of case management on the use of r health services by rural clients in substance abuse treatment. *J Drug Issues.* 2000; 30(2):435.464.
26. Minkoff K. Comprehensive continuous integrated systems of care and psychopharmacology practice guidelines for individuals with co-occurring psychiatric and substance use disorders. Behavioral Health Recovery Management website. 2005. Available at: http://www.bhrm.org/guidelines/psychopharmacology.pdf. Accessed August 28, 2009.
27. Boyle MG, White WL, Corrigan PW, Loveland DL. Guidelines for linking primary care. Behavioral Health Recovery Management website. Available at http://www.bhrm.org/guidelines/BHRM%20Primary%20Care%20Integration.pdf. Accessed August 30, 2009.
28. Granfield R, Cloud W. Social context and "natural recovery": the role of social capital in the resolution of drug- associated problems. *Subst Use Misuse.* 2001; 36(11): 1543–1571.
29. Cunningham JA, Koski-Janees A, Toneatto T. Why do people stop their drug use? Results from a general population sample. *Contemp Drug Probl.* 1999; 26:695–710.
30. Cunningham JA, Breslin FC. Only one in three people with alcohol abuse or dependence ever seek treatment. *Addict Behav.* 2004; 29(1):221–223.
31. Sobdell LC, Cunningham JA, Sobdell MB. Recovery from alcohol problems with and without treatment: prevalence in two population surveys. *Am J Public Health.* 1996; 87(7): 966–972.
32. Larimer ME, Kilmer JR. Natural history. In Zernig G, Saria A, eds. *Handbook of Alcoholism, Pharmacology and Toxicology.* Boca Raton, Fl: CRC Press; 2000:13–28.
33. Smart RG. Natural recovery or recovery without treatment from alcohol and drug problems as seen from survey data. In Kingemann H, Sobdell LC, eds. *Promoting Self-Change from Addictive Behaviors: Practical Implications for Policy, Prevention and Treatment.* New York: Springer; 2007.
34. Carbello JL, Fernández-Hermida JR, Secades-Villa R, García-Rodríguez O, Sobdell LC. Natural recovery from drug and alcohol problems: a methodical review of the literature from 1999 through 2005. In Klingerman H, Sobdel LC, eds. *Promoting Self- Change from Addictive Behaviors: Practical Implications for Policy, Prevention and Treatment.* New York; Springer; 2007:87–101.
35. Cloud W, Granfield R. Natural recovery from substance dependency: lessons from treatment providers. *J Soc Work Pract Addict.* 2001; 1(1):83–104.
36. White WL. The mobilization of community resources to support long-term addiction recovery. *J Subst Abuse Treat.* 2009; 36:146–158.
37. Vanderplasschen W, Rapp RC, Wolf JR, Broekaert E. The development and implementation of case management for substance use disorders in North America and Europe. *Psychiatr Serv.* 2004; 55:913–922.
38. Cox GB, Walker RD, Freng SA, Short BA, Meijer L, Gilchrist L. Outcomes of a controlled trial of the effectiveness of intensive case management for chronic health problems. *J Stud Alcohol.* 1998; 59:523–532.
39. McClellan AT, Hagan AT, Levine M, Meyers K, Gould F, Bencivengo M, Durell J, Jaffe J. Does clinical case management improve outpatient addiction treatment? *Drug Alcohol Depend.* 1999; 55:91–103.
40. Godley MD, Godley SH, Dennis M, Funk R.R., Passetti LL. The effect of assertive continuing care on continuing care linkage, adherence and abstinence following residential treatment for adolescents with substance use disorders. *Addiction.* 2007; 102(1):81–93.

41. Rapp RC, Siegal HA, Li L, Saha P. Predicting post primary treatment services and drug use outcomes: a multivariate analysis. *Am J Drug Alcohol Abuse*. 1998; 24:603–615.
42. Siegal HA, Rapp RC, Li L, Saha P, Kirk KD. The role of case management in retaining client in substance abuse treatment: an exploratory analysis. *J Drug Issues*. 1997; 27(4):821–831.
43. Schwartz M, Baker G, Mulvey KP, Plough A. Improving publicly funded substance abuse treatment: the value of case management. *Am J Public Health*. 1997; 87:1659–1664.
44. Siegal HA, Fisher JH, Rapp RC, et al. Enhancing substance abuse treatment with case management: its impact on employment. *J Subst Abuse Treat*. 1996; 13:93–98.
45. Siegal HA, Li L, Rapp RC. Case management as a therapeutic enhancement: impact on post-treatment criminality. *J Addict Dis*. 2002; 21(4):37–46.
46. Conrad KJ, Hultman CL, Pope AR, et al. Case managed residential care for homeless addicted veterans: results of a true experiment. *Med Care*. 1998; 36(1):40–53.
47. Friedmann PD, Hendrickson JC, Gersterin DR, Zhang A. Designated managers as facilitators of medical and psychosocial service delivery in addiction treatment programs. *J Behav Health Res*. 2004; 31(1):86–97.
48. Kirby MW, Braught GN, Brown E, Karane S, McCann M, Van DeMark N. Dyadic case management as a strategy for prevention of homelessness among chronically disabled men and women with drug dependence. *Alcohol Treat Q*. 1999; 17:53–71.
49. Hall JA, Carswell C, Walsh E, Huber DL, Jampoler JS. Iowa case management: innovative social casework. *Soc Work*. 2002; 47:132–141.
50. Blomqvist J. Paths to recovery from substance misuse: change of lifestyle and the role of treatment. *Subst Use Misuse*. 1996; 31(3):1807–1852.
51. Boyle MG, White WL, Corrigan PW, Loveland DL. Behavioral health recovery management: a statement of principles. Behavioral Health Recovery Management website. Available at http://www.bhrm.org/papers/principles/BHRMprinciples.htm. Accessed November 20, 2009.
52. Loveland DL, Boyle M. *Manual for Recovery Coaching and Personal Recovery Plan Development*. Behavioral Health Recovery Management website. Available at http://www.bhrm.org/guidelines/addguidelines.htm. Accessed November 20, 2009.
53. Miller WR, Rollnick S. *Motivational Interviewing (2nd Ed)*. New York: Guilford Press; 2002.
54. Meyers RJ, Smith SE. *Clinical guide to alcohol treatment: the community reinforcement approach*. New York: Guilford Press; 1995.
55. Godley M. Assertive approaches to continuing care among youth. In Kelly J, White W, eds. *Addiction Recovery Management: Theory, Science and Practice*. In Press
56. Bond GR, Vogler KM, Resnick SG, Evans LJ, Drake RE, Becker DR. Dimensions of supported employment: factor structure of the IPS fidelity scale. *J Ment Health*. 2001; 10(4): 383–393.
57. Bond GR, Becker DR, Drake RE, Rapp CA, Meisler N, Lehman AF, Bell MD, Blyer CR. Implementing supported employment as an evidence-based practice. *Psychiatr Serv*. 2001; 52:313–322.
58. McClellan AT, Carise D, Kieber HD. Can the national addiction treatment infrastructure support the public's demand for quality care? *J Subst Abuse Treat*. 2003; 25:117–121.
59. O'Farrell TJ, Fals-Stewart W. *Behavioral Couples Therapy for Alcoholism and Substance Abuse*. New York: Guilford Press; 2006.
60. Ling W, Amass L, Shoptaw S, et al. A multi-center randomized trial of buprenorphine-naloxone versus clonidine for opioid detoxification: findings from the National Institute on Drug Abuse Clinical Trials Network. *Addiction*. 2005; 100–1090–1100.
61. Substance Abuse and Mental Health Services Administration. Alcohol treatment need, utilization and barriers. *The National Survey on Drug Use and Health (NSUDH) Report;* 2009.
62. Smith JE, Meyers RJ. *Motivating Substance Abusers to Enter Treatment: Working with Family Members*. New York: Guilford Press; 2009.
63. Prindle JC. Albert Einstein quotes. Albert Einstein Institute website. Available from http://www.alberteinsteinsite.com/quotes/einsteinquotes.html#general. Accessed on November 20, 2009.

Chapter 14
Peer-Based Recovery Support Services Within a Recovery Community Organization: The CCAR Experience

Phil Valentine

Abstract The Connecticut Community for Addiction Recovery (CCAR) has a rich history as a lead Recovery Community Organization. This chapter describes CCAR's evolution from a pure advocacy organization to a provider of peer-based recovery support services. A key part of this story is the development of recovery community centers (RCCs) that are a grassroots model, conceived in the idea of a "field of dreams – build it and they will come." CCAR's experience has certainly proved this to be true. And powerful. RCCs have served as the hubs where an impressive array of peer-based recovery support services were designed and delivered. For example, in 2008, 276 volunteers contributed more than 13,000 h of service mostly within the walls of RCCs. 24,951 outbound phone calls were made by Telephone Recovery Support Calls to 1,285 recoverees. As the CCAR Recovery Coach Academy continues to graduate more and more recovery coaches, the impact on local communities and Connecticut's recovery-oriented system of care will grow through the continued infusion of the language, culture, and spirit of recovery from alcohol and other drug addiction. The chapter will close on CCAR's observations and experience with the healing power within communities of recovery.

Introduction

Peer-based recovery support services are activities provided by a volunteer force dedicated to helping and facilitating recovery from alcohol and drug addiction. During the past 12 years, our Connecticut organization has taken significant strides in designing, developing, and implementing these services to the point that in 2009, 268 volunteers contributed 14,697 h of service, and made 36,865 outbound support calls to 1,420 recovering persons, contributing the equivalent of $378,448 in service provision. This chapter describes in detail the origins, growth, and impact of this

P. Valentine (✉)
Connecticut Community for Addiction Recovery, Hartford, CT, USA
e-mail: ccar2005@ccar.us

J.F. Kelly and W.L. White (eds.), *Addiction Recovery Management: Theory, Research and Practice*, Current Clinical Psychiatry, DOI 10.1007/978-1-60327-960-4_14,
© Springer Science+Business Media, LLC 2011

recovery community organization – the Connecticut Community for Addiction Recovery (CCAR). First, the spark that started this enterprise is described, followed by a brief history of how initial grassroots advocacy grew into vital and meaningful service provision in the heart of the community. This is followed by a description of the Recovery Community Center (RCC) and its ingredients and activities and how such centers can serve as a powerful adjunct to formal treatment services at the local and state level.

The Beginning

I have a dear friend, his name is Arno, and I have dubbed him Shortcast because he doesn't cast very far when he's fishing. He fishes in the first wave or just beyond and (I'd never tell him this), he usually catches more fish than me. Every October my buddy Shortcast and I head to the hallowed fishing rounds of Race Point, Provincetown at the end of Cape Cod to get in on the fall migration of the famed striped bass. I left last Saturday afternoon and returned Wednesday. The fishing was spectacular and the weather even more so.

Seems that with our impeccable timing (I say sarcastically), we chose a few days when a couple of tropical storms merged in the Atlantic and descended upon the Cape. One day, we had driven oversand out to the point. Race Point is a huge sand bar and the water moves quickly past it at all times, now add those high winds and you have some torrents! It was frothy, foamy, wild, wild water... I have never seen conditions like this, before or since. Twenty foot rollers steamed by. Rain and sand blasted the truck as it shook in the wind. Arno and I are very bright, intelligent fisherman, deeply devoted to our passion. I looked at Arno and said, "I ain't going out there." He said, "Me either." He turned on the radio.

There was only one other truck foolish enough to be on that tiny strip of sand. We watched in amazement as some very old guy struggled to open the truck door, grab a rod, and fight his way to the edge of the raging torrent. Crap, we're going to have to rescue him. With great effort, he made a cast, and as soon as his lure hit the water, he hauled back. Fish on! Arno and I looked at each other and being brilliant fisherman, we both yelled "Let's go!" We caught fish for hours and hours. As other guys drove up and saw us catching, they too, started reveling in the fantastic fishing. We remember it now as one of the best days of surf fishing we have ever experienced.

The CCAR would never have started if some guy did not test the water and take the first cast. That man, a pioneer in the field of establishing recovery community organizations, is Bob Savage. Bob founded CCAR. He had a 30-year career in Connecticut's state treatment system and when he retired, he set out to answer a couple questions that had nagged him while in public service.

1. Where are the people in recovery when we are making critical decisions concerning them?
2. Can the recovery community be organized to advocate for issues of importance to them?

Working from his home and having his expenses covered by the New England Institute of Addiction Studies (NEIAS), Bob traveled all over Connecticut and New England, speaking wherever he could to rally the recovery community. He began holding monthly Chapter meetings in Connecticut that ultimately evolved into CCAR, while also getting the New England Alliance of Addiction Recovery (NEAAR) going as well. With this effort, he garnered funding from the CT Department of Mental Health and Addiction Services (DMHAS), and then was able to write a successful grant to the federal government for a Recovery Community Support Program (RCSP) under the Center for Substance Abuse Treatment (CSAT), Substance Abuse Mental Health Services Administration (SAMHSA).

Bob was vital to the development of the recovery advocacy movement in New England. The Savage legacy leaves behind many lessons that are still guiding CCAR today: Pick a few things and do them very well. Don't try to do everything. Quality counts.

- Family, family, and more family. Family members have the potential to be the recovery advocacy movement's most powerful constituency.
- Be an ally of the Single State Agency. Work with them, not against them.
- Pay people in recovery well. Value their experience. If a recovery community organization doesn't pay people in recovery well, who will?
- We have a right to be heard and to speak even when it's uncomfortable to voice our opinions.
- Tenacity works.
- Integrity matters.
- Treat your Board with utmost respect.
- Hire carefully and take your time when hiring.
- Address all personnel situations in reasonable time frames. "20 min of intense discomfort is a small price compared to months, or years, of prolonged pain."
- Seek help on special issues from people who have more experience than you in a given area.
- Share your challenges as well as your successes.
- Surround yourself with great people.
- The art of true delegation – give someone a task or a project and let them do it.

As CCAR grew, Bob began hiring people as funding allowed. In January 1999, I, Phillip Valentine, was CCAR's first hire and started as the Associate Director. I think my story of how I was hired lends itself to the spiritual component inherent in this movement. A few months before I heard about the CCAR job, or a new recovery movement, there was a crisis in my marriage. I had been out of full time work for more than 2 years, staying at home with two very young children, while Sandy was working full time at a major insurance company. The crisis was that she wanted to be home with the kids. We sought out marriage counseling to sort out how we were going to do this and the marriage counselor asked me a very provocative question that changed the course of my life. She said, "Phil, you have about 30 good years left, what are you going to do with them?" I started looking hard for a job, any job. I was working the floor at Dick's Sporting Goods when I interviewed with CCAR. I was hired even though I had little knowledge of treatment or recovery advocacy. All the acronyms baffled me. I quickly absorbed everything I could and discovered that my personal experience with recovery (largely outside of any formal treatment setting) was a valuable and desperately needed voice. This was driven home on my very first day on the job. Bob wanted me to go to the LOB and attend a parity meeting. First, I sheepishly asked, "What's the LOB?" The Legislative Office Building. "Oh, where's that?" Next to the Capitol. "Oh, I know where that is... what's parity?" I made the meeting, quite nervous and insecure not knowing what to expect. There were many people with suits and long initials after their names. The conversation turned to recovery support services and the chair asked me what I thought. I said, "Well in my recovery program, we're told to go to 90 meetings in 90 days." I looked around and people were furiously writing. Then they wanted to know more and as I answered their questions, it became apparent that not only did I personally have something to offer, the recovery community needed to be at these tables.

The Early Years: Planning and Organizing

In the early years, we spent all our time organizing. This is a key point. Bob had traversed the state for 2 years and then I joined him. We talked to individuals, groups, sat in on all types of meetings and we gradually established a solid group of volunteers who formed our core and were instrumental in "putting a face on recovery." CCAR continues to be successful with our advocacy efforts that were started in the formative years.

Frequent speaking engagements – CCAR makes presentations to a variety of audiences such as community organizations, treatment providers, prisons, the legislature, state agencies, etc. The presentations demonstrate to the public that people in long-term recovery do exist. We hold jobs, pay taxes, raise families, and have a voice when it comes to the public's perception about alcohol and other drug addiction. These presentations also serve as outreach to those who may need recovery support services early in their recovery and to attract persons who may want to volunteer their services for CCAR.

Recovery poster series – Posters were developed using with recovery messages such as "Harvesting the Power of Recovery," to show the positive aspects of a life without alcohol or other drugs.

Cable public access TV shows – CCAR began using local resources, i.e., local public access TV in 2005 and has aired hundreds of personal stories of recovery.

DVDs, videos – CCAR has developed three video series that capture the lives of persons in recovery. Our first video, *Putting a Face on Recovery,* featured CCAR members telling their stories of recovery. The second, *The Healing Power of Recovery* answered the question "Would it be possible to capture the healing power of recovery on video?" This was the question CCAR asked us after the tremendous healing experience of Recovery Walks! 2001, held just 5 days after the now infamous 9/11. On September 16, 2001, over 2000 people gathered at Bushnell Park in Hartford and initially shared their confusion and grief over the tragedy. Yet, as the day progressed, the hope and resiliency of recovery surfaced and brought the walk experience into a dimension of quiet determination and community healing. Our latest project, *The Legacy of Hope: Recovery Elders Video Project*, documents the lives and recovery stories of people in ultra long-term recovery; i.e., people with 20, 30, 40, or more years.

Recovery Walks!, Rally for Recovery [Faces and Voices of Recovery (FAVOR)] – Every year CCAR hosts a Recovery Walks! event in Bushnell Park, in downtown Hartford. From 700 our first year, to almost 2,000 last year (2009), people are taking notice! The message that "Recovery is possible" is gaining momentum in Connecticut and influencing citizens, legislators, and most importantly, those with addictions. Faces and Voice of Recovery helps raise the national profile of the recovery community by supporting these Recovery Month events collectively called, "Rally for Recovery" where many thousands support recovery from alcohol and other drugs.

CCAR website http://ccar.us – Our website updates information regularly on purpose of a recovery community organization, trainings, events, and resources.

Today, our elevator speech has evolved to this: CCAR organizes the recovery community to: (1) put a face on recovery and (2) provide recovery support services. CCAR has a rich history of advocacy in that we

- Wrote the Recovery Core Values along with Advocacy Unlimited that became the foundation for the Commissioner's Policy # 83: Promoting a Recovery-Oriented Service System.
- Helped turn "Heroin Town," a negative Hartford Courant newspaper series, into "Recovery Town."
- Educated the legislature about the Pardons Process where significant changes have been made.
- Assisted DMHAS through some "Not in My Back Yard" (NIMBY) housing issues associated with Access to Recovery (ATR).
- Involved in FAVOR issues – restoration of RCSP funding, HBO Addiction documentary, insurance discrimination.

About 4 years into our existence, our federal grant program shifted its focus from Recovery Community *Support* to Recovery Community *Services*. One wonders if our collective advocacy effort worked so well that the government felt the pressure and shifted to recovery support services. The shift proved to be a blessing. At the time, we were wrestling with a very simple but deep question asked by our membership, "what can I do?" We were often stretched to find something meaningful. They could tell their story (when and where?), or they could attend a Chapter meeting (and then?), etc. You catch the drift. There was also a segment of our membership that wanted to be of service, they wanted to provide support, give rides, lend a listening ear, mentor, etc., and we didn't have those opportunities available. So when the Recovery Community Services Program (RCSP) switched from Support to Services, we resisted at first and then began to see how this could really be of benefit. We started slowly and as we grew into the delivery of support services, they became much more defined. Now we have volunteer opportunities for those who are wired for advocacy and those who are wired for service. You may describe advocacy as peanut butter, services as jelly – separate, they are each very good, put them together and you have something special.

Foundational Principals

As CCAR developed, an ethical framework gradually emerged that we refer to as "foundational principals," that steers our work. They are given below.

You Are in Recovery if You Say You Are

Early on CCAR held a series of day-long planning meetings once a month on Saturdays. We debated how CCAR would define recovery and tried to answer questions like "Is abstinence a requirement of recovery? What about medication? What about methadone? Should there be an amount of clean time required for participation and/or membership? How would we determine who was clean and who was not? Drug tests? (we think not). At times, these issues elicited strong, emotional responses. Someone suggested that we base our definition of recovery somewhat on the definition of membership put forth by Alcoholics Anonymous – "all that is required for membership is a desire to stop drinking." Who determines if a person has the desire? The person. Who determines if a person is in recovery? The person in recovery. Finally, we concluded that "you are in recovery if you say you are." When I mention that definition to researchers they scoffed and dismissed it, but there's a lot more to it than would seem apparent at first blush. This definition has served CCAR well over the years. Not to say that it hasn't been tested. What do you do when a person volunteering at one of our Centers seems to be under the influence (odor) but insists that they are in recovery and their behavior is appropriate?

On the same track, CCAR has never formally defined membership. Our members are people who have agreed to be on our mailing list. Paid membership was something we batted around, but never saw a way to do it. Paid membership also seemed to run contrary to many of our recovery backgrounds. Recovery is free. We decided as an alternative that running an Individual Giving Campaign would give those who wanted to contribute financially the opportunity to do so. We did not want "money" to define membership. We also believe that "you're a member if you say you are." Our vision and mission portrayed through frequent presentations attract many people to our organization.

There Are Many Pathways to Recovery

I admit it, I didn't always believe this. As I mature in recovery, or maybe just mature, I have become much more receptive to alternative pathways. I have seen this on many instances, one experience still resonates. I was facilitating a training, *12 Steps and Religion: Adversaries, Strangers, or Friends*, and we had a very diverse audience. There were two African American women in attendance who during introductions said they were in recovery for more than 20 years each. Their eyes were lit up and they talked about the recovery ministry they were leading at their church. As the discussion ensued, a man from a 12-step program challenged them that they were not really in recovery because they hadn't attended any meetings in many years. Their pathway was the church and as far as CCAR is concerned they are in recovery because... they say they are!

The CCAR philosophy is that "our tent is big enough for everyone." We don't really pay attention to what your illness is, your drug of choice, your recovery support, the medication you may be on (or not on), etc. "You are in recovery if you say you are" and you are welcome. Our thriving all-recovery groups support this notion. As a result, we have become an incredibly diverse organization.

Focus Is on the Recovery Potential, Not the Pathology

People that frequent the CCAR RCCs do not go through a formal assessment process of any kind. When someone enters they usually find a volunteer, or other person in the Center, and have a conversation. "What's going on? What are you looking for? How can we help you?" CCAR's intention is to help move someone along the road of recovery. We don't ask what they are recovering from. In 2007, DMHAS was convening a co-occurring conference and was looking for people with co-occurring disorders to speak. A flyer was posted in the Hartford Center. Six people, all regular CCAR volunteers, signed up. We had no idea they were "co-occurring." They were here working on their recovery while serving and helping others.

Err on the Side of the Recoveree

This is the essence of a person-centered approach. Do you strictly follow the established policy or do you do what you believe is best for the individual knowing that it goes against a policy? Methadone clinics are often forced to choose between these two. CCAR introduced the term recoveree (refugee, employee), coined by Melissa Scheffey, an Administrative Assistant in the early years, to describe a person in recovery. We refrain from using terms like client, patient, consumer, etc.

Err on the Side of Being Generous

When on the fence about making a decision, CCAR asks what the generous thing to do is and that often steers us in the right direction. This principal also supports a person-centered approach. A CCAR staff member (also a person in recovery) says, "I refer often to the "Am I being generous?" question when working with recoverees both in my personal life as well as in CCAR. The easier decision is to play it cautious when faced with a decision if I am concerned someone might be taking advantage or if I question what I suspect might be their real motive. I know what kind of thinking can be behind the actions of recoverees because I *am* a recoveree. However, when I err on the side of being generous I am giving someone the chance that was afforded to me to do the next right thing. In the process I am changing my own thinking to that of optimism and hope rather than pessimism and doubt. I am also subscribing to the belief that good works multiply."

Before we discuss specific services CCAR has developed we offer this abbreviated table of Milestones to give you an idea of our evolution (Table 14.1).

The Recovery Community Center

As CCAR shifted from all advocacy to delivering peer-based recovery support services, it became rapidly apparent that we needed a place to operate from. Many of us had seen the movie "Field of Dreams" where Kevin Costner's character heeds a spiritual whisper "build it and they will come." We listened to the voice of the recovery community and built our first one in Willimantic, opening up the first floor of a multipurpose house on Main Street. And they started to come. In our first year of operation, our log book had more than 10,000 sign-ins. This is a duplicated number, but is an excellent indicator of the amount of foot traffic this Center generates. In 2009, our four sites drew more than 35,000 visits. So what is a RCC? CCAR was asked this question a lot, in fact, several states have traveled to Connecticut to experience our model. In response to the question, CCAR developed the Core Elements below.

Core Elements of a RCC: Overview

A RCC

- Is a recovery oriented sanctuary anchored in the heart of the community.
- Is visible so local communities of recovery can actively put a face on recovery.
- Serves as a physical location where CCAR can organize the local recovery community's ability to care, specifically through the provision of a variety of recovery support services.
- Provides peer-based recovery support services using a volunteer force to deliver a vast majority of these services.

Table 14.1 CCAR milestones

1997	CCAR holds Connecticut's first Recovering Community Organization meeting
1998	Receiving funding from CSAT's Recovery Community Support Program laid a financial foundation that was later supplemented by funding from the Connecticut Department of Mental Health and Addiction Services (DMHAS)
2000	Our first Recovery Walks! held in 2000 was another early milestone and an idea that came from the recovery community. We had never heard of a walk in support of recovery from alcohol and other drug addiction. We did some internet research and found one walk/run for a treatment center in the DC area, so we decided that if we held a walk and 50 people showed up, we would be successful. 700 showed up for that first walk. Currently walks for recovery are held coast to coast. That's an incredible breakthrough. Recovery is truly becoming more visible
	We wrote the Recovery Core Values in collaboration with mental health recovery advocates that became the cornerstone of Tom Kirk's (DMHAS Director) policy on a Recovery-Oriented System of Care that has become a national model
	We produced a couple videos that are still pertinent and powerful today – Putting a Face on Recovery and The Healing Power of Recovery
	We held our third Legislative Day and a few legislators revealed for the first time publicly their own personal recoveries
2004	Opened our first Recovery Community Center in Willimantic. This was in response to a high profile series of newspaper articles in the state's largest paper, *The Hartford Courant*, labeling Willimantic "Heroin Town." We like to say that a few years later, CCAR has had a hand in turning Heroin Town to Recovery Town
2005	New London Recovery Community Center opened (#2)
	Another milestone was starting our Recovery Housing Project that inventoried the state's independently owned, privately operated sober houses, established a coalition, wrote standards, and delivered training
2006	Bridgeport Recovery Community Center Opened (#3)
	Hartford Recovery Community Center opened (#4)
2007	Telephone Recovery Support Program funded. Recoverees receive a phone call from a trained CCAR volunteer once a week for 12 weeks to support the recoveree's progress. The average time period that each recoveree is involved in Telephone Recovery Support is 20 weeks
2008	CCAR formed the Recovery Technical Assistance Group (RTAG) to provide consulting, technical assistance to recovery community organizations and other entities
	The first Recovery Coach Academy was held, a 7-day training that drew 30 participants in a "learning laboratory" model
2009	Held the fourth annual Volunteer Recognition and Celebration dinner with Mark Lundholm. 209 people attended, 108 of them volunteers, and 27 Presidential awards were given
	CCAR earned a $100,000 contract from the CT Department of Correction for the Re-entry and Recovery Project for people in the Hartford parole district
	Recovery Walks! celebrated its tenth anniversary

- Attracts people in recovery, family members, friends, and allies to serve as CCAR volunteers, who in turn help those coming up behind them.
- Fosters the inherent nature of the recovery community (people in recovery, family members, friends, and allies) to give back.

- Functions as a recovery resource for the local community.
- Is a location where, sometimes, people still struggling with addiction will enter and the RCC will help them navigate the system.
- Is a place to find workshops, training and educational sessions to enhance one's own recovery.
- Maintains a structured schedule of recovery-related workshops, trainings, meetings, services, and social events.
- Hosts and promotes recovery social events.

It's important to note what an RCC is not. An RCC is not a treatment agency – no clinical services are provided. An RCC is not a 12-step club. An RCC is not a drop-in center. An RCC is not a place for people to simply hang out, watch TV, and play cards/pool. CCAR is not seeking to duplicate existing resources. Recoverees in the Center are actively working on their recovery, or helping another person with theirs.

CCAR developed these Core Elements of a RCC based on our vision and experience.

Site

- A RCC should be at a minimum 2,500 square feet and have these standard areas:
  - Group/Training room that seats a minimum of 50
  - Computer room that can comfortably hold at least four computers (high-speed internet capable)
  - Two offices: one for the RCC Manager and the other for additional staff
  - Reception area
  - Telephone Room, private for making Telephone Recovery Support calls with at least three phones and phone lines
  - Lounge area for reading, socializing
  - Kitchen area
- Location. CCAR believes by having a prominent, visible location whose sole purpose is to promote recovery, we literally bring recovery from church basements onto main street. The location should also be easily accessible to those without personal transportation.
- An RCC should be handicapped accessible.

Administration

- At a minimum, an effective RCC needs the following staff:
  - One full time RCC Manager. Ideally, this person will be intimately familiar with the local recovery community and knowledgeable of all local social services, businesses, faith organizations, and neighborhoods.

- One RCC Assistant Manager (note: CCAR received a Connecticut State grant to provide Telephone Recovery Support so this position is filled by the Telephone Recovery Support Coordinator)
- One Administrative Assistant
- The RCC Manager will be given an annual budget to provide programming, training, workshops, and social events.
- The staff and selected volunteers of an RCC will participate in local and statewide fundraising activities.

Programming

- All program efforts at an RCC are overseen by the CCAR paid staff and volunteer force, and significant input is gathered from the recoverees at the RCC, the volunteer force, the RCC Advisory Council and the local recovery community.
- Programming is determined through three sources:
  - CCAR Management Team
  - CCAR staff
  - The Advisory Council representative of the local recovery community
- Currently, programming coming from the Central Office consists of
  - Telephone recovery support
  - Recovery-oriented employment services
  - Referrals to recovery housing
  - Recovery and re-entry services (Department of Correction)
  - All-recovery groups
  - Volunteer trainings
  - Recovery training series
  - Family/community education
  - Family support groups
  - Recovery coaching
- Recovery coaching that includes peer one-on-one interaction should be an integral part of every RCC.
- An RCC will provide support of recovery housing through knowledge and application of the Recovery Housing Project database.
- An RCC will provide employment support to recoverees to help build personal recovery capital.
- An RCC will deliver the CCAR Recovery Training Series using peer volunteers and outside facilitators who have been trained to conduct such education programs.
- An RCC will organize and/or host social activities that are member and committee driven and supported by peer volunteers.
- An RCC is welcoming to mutual aid societies (i.e., 12-step), community organizations, recovery-oriented agencies, etc. to host their meetings and/or events at the RCC.

- An RCC will publish a monthly schedule of activities. This schedule will be posted prominently in the RCC itself and available on the internet.

Volunteers

- Volunteers are CCAR's number one resource and must be treated as such. Each RCC will make an outstanding effort to recruit, train, engage, supervise, and recognize CCAR volunteers.
- All programs and services in an RCC are best implemented by volunteers who are trained and supported through the Volunteer Management System (VMS). Staff is paid to support the volunteers.
- A statewide Volunteer Manager will work with the staff of each RCC and the CCAR Management Team to achieve the goals and objectives of the VMS.

General

- An RCC must be volunteer driven, member-inspired, and premised on peer support.
- An RCC must have clear Policies and Procedures that are readily available to the membership and reviewed every year.
- An RCC will have Rules of Conduct clearly posted.
- Ideally, an RCC would have a van to transport people and to help with access to peer-based recovery support services.
- An RCC will have computers for individuals in recovery with connections to printers and high-speed internet.
- An RCC will have at least one large screen TV, DVD player, and VCR for training, workshops and seminars. The TV will not be hooked up to cable, dish or any other connection that allows for multiple channel TV viewing.
- All RCC staff and appropriate volunteers will be trained to use the online databases and the internet to access services for recoverees. Every RCC will have a Community Resource Book with pertinent forms and applications that is updated quarterly.
- In general, An RCC will not be open on Holidays. Holidays are times for paid staff and dedicated volunteers to take time away for rest and rejuvenation. CCAR understands that Holidays may be a tough time for some individuals and will rely on other natural recovery supports to assist those individuals.

Volunteer Management System

As a person in recovery I have benefited immensely from volunteering at the Hartford Recovery Community Center (HRCC). Whether making Telephone Recovery Support

(TRS) calls or recovery coaching I have been given countless chances to promote and enhance recovery in the lives of others. CCAR has afforded me so many opportunities to give back to the recovery community.
CCAR Volunteer

I lost my job just about a year ago and started using the research room at New London Recovery Community Center for job searching. After frequenting the Center for a couple of months, and job searching to no avail, I began to think it was a prime opportunity for me to turn my situation around and give back to the community. I was trained as a TRS caller and started reaching out to others who were in need of support in their recovery. By doing so it has given me back my integrity and purpose in life while maintaining my own sobriety through this rough time. Although I have yet to find a job, once I do, I will continue to give my time and support to others in need because the feeling of knowing that I am helping someone else through their journey in recovery is priceless. Thank you CCAR for being there for me through this rough time in my life. I am forever grateful. God Bless . . .
Kathy James, CCAR Volunteer

In 2005, CCAR made a conscious decision to move to an organizational culture that completely embraced volunteerism. We hired a full-time Volunteer Coordinator, Normajean Cefarelli and she has been instrumental in CCAR's success. After researching many venues, we modeled our VMS after large hospitals including applications, interviews, background checks, job descriptions, training, supervision, and celebration. Early on CCAR encountered some resistance to the idea of performing background checks on our volunteers. People argued that most of the people we work with and who were currently helping out with CCAR had a criminal record so they would be disqualified from volunteering. Management assured that this would not be the case. Long criminal histories could be viewed not as liabilities, but as resumes. We also knew that it was important to protect volunteers from situations that might pose a threat to their safety, public safety, and CCAR's safety. An example would be ensuring that volunteers assigned to working with children at a CCAR event do not have a criminal record involving minors.

Why volunteerism? Simply put, an active volunteer force can generate more positive results than a paid staff could possibly accomplish alone. At CCAR, we focus all our staff efforts on supporting our volunteers. We, then, substantially increase the person-power behind our mission. This also taps into the time-honored recovery principle, "You can't keep it unless you give it away." The table below indicates the growth of the CCAR volunteer system (Fig. 14.1).

Telephone Recovery Support

I have volunteered at CCAR since August 2008 as a Telephone Recovery Support person. I have talked to hundreds of people and have heard as many stories. All the recoverees have been unanimous on two counts about their addiction and CCAR. First, they are in recovery now because they absolutely could NOT live their lives as addicts anymore. They all express the strongest desires to have a quality life that allows them to feel emotions, to care for their children and families, and to lead healthy, productive lives. Second, they look forward to receiving the TRS phone call once a week. Some recoverees have developed special bonds with certain TRS volunteers and others simply like to know that someone out

Volunteer Hours

- In 2005, 90 CCAR Volunteers contributed 3,450 hours
- In 2006, 204 CCAR Volunteers contributed 5,328 hours
- In 2007, 304 CCAR Volunteers contributed 8,078 hours
- In 2008, 276 CCAR Volunteers contributed 13,080 hours

Using the Connecticut Volunteer Rate, the monetary value contributed in each year

- In 2005: $74,870
- In 2006: $155,612
- In 2007: $175,293
- In 2008: $336,797

Fig. 14.1 Growth of the CCAR volunteer system

there cares about them. In my experience, TRS is tantamount to the all-recovery meetings, RCCs, and the social events because it delivers support to the recovery on an intimate, nonjudgmental level.

TRS volunteer

When asked if I find the TRS calls helpful I can't say yes enough. There's something so supportive about knowing that no matter what happens in my life there's someone who genuinely cares about how my recovery is going. My volunteer has shared in every victory I have had in my recovery since the calls began. I hope to continue receiving these calls for a long time to come.

TRS recoveree

Out of all of the commitments I've had – TRS is my favorite way of giving back. Honestly – it's a toss up as to who gets more out of it. . .me or them.

TRS volunteer

When I was using my phone never rang and I wanted it to. I remember just sitting there, staring at the phone wishing someone would call me, talk to me. . .possibly help me. Now I'm in recovery, for me this is the perfect way of giving back. . . being that phone call that I never got.

TRS volunteer

In this CCAR program, a recoveree receives a phone call from a trained CCAR volunteer (usually a person in recovery) once a week for a minimum of 12 weeks to check-in on the recoveree's progress. Recoverees have the option of continuing with the phone calls after the 12 weeks and many of them do. Calls are made in English and Spanish. The average length of enrollment for all participants is just under 20 weeks, with one receiving calls for more than 3 years. When a recoveree moves, CCAR keeps calling: for example, three recoverees are receiving calls while residing in Puerto Rico. Our internet-based phone system allows us to do this without additional cost.

The program also resonates with me personally. I recall that back in the early days of my recovery, I was told to get phone numbers. And get phone numbers I did. I had a book full of them. However, I don't recall being told to actually *use* the numbers. Now, I know this is probably not true, but I do know that it was very difficult for me to pick up the phone, but when someone called me, I would talk and talk and talk. This is proving to be true as CCAR outreaches to those new in recovery.

As of January 2009, CCAR enrolled 1,285 new recoverees into Telephone Recovery Support that were referred by 37 different providers across the state. 45% of the referrals to TRS come from recovery houses through the Recovery Housing Coalition of Connecticut. Intake is simple, one signed form faxed to a main number. The recoveree is called within 24 h. In 2008, CCAR volunteers placed 32,830 outbound calls to recoverees across the state. Of those calls, we talked to someone 9,046 times. This is a number that usually causes me to pause and comment. Connecticut is a small state, so more than 9,000 connections made by our volunteers, makes me wonder about what that infusion of love, concern and care means. And how do you measure something like that? It's like a steady pulse of healing electricity that stimulates recovery.

McKay and colleagues [2] provide documentation for Telephone Recovery Support as an evidence-based practice. Their study showed that telephone-based continuing care, in which an addiction counselor supports patient recovery with 15-min calls once a week, can be as good as or better than face-to-face care at helping most patients maintain abstinence after intensive outpatient treatment (IOP). In another NIDA-funded study [3], the benefits of telephone support were evident nearly 2 years after the last call for all but 20% of patients with severe addiction problems that did not resolve during IOP.

CCAR has also had several instances where the call came at the exact right time. For example, in the 2008 CCAR Annual Report, Kevin Hauschulz, lead Telephone Recovery Support coordinator, reported "One volunteer helped to save one of our recoveree's lives. In this situation, the recoveree said he was having suicidal thoughts, and after conferring with me, the volunteer called Mobile Crisis and told them the situation. After Mobile Crisis, the house manager, and my volunteer talked with the individual, it was determined that this individual needed a higher level of care temporarily. The individual was so grateful that someone actually cared about him, and was very grateful to be a part of Telephone Recovery Support. Subsequent calls to this recoveree have shown him to be in a much better space after a brief hospitalization."

At each of our RCCs, the volunteers have access to a comprehensive book of recovery-related resources. The book contains support meeting listings and phone numbers for all the treatment providers. Beyond those listings, it contains other system related resources including key local contacts from many of the state agencies like the Department of Social Services, Department of Children and Families, Department of Correction, Department of Labor, etc.

Recovery Coaching

Recovery coaching promotes recovery by helping people overcome barriers to their recovery and develop "recovery capital." Recovery coaching is provided primarily by a Recovery Coach, a position within the CCAR VMS. Recovery coaches are trained through a 5-day experiential course at the CCAR Recovery Coach Academy, where they learn to become resource brokers, role models, mentors, motivators and cheerleaders, allies and confidantes, problem solvers and truth tellers, advocates and community organizers, friends and equals [4]. The Academy also trains participants in the basics of behavioral health disorders, crisis intervention, communication skills, motivational enhancement, recovery wellness planning, cultural competency, and recovery ethics. Participants learn about some of the components, core values and guiding principles of recovery; build skills to enhance relationships; discuss co-occurring disorders and medicated assisted recovery, learn the stages of change and their applications, and experience wellness planning.

Recovery coaches work with recoverees to develop a Recovery Wellness Plan designed specifically for the Recovery Coach Academy and based on the work of Calori and Wuelfing. Through working this plan, recoverees develop personal goals in regard to connectedness to the recovery community; physical, emotional health, spiritual health; living conditions, education, employment, and daily living management. They list the steps it will take to reach their goals, people they may need to help them, and timelines for achieving goals. The Recovery Wellness Plan helps recoverees take the next steps in their recovery journey and monitors progress made. It also supports personal responsibility, strengths, and resilience of the recoveree.

CCAR trains more than 100 people annually through the RCA with people from many states attending. CCAR has also taken the RCA to other states. If they are being trained to serve as a CCAR volunteer, participants sign an agreement to give 50 h of service upon completing the course. The RCA provides a classic win–win scenario: volunteers give back through recovery coaching activities and, thereby, and if they are in recovery themselves, reduce their own risk of recidivism. It is not a requirement that you be in recovery in order to be trained as a recovery coach. Recovery coaches interact with new recoverees instilling hope and a desire to strive for something better. CCAR works to have a diverse pool of recovery coaches from which the recoveree may choose. In addition, Spanish-speaking recoverees can connect with Spanish-speaking coaches. We have seen new recoverees come full circle when they attend the RCA and become recovery coaches themselves (Fig. 14.2).

In general, recovery coaches can be placed somewhere along a continuum with case manager at one end and 12-step sponsor at the other, with CCAR recovery coaches falling much closer to the sponsor side. Recovery coaches fulfill many of the case management roles described in the SAMSHA/CSAT Treatment Improvement Protocol (TIP) 27, *Comprehensive Case Management for Substance Abuse Treatment*. In addition to being delivered by people in recovery and therefore qualifying as an additional peer support role, recovery coaching has been suggested and evaluated in relation to individuals with serious mental illnesses by the Yale Program of Recovery and Community Health (PRCH) faculty [1].

CCAR recovery coaches, other volunteers and staff are charged with helping people along their chosen recovery pathway. Besides one-on-one support and

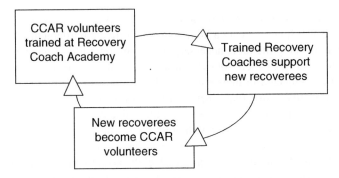

Fig. 14.2 The cycle of recoveree to recovery coach as a function of the RCA

encouragement, they have a variety of other peer-based recovery support services to work with. They help new recoverees make informed choices as to what may work best for them.

One of the functions a recovery coach may take on with a recoveree includes navigating the system. Connecticut has one of the best systems in the USA for treatment of alcohol and other drug addiction. Yet, our system can still be daunting for someone new to it. Many of the CCAR recovery coaches, other volunteers and staff have extensive experience with the system, whether it is as clients or years of advocating for individuals to receive the appropriate treatment. A lot of our success working within the system has been our ability to work with the treatment providers. Early on, there was a notion out there that CCAR would be a competitor with treatment providers for a shrinking pool of money. Our recovery community organization utilizes a tiny percentage of the overall dollars and the value added far exceeds, especially for providers, the dollars allocated. For example, the recovery community has more weight with legislators and policy makers, than treatment providers who are sometimes seen as self-serving. The face and voice of recovery is a powerful influence when telling a story of personal transformation. We have seen time and time again, that when someone introduces themselves as a person in recovery, the audience immediately pays attention. As the story is told, often times, a clinical treatment setting was where this person's recovery was initiated. Discerning providers then see how this advocacy will benefit their work.

Recovery Housing Project

In 2004, following Preliminary meetings and conversations between CCAR staff and the owners of independently owned, privately operated sober houses, it became clear that sober houses filled an important need in Connecticut's treatment/recovery system. Across the state individuals and couples in recovery quietly opened a number of dignified, safe, and sober recovery environments where people, in early recovery as well as those who have a history of recovery, take the time to rebuild their lives. Sober houses create a homelike, supportive environment where people can not only develop the tools necessary to embark on a life of recovery, but also increase the quality of their sobriety in a safe, secure place for people who are committed and engaged in their recovery. These houses have two things in common; first, they make sure that a person who is in recovery lives in a place that is free from alcohol and drug use and second, the residents themselves reinforce their recovery though support from and with other recovering persons. This environment provides a very important support group function. Residents generally are encouraged to live in the home for as long as they feel the need for group support. There is usually an on-site, live-in manager or couple who are in sustained recovery and responsible for the supervision of residents and adherence to the house rules.

Sober houses are self-supporting as rent collected from the housing residents covers operational expenses and provides income to the individuals who own/operate the house. Sober houses often help to provide transportation for persons seeking or going to work, receiving medication, obtaining proper identification papers, etc. These additional supports often are usually offered on an individual, as-needed basis without an additional charge. CCAR determined that a considerable number of these sober houses were operating across the state yet no one knew how many. With funding from the state, CCAR established the Recovery Housing Project that (1) maintains an inventory of all sober housing in the state, (2) staffs the Recovery Housing Coalition of Connecticut, and (3) provides training to those interested in opening sober housing.

At the end of 2009, CCAR has access to 158 houses with 1,474 beds, and makes about 25 referrals to recovery houses weekly (~1,200 annually). With this capability, CCAR has always been able to find people places to live across the state. We operate a website findrecoveryhousing.com where anyone can search our database. The Recovery Housing Coalition has established standards for sober housing that was particularly useful to the state during the ATR years. CCAR delivers four trainings annually, "So, you want to open a recovery house?" So far, we estimate more than 50 new houses have opened as a result of this training.

Recovery-Oriented Employment Services

In 2008, in collaboration with ADRC, a Hartford-based addiction treatment provider, CCAR established Recovery-Oriented Employment Services (ROES). CCAR's role is to deliver comprehensive vocational training incorporating recovery principles, establish a recovery-friendly employer database; and train employers on becoming more recovery friendly. CCAR's in-depth written curriculum helps recoverees build the life skills and attitudes needed to secure employment. Modules include financial basics and time management, employment risks in early recovery, developing a skills inventory and making your cover letter/resume stand-out, internet job searching, work challenges, interview skills, integrating recovery thinking into workplace ethics, and sustaining employment. The ROES curriculum is consistent with the best practices outlined in TIP #38, *Integrating Substance Abuse Treatment and Vocational Services.*

All-Recovery Groups

A peer-led recovery support group is offered in all our RCCs. The idea for the group originally came from communities of recovery in the Willimantic area, where people wanted an open group welcoming recoverees, family members, friends, and allies to talk about their common goal of recovery. These groups, which are well attended, meet several times weekly in each RCC, and all are welcome to attend.

Winners Circle Support Group

Winners Circle is a peer-led, peer-driven support group designed to address the special needs of formerly incarcerated men and women in recovery and their family members, friends, and allies. The only criteria are a desire to participate in one's own healing and recovery, and to aid others' by providing encouragement and support. Winners Circle events, held weekly in each RCC, enable participants to interact in a positive social setting in which they feel free to investigate and develop new life skills.

Family Education and Support

Family Night is an alcohol/drug addiction education and support program for community members, people in recovery, and their families. Recoverees and family members can access information about addiction and recovery and share their experience, strength, and hope through this five-part series.

Recovery Training Series

CCAR hosts a variety of popular workshops, trainings, and conferences to promote recovery and communities of recovery. The following can be scheduled according to need: GED, the Pardons Process; Financial Management; Smoking Cessation; Understanding Addiction and Recovery; Relationships in Recovery; Nutrition and

Recovery; 12 steps and religion; Women in Recovery through Enhanced Design (WIRED); Yoga; "Our Stories Have Power" from FAVOR; Hepatitis C Information and Education; and Double Trouble: 12 Steps Meetings for Co-occurring Disorders.

Peer-Led Recovery Social Activities

The recovery community knows the importance of hosting alcohol and drug free social events to maintain and sustain recovery. CCAR activities include comedy nights, open mike nights, spaghetti dinners, super bowl parties, and holiday parties. CCAR recoverees have the opportunity to attend events where they will see that people do have fun in recovery and to help plan and implement them.

Integrating CCAR Activities with Addiction Treatment

CCAR has excellent relationships with a vast majority of the addiction treatment providers in Connecticut. In fact, 57 different providers referred people to our Telephone Recovery Support service. Five of nine Board members work in a clinical addiction treatment setting. CCAR bridges the gap between treatment and sustained recovery. Often, insurance will provide several days of detox and then refer clients to a "partial hospital program" in which they attend Monday–Friday for about 5 h of counseling and groups. After a few weeks, this drops to "outpatient" which consists of several days a week for up to 3 h. The 28 day or longer programs are dwindling with the high cost of inpatient stays unless the individual has the resources to pay privately. Most cannot afford the $1,000 or more per day stays for these programs. CCAR has worked to develop solid relationships with most treatment providers in Connecticut and they refer clients to us for recovery support knowing that detox or treatment is just a beginning. CCAR staff also make regular presentations at treatment programs, sober houses, residential programs, half way houses, and homeless shelters educating both staff and recoverees of the recovery support services we offer. Many are enrolled into Telephone Recovery Support while still in treatment so they can begin receiving phone calls immediately upon discharge. The Recovery Support Services offered by CCAR are not a substitute for clinical treatment but an adjunct. In some cases, recoverees have not received treatment and use the recovery support offered by CCAR to sustain their recovery. Long-term recovery must be accomplished while facing the everyday challenges of work, relationships, family, with recoverees learning how to handle these daily stresses without turning to alcohol or other drugs. CCAR provides some of these tools for as long as recoverees need them, free of charge. People in recovery know we must give it away. . .in order to keep it.

Key Points

1. This may seem simplistic, but many miss this point: the first step in forming a recovery community organization is organizing the recovery community.
2. Listen to the people you serve. Listen.
3. The organizational culture of a successful recovery community organization is one of service and volunteerism.
4. Telephone Recovery Support is a thriving example of "Keeping It Simple."
5. Recovery coaching meets many needs of the person (and family) new to recovery and the demand for this service will only continue to grow.
6. Honesty, integrity, and transparency above all things.
7. Err on the side of the recoveree and generosity.
8. Focus on the recovery potential, not the pathology.
9. Hope is the spark that ignites the recovery process. Transmit hope in all you do.
10. Lead by example – expressions of love and kindness will foster an organizational culture of recovery and service.

References

1. Davidson L, Tondora JS, Staeheli MR, O'Connell MJ, Frey J, Chinman MJ. Recovery guides: an emerging model of community-based care for adults with psychiatric disabilities. In: Lightburn A, Sessions P, editors. Community based clinical practice. London: Oxford University Press; 2006. p. 476–501.
2. McKay J, Lynch K, Shepard D, Morgenstern J, Forman R, Pettinati H. Do patient characteristics and initial progress in treatment moderate the effectiveness of telephone-based continuing care for substance use disorders? Addiction. 2005;100(2):216–26.
3. McKay JR, Lynch KG, Shepard DS, Pettinati HM. The effectiveness of telephone-based continuing care for alcohol and cocaine dependence. Arch Gen Psychiatry. 2005;62(2):199–207.
4. White W. Recovery coaching: A lost function of addiction counseling? Counselor. 2004;5(6):20–2. http://www.williamwhitepapers.com/pr/2004. Retrieved Jan 2010.

Chapter 15
The Physician Health Program: A Replicable Model of Sustained Recovery Management

Gregory E. Skipper and Robert L. DuPont

Abstract Physician Health Programs (PHPs) in the USA have evolved over the past 3 decades as models of recovery management. They encourage early referral, sophisticated evaluation, and active long-term monitoring and care management of troubled physicians, especially those with substance related disorders. There are many benefits to these unique programs. Early detection of potentially impaired physicians not only protects patients but also saves physicians' careers. Additionally, when addressing these problems clinically, rather than awaiting a crisis necessitating disciplinary action, complex and prolonged legal battles are avoided. PHPs safeguard both patients and physicians, and in the process they have developed one of the most successful models of recovery management.

The strongest incentive for early referral is the opportunity for confidential care and advocacy for physicians who cooperate with their PHPs. PHPs have proven successful with reports of 5-year abstinence rates of 79%, return to work rates of 96%, and virtually no evidence of risk or harm to patients from participating physicians.

Can the principles used by PHPs be transferred for use by other patients? Compared to other patients with addictions, physicians are an affluent and usually highly motivated group; however, there is evidence that their addictions are as severe as or worse as those of the general population. Certainly their access to drugs of abuse is greater than the general population. Many elements of PHP care management can be transferred, in whole or in part, to others offering the promise of substantial improvements in long-term outcomes.

Keywords Addiction recovery management · Physician Health Programs · Abstinence-based recovery · Physicians · Alcoholics anonymous

G.E. Skipper (✉)
Alabama Physician Health Program (Medical Director),
Medical Association of the State of Alabama,
19 S. Jackson St, Montgomery, AL 36104, USA
e-mail: gregory.skipper@gmail.com

J.F. Kelly and W.L. White (eds.), *Addiction Recovery Management: Theory, Research and Practice*, Current Clinical Psychiatry, DOI 10.1007/978-1-60327-960-4_15,
© Springer Science+Business Media, LLC 2011

The PHP Concept and Its Applicability to the General Population

PHPs in the USA evolved over the past 3 decades under the authority of medical licensing boards, with the sustained support of the American Medical Association (AMA), to encourage early referral and long-term intensive management of behaviorally impaired physicians. Although the initial focus of PHPs was solely on alcohol and other substance use disorders, in recent years their focus has expanded to include a wide range of potentially impairing physical and mental disorders. The overriding PHP concept is to promote early detection and referral of treatable disorders that often cause impairment. This usually includes substance-related disorders and psychiatric disorders, but increasingly includes degenerative physical or neurologic diseases, disruptive behavior, and professional sexual misconduct. The motivation for early referral is greatly enhanced when PHPs offer confidentiality. In this chapter, we focus on the concepts developed by PHPs for care management of substance use disorders.

The state PHPs grew out of the earliest Employee Assistance Program model of work-related alcohol and substance use problems with the twin goals of saving physicians' careers, and also protecting the public and the public's confidence in their physicians. PHPs have a high expectation for successful abstinence-based recovery and have developed their programs to help physician participants achieve this goal. From the beginning, these programs have been led by a remarkable group of highly dedicated physicians, many of whom were themselves in recovery from serious substance abuse disorders. These program leaders networked together as the programs evolved to create a unique care management system. A parallel evolution took place with commercial airline pilots, supported and encouraged by the Federal Aviation Administration. This program, the Human Intervention Motivation Study (HIMS) [1], has similar dual objectives – saving pilots' careers, and protecting the public and the public's trust in their pilots.

Today the nation's PHPs provide a remarkable model of actively and intensively managing the care of recovering physicians over extended periods. They treat addictions as long-term chronic disorders. The PHPs evolved entirely empirically, without theoretical foundation, adopting policies that worked and discarding those that did not, over decades. In this process, they have set a new and far higher standard for outcomes. Our hope is that examining PHPs and their approach can provide inspiration and direction for the improvement of the treatment of all people suffering from substance use disorders.

The primary assumption on which medical licensing boards base their support for PHPs is that the early detection of, and active long-term management of, potentially impairing behavioral problems in physicians protects patients. Additionally, when substance abuse problems are addressed clinically, rather than awaiting a crisis necessitating disciplinary action, complex, expensive, and prolonged legal battles are avoided, intervention occurs more rapidly and careers and lives are preserved.

Physician Health Programs (PHPs) today are endorsed by medical licensing boards and without their support the task of PHPs would be more difficult, if not impossible. Based on experience now extending over 3 decades, medical licensing boards have recognized that PHPs can often act more rapidly to recommend discontinuation of practice and entry into a definitive evaluation, and when needed treatment and monitoring, because unlike boards, PHPs are not constrained by due process and other legal impediments to action. Regulatory boards, as legal entities, are usually required to conduct an investigation, develop a case, give notices, conduct due process and judicial hearings, and allow appeals. This process regularly takes months or even years to resolve. In contrast, PHPs only need credible symptoms (and not probable cause) to recommend discontinuation of practice and thorough evaluation. PHPs can only recommend because they have no direct authority over licensure. However, in most cases, physicians comply with PHP recommendations to avoid the risk of formal notification of the board. PHPs, in contrast to board action, can often have a physician in treatment the very day of initial referral. The public is well served and protected when PHP services are readily available.

It is not surprising that controversy has arisen in some states regarding the role of PHPs. In 2008, the California Medical Board discontinued the PHP (called the California Diversion Program). This was the result of media-fanned public controversy over the potential for substance abusing physicians to cause harm to patients. In California, this concern was vocally raised by an attorney representing a citizen's advocacy group. As in California, in 2008, the media periodically highlight unusual cases where addicted physicians cause patients harm. In most cases, however, the harm to patients caused by addicted physicians occurred prior to referral to PHP care. There are few recorded cases of patient harm following referral for PHP care. Nevertheless, the stigma of addiction and the sensationalism of the media combine, in the case of addicted health professionals, to create a volatile opportunity for headlines, such as "Doctors on Drugs." It is ironic that PHPs are attacked for "hiding the addicted physicians" when the very process of early detection, based on confidential referral, is essential to protecting the public because it encourages early intervention and continued participation of physicians eager to protect their ability to practice medicine.

Most PHPs do not provide direct treatment services themselves. Instead they oversee and manage care, utilizing carefully selected existing local and national evaluation and treatment resources. PHPs have refined the art and application of recovery management. In essence, PHPs have developed a primary care paradigm for substance-use disorders, one where early detection is encouraged, nonconfrontational interventions are performed with dignity and care, thorough evaluation and treatment are obtained, and long-term monitoring with contingency management are carried out. The concept is elegantly simple even if the execution is often complex. This concept mirrors the traditional success of primary care management for general health disorders, a phenomenon that has been surprisingly lacking in the mental health field. PHP care and monitoring are a successful example of the management of addictions as chronic illnesses.

PHPs encourage early referral through active, widespread education of physicians and of health care institutions regarding the opportunity and importance of confidential reporting. Colleagues who are unwilling to "snitch" on a colleague to the licensing board are willing to refer a colleague for confidential medical care. After physicians are referred because of concern over possible substance use disorders, intervention to formal, usually in-patient, evaluation rapidly follows. At the completion of the evaluation, when appropriate, treatment and long-term contingency monitoring are begun. Throughout this process co-occurring disorders are identified and treated. If relapses occur, the most frequent response is renewed evaluation and intensified treatment and monitoring. In cases where relapse is associated with an active risk to patients, most PHPs immediately report the participant to the licensing board. Overall, PHPs have proven successful with reports of 5-year abstinence rates for substance-use disorders of 79%, return to work rates of 96%, and little or no evidence of serious risk or harm to patients [2].

Many aspects of PHP care relate to subtle issues, such as the dedication and sense of mission of the PHP staff, who defy facile description. There are many variations from one PHP to another, but there is also a core system and strategy that we are describing here. The basic transaction of the PHP with the physician participant is that the PHPs offer physicians confidential support in dealing with threats to their license in return for the physicians' commitment to adhere to the agreed upon treatment and monitoring. In order for the public to be protected, however, there must also be a limit to confidentiality, usually worked out in detail between the PHP and the licensing board. In some cases, all relapses are reported and in others, the PHP only reports the physician who becomes a danger to patients (most relapses occur outside the context of patient care, e.g., drinking beer during a party over a weekend). In any case, relapses are dealt with in a decisive manner. The conditions of the physicians' relationships with the PHP are clearly detailed in simple language in an agreement between the PHP and the physician and signed by both. These agreements, based on recommendations from evaluation and treatment providers, detail each participant's individualized, highly specific treatment and monitoring plan.

In this process, PHPs set a uniquely high standard, absolute abstinence from any use alcohol or other drug of abuse for the entire duration of their care and monitoring, typically lasting 5 years or longer. Any unauthorized use of alcohol or other drugs is considered a relapse and is taken very seriously. Many programs even consider behaviors in violation of agreements (i.e., failure to attend required meetings or dishonesty), short of actual drug use also a relapse.

Whether for initial evaluation or reevaluation, PHPs usually utilize highly qualified evaluation programs for assessments, often on a residential basis, not only to identify any substance abuse problem but also to identify co-occurring disorders that might complicate treatment or decrease chances of successful outcome. As a result of in-depth evaluation, an active treatment plan is developed to address each and every one of the identified problems. The PHPs use the highest level of evaluation and treatment available, allowing participating physician patients to choose only from among a small group of providers approved by the PHP, providers who are well known to the PHP for their outstanding work. The quality of these providers is enhanced as they compete for referrals because of the prestige of being selected by PHPs as one of the best providers of treatment and monitoring.

The contrast between this form of care and that received by the general public is profound. Most patients treated for addictions do not receive adequate independent evaluations to carefully identify co-occurring disorders. Most patients also do not receive a comprehensive and customized treatment plan. In fact, whether abstinence-based treatment is attempted at all, especially with regards to opioid addiction, depends greatly on the services the patients select rather than a medical recommendation based on evaluation. Often the choice of treatment modality is governed more by accident or geography than by the addicted patients' needs. In the world of substance abuse treatment for the average person, it is sad to note that the standard of care is not high. In fact, there is a national cynicism and self-fulfilling negative prophecy regarding poor outcomes for most abstinence-based treatment. Routine random drug testing is almost nonexistent in treatment outside PHPs. Most substance abuse treatment is brief. Aftercare, such as it is, is almost always voluntary and seldom prolonged, if it exists at all. Few patients have the benefit of ongoing testing or contingency management. Can anyone wonder why substance abuse treatment outcomes are poor?

While not related to the evolution of the PHP model, an important but largely obscure body of academic literature has emerged regarding "contingency management." Typically these experiments use small positive rewards (i.e., an allowance, a chance to participate in a raffle or enhanced driving or in pharmaco-therapy take-home privileges) for negative drug tests. When patients fail, there are negative rewards (i.e., forfeiture of privileges or fines). The results of these research-based contingency management studies have been strikingly positive even with these modest, even trivial, rewards and punishments [3]. This growing body of academic knowledge regarding contingency management lends credence to the idea that PHP-type care could be applied widely in substance abuse treatment

Cost is an important consideration when thinking about extending the PHP model more widely. The cost of running a PHP on average is $2,300 per year per monitored participant; however, since most PHPs are subsidized by their licensing boards, the costs are shared by all licensed physicians. This cost per licensed physician averages $23 per year, not an excessive cost when one considers the considerable benefits.

The bottom line is that components of these highly successful programs for airline pilots, attorneys, and other health professionals should be more widely used for all patients with substance-use disorders.

History of PHPs

Physicians have a long and colorful history of substance abuse in America. Addiction touched the lives of some of the nation's most prominent practitioners, including Dr. William Halsted (1852–1922), the father of modern surgery, who was addicted to cocaine and morphine. One of the cofounders of Alcoholics Anonymous (1935) was a physician, Dr. Robert (Bob) Smith, a proctologist. An organization of recovering physicians, the International Doctors in A.A. (IDAA), was founded in 1949 by Dr. Clarence Pearson and has continued to thrive. Recovering doctors continue to play an important role in the development of the broader field of addiction medicine.

PHPs began to emerge in the late 1970s in response to two primary factors. (1) Medical regulatory licensing boards had begun to investigate complaints of all types, including those related to suspected substance abuse, from the public (leading to a heightened necessity to deal with problem doctors). Prior to that time, boards had assumed the role of confirming that doctors had graduated from medical school and/or, beginning in the 1950s, that they had passed the required tests (national boards) to ensure adequate knowledge-base prior to licensure. It was not until the 1970s, however, that regulatory boards generally began accepting the role of "policing" the profession. Once this began, it became clear that exclusive reliance on disciplinary action was not the best approach to illness [4]. (2) In 1973, the Journal of the American Medical Association (JAMA) published the seminal paper "The Sick Physician. Impairment by psychiatric disorders, including alcoholism and drug dependence" and the AMA actively began to encourage the development of PHPs to address the need for early detection and treatment of troubled doctors [5].

The AMA held its first conference on physician health in 1975 and has continued every 18 months since. State medical societies began to organize volunteer committees on physician "impairment" and this momentum eventually coalesced with support from regulatory boards, and the result was the state-by-state emergence of professional PHPs. Currently, all but four states in the USA have formal PHPs, ranging in size from one employee and a $20,000 budget to a 1.5 million dollar budget and 19 full-time employees [6]. It is estimated that over 9,000 physicians are now in PHP monitoring in the USA [7].

During the time of their development, from the late 1970s and continuing to the present, several trends can be observed. (1) An initial focus on substance abuse disorders gradually broadened to other psychiatric disorders, disruptive behavior, professional boundary issues, physical disabilities, and cognitive disorders. Most PHPs have evolved to recognize their role as addressing any remedial impairment-related disorder. (2) An initial focus on physicians has gradually broadened so that most PHPs work with other health care professionals (dentists, veterinarians, pharmacists, etc.). (3) The Federation of State Physician Health Programs emerged in the early 1990s to provide encouragement sharing of ideas, support, and refinement of approaches to education, interventions, sources for evaluation and treatment, and methods of monitoring for PHPs.

Care Management

"Care management" is the term used to describe the process utilized by PHPs. Care management represents a dynamic combination of ambitious and sustained empathy and case management. Research in the mental health field has shown that these are the two most important determinants of best outcomes for the treatment of complex mental health disorders: case management, and the presence of a "positive relationship between the participant and a primary healthcare provider." When these two are present, chances for successful outcomes are maximized.

Just as a "case manager" oversees and supports the patient throughout the process of treatment, the PHP oversees and supports the patient throughout the entire course of their recovery, from evaluation, through treatment, and then as an intensive and supportive monitor for years into recovery. During the monitoring phase, if the patient shows laxity or irregularity in his or her recovery activities that might lead to relapse, the PHP initiates an intervention to correct the behavior and/or move the patient toward reevaluation and possible further treatment.

The PHP coordinates the entire process, consulting experts and key service providers, as well as with family members and workplace associates of participating physicians, to ensure that the plan is developed appropriately and monitored to achieve optimal outcomes. The PHP also helps obtain the best specialist services, during and following treatment, to address particular needs of the participant. This care management approach promotes participants use of skilled services to deal with complex and multiple needs from a range of service providers. The goal of care management is to achieve seamless competent service delivery.

Care management ensures service provision that is participant rather than organizationally driven. PHPs serve as a resource, coordinating specialized activities that flow from the particular setting and evaluation or treatment program, while building a genuine trusting but accountable relationship with the participant. PHPs directly provide the following core services: screening, assessment/risk management, care planning, implementing service arrangement, monitoring/evaluation, and advocacy. This care management is clearly contrasted with typical managed care, which seeks to minimize costs. In PHP care management, the primary effort is to promote the best long-term outcome, not to achieve the lowest cost.

For these processes to be effective, policies must be developed and the PHP supervised, optimally by an oversight committee. Policies, to which the PHP staff adhere, provide a framework to set limits on participants' behavior. The committee that oversees the program and policies provides important backup and support for the PHP.

The PHP Model

Modern PHPs typically provide a range of services including (1) educational programs that promote early referral, (2) professional intervention services, (3) referral to formal evaluation, (4) referral to formal treatment, and (5) long-term monitoring.

Educational programs: Educational programs provide an excellent opportunity to encourage early referral by emphasizing the confidential clinical nature of the programs and for the PHP staff to become known and trusted. In these meetings, the PHP staff explain who, how, and when to refer physicians with possible behavioral problems, including substance use disorders. Early referral of physicians with substance use problems before actual impairment and patient harm occurs is the goal. Providing copious education to every willing hospital, medical group, county medical society, etc. is an excellent way to spread the word about the PHP program.

Professional intervention services. When a physician is referred to a PHP, a preliminary assessment is performed to verify that the referral is legitimate and appropriate. Illegitimate referrals are rare but can occur from disgruntled spouses or political enemies. Once a referral is deemed legitimate a professional intervention is conducted, often within hours of initial referral. It is of note that interventions utilized by PHPs are not similar to the Johnson-model interventions performed by groups. PHP staff have perfected the art of professional intervention. A professional intervention is simply one in which physicians are presented with information about the PHP, the fact that concerns have been raised about their behavior, the concerns appear legitimate (even if not accurate), and a formal evaluation is strongly recommended to determine if a real problem exists. PHP procedures and policies provide protection and advocacy for the physician, if the physician voluntarily follows the PHP's recommendations.

Referral to formal evaluation. PHP policies usually specify that a formal evaluation at an authorized evaluation site is the next step. Most PHPs provide a list of authorized sites that have been screened and meet criteria established by the PHP to conduct evaluations. If the evaluation fails to identify a problem, this fact can be used to exonerate the physician by the PHP and to squelch the original complaint – a situation that while rare does occur thus validating the PHP evaluation process. Whatever the outcome of the evaluation, the PHP assists the physician by documenting the findings. Many PHPs actually participate in the "end of evaluation" summary, often by conference call. During this summary, the evaluating programs present their findings. The PHP staff can then answer questions for participants regarding their options, consequences for noncompliance, where to continue treatment, etc. Participants are always given options and are always treated with respect and dignity.

Referral to formal treatment. PHPs assure that physicians receive credible care by referring them to competent patient-oriented treatment centers. Most PHPs maintain criteria for placing evaluation and treatment programs on their "authorized" lists. Participants are allowed to choose among the options. Participants are given, usually in writing, a limited time in which to make their decisions regarding entering treatment. Once treatment begins, treatment centers are asked to provide regular, at least weekly, updates so that PHP staff can be involved in the treatment process. PHP staff often communicate with the workplace (where the participant is expected to return following treatment), the participants' families, and others.

Long-term monitoring. PHPs conduct long-term monitoring, utilizing random drug testing, reports from a worksite monitor, group attendance with the documentation of attendance, and other recovery oriented activities. The benefits of long--term monitoring are numerous including the ability of the PHP to advocate on behalf of the participant. This becomes a positive experience, when the PHP can document proof of recovery and applaud the recovering doctor for their success.

Key Ingredients

Studies have yet to be conducted that definitively isolate the most potent ingredients of PHP care management; however, we have identified eight practices that addiction counselors and the treatment programs could incorporate into their own work.

Find a motivational fulcrum. The PHP utilizes a crisis-induced window of opportunity to transition those they serve from the experience of pain to the experience of hope. The common message is, "You are in a bind. We can help you now because we represent a legitimate process and a group of physicians who have escaped the very pain that you are now experiencing." The PHP intervention focuses on the arena in which the physician's identity is most enmeshed, the status-imbued practice of medicine and the potential loss of identity, income and social standing that would follow license revocation. Even where contact with the PHP is voluntary, these potential realities remain an omnipresent subtheme of the assistance process. What counselors can take from this is the importance of contingency management, i.e., linking recovery to meaningful positive rewards and relapse to negative consequences that are serious and likely to be imposed. Establishment of a behavioral contingency agreement, on paper, clearly identifying required aftercare activities and a commitment to regular drug testing – a tangible measure of sobriety and of relapse. This reinforces important mediums of continued recovery and provides a source of support and remotivation, which is especially important during early recovery. The stakes involved in this contingency are best, if they are specific and serious, for example, loss/retention of intimate relationship, job/career, children, freedom, or privileges. Counselor folklore is replete with admonitions that no one can get sober except for themselves, but lighting the sobriety fire requires kindling and a source of ignition that is specific to each patient. Contingency management techniques are becoming more widely accepted and their effectiveness is well documented [2].

Provide comprehensive assessment and treatment. Another key component used effectively by PHPs is the provision of comprehensive formal evaluation and high-quality treatment that addresses the full scope of identified problems. What the mainstream substance abuse treatment system can take from this is the need to provide patient-oriented treatment rather than having a fixed program to which patients must adapt. What distinguishes the settings in which doctors are treated from the most common forms of substance abuse treatment is not that the treatment for physicians is more expensive (a factor that does not always translate to better quality), but that it is far more intensive and comprehensive, e.g., more likely to be prolonged (if needed) and to include concurrent psychiatric evaluation and treatment plus rigorous family programs and treatment of any other problematic condition (i.e., chronic pain, sexual disorders, etc.) [8].

Provide the care management oversight role. PHPs oversee and guide care, utilizing well-established best providers. PHPs create structure and accountability. The role of the PHP is similar to that of the coordinating role of a primary care physician who helps to select specialists and other resources, acting as a guide through the complex maze of healthcare. Likewise, PHPs direct care for troubled physicians, helping them to select appropriate resources and conducting long-term monitoring. Similar long-term oversight, coaching, directing, and monitoring could be provided for all patients.

Have a high expectation for abstinence-based recovery. PHPs expect each physician participant to maintain lifelong abstinence from alcohol and drugs. Relapses are seen as temporary setbacks or learning experiences. Reevaluation and, commonly, further treatment are constructive responses that reinforce the goal of long-term recovery. The goal is to set physicians up for success – both in their recovery and their practices. This approach can inspire higher expectations for success for all substance abuse patients. Good care management involves continued pursuit of whatever treatments or changes in care are necessary for long-term recovery.

Assertively link to recovery support groups. PHPs rely on active (linkage to a particular person/group/meeting) rather than passive (verbal encouragement for participation) referrals to 12 step and other recovery-focused mutual aid groups. They also link each member to professionally directed group therapy with other physicians in recovery and monitor physician attendance at such meetings. The PHP encourages participation in peer-based recovery support groups, e.g., Caduceus Meetings or International Doctors in Alcoholics Anonymous. The goal is to link each individual participant with people who will reinforce their identity as a recovering physician and to lead these same individuals into sustained relationship with the larger recovery community.

Sustain monitoring and support and, when necessary, reintervene. Posttreatment monitoring and support enhance long-term recovery outcomes [9]. PHPs are unique in the length of time they monitor and support persons in recovery. The monitoring function involves periodic interviews as well as random urine and hair testing for 5 years or longer. PHP staff members respond immediately and vigorously to any positive drug screen with an appropriate level of reevaluation, encouragement to seek further treatment if needed, and the ever present potential, if warranted, of referral to the licensing board if recommendations are not followed. Every participating physician knows that referral to the licensing board could result in loss of license.

This high level of surveillance and support does not eliminate relapse. Studies reveal that up to 25% of physicians in PHPs experience at least one relapse [10]. Nevertheless, the results of PHP care management set the standard for low levels of relapses over very long periods of time. With active monitoring and reinterventions, most participating physicians eventually establish stable recovery, thus avoiding posing threats to the safety of their patients, and retaining their licenses to practice medicine. Active and sustained monitoring insures early identification of relapses, which in PHPs typically lead to increased support and reintervention. This may be the component that most distinguishes PHPs from many mainstream addiction treatment programs, other employee assistance programs, drug court and other criminal justice programs, and intervention programs in the child welfare system, none of which offer this high level of prompt rigorous and enduring monitoring and support.

Reintervene at a higher level of intensity. Another distinguishing feature of PHPs is that relapse and reintervention are followed by reevaluation and the possibility of more intensive, prolonged, and specialized treatment rather than a readmission and replication of the same treatment that was provided earlier. This blend of support and accountability, alliance and toughness distinguishes PHPs from other interventions that seek but too often fall short of creating and sustaining these important ingredients.

Integrate these elements, where possible, within a comprehensive program. Many persons achieving successful recovery experience elements of what we have described here, but the PHPs are distinguished by their inclusion of these elements within an integrated and long-sustained program. The level of cohesion and coordination that comes from such integration may itself contribute to the PHP's high, long-term recovery rates. The best drug courts and the more innovative programs in the child welfare system share similar direction and integration but seldom have the intensity or duration that is typical of PHP care management. Where such elements are lacking, counselors could better serve their clients by providing the leadership within a multiagency intervention model that utilizes an integrated service plan and contains the potent ingredients that are common in PHP care.

Summary of Results of a National Study of PHPs

In 2006, the first national study of PHPs was conducted in two phases with the active support and participation of the Federation of State Physicians Health Programs (FSPHP). Phase I consisted of a survey to identify which states had functioning PHPs and to explore their structure and function. Phase II was an assessment of outcomes utilizing record reviews of participants who had been in the PHP 5 years or more. Results of this study are summarized.

Phase I

Each state and the District of Colombia were surveyed identifying 49 PHPs. Nebraska and North Dakota had none. Georgia was excluded from analysis, as its PHP was essentially nonexistent (three participants) and was not officially recognized by its board. Of the resulting 48 possible states, 42 (86%) participated in the Phase I survey.[1]

---

[1]Since 2006, two additional states have lost their PHPs, California and Wisconsin.

One hundred percent of respondents claimed to have a defined relationship with their regulatory boards and most were primarily funded by the regulatory boards (average funding from boards for all PHPs was 50%). Other sources of funding included participant fees, hospitals, medical association or societies, etc. The majority of PHPs (54%) were setup as nonprofit foundations and the remainder were either run within the state medical association (35%) or were part of the regulatory board (13%).

Seventy-six percent of programs maintained a list of authorized evaluation and treatment providers and 48% based this list on specific written criteria. Ninety-five percent of programs required weekly updates from treatment providers. There is little doubt that evaluation and treatment programs actively compete for this PHP business, which may stimulate a healthy competition that could improve the quality of care offered by these programs. All but one PHP required a 5-year monitoring agreement for substance use disorders. The most common components of care specified in monitoring agreements were 12-step group attendance (95%), worksite monitor (71%), and drug testing (100%). There were numerous other commonly offered components of care including group therapy, aftercare, individual therapy, monitoring physician, visits with the PHP staff, etc.

Regarding drug testing, urine is the most common matrix tested; however, hair, breath, and saliva are also utilized occasionally, and there is a growing trend to increase the use of these alternatives to urine testing. The panel most often performed was a 20+ drug health professional drug panel, in contrast to the five-drug (or less) panel commonly used in most monitoring programs. The average participant received weekly random drug testing for the first 6 to 12 months followed by once or twice per month for the remainder of the agreement. The testing was random, meaning that typically every day of the work week the physician participants called a phone number to see if that day they needed to submit a sample for testing. Even if they had been tested the day before, they could be tested next. The frequency of testing varied over time, depending on the physicians' performance, but the random testing continued throughout the extended period of PHP care. Testing was not only for drugs of abuse but also for alcohol use. If problems emerged, frequency of random testing was substantially increased. All agreements included total abstinence, including alcohol abstinence, and 61% of programs routinely used ethylglucuronide (EtG) testing to better detect alcohol use.

Phase II

Phase II of this national study of the state PHPs involved reviews of PHP participant records of physicians who had signed monitoring contracts 5 years prior to when the study began. Sixteen state PHPs participated in this phase of the study and 904 records were reviewed.

Most of the agreements of the 904 subjects were for substance dependence (88%). The remainder was for substance abuse. The most common primary substance of abuse was alcohol (50%), followed by opioids (36%), and stimulants (8%). The remainder included marijuana, sedatives, and hallucinogens. Fourteen percent of physicians admitted intravenous drug use, 17% had been arrested (mostly for driving while intoxicated, DWI), and 9% had been convicted of a crime related to the substance use.

Regarding various specialties, anesthesiology, emergency medicine, psychiatry, and family practice were overrepresented compared to what was expected from their relative prevalence among all physicians. Pediatrics, surgery, and pathology were underrepresented. The most common source of referrals were the regulatory boards (22%), a hospital (18%), self-referral with coercion (14%), a colleague outside the hospital (14%), self-referral without apparent coercion (11%), or a substance abuse treatment center (7%). All these physicians faced serious problems that they considered would jeopardize their practice of medicine.

Evaluations on the 904 physicians were usually conducted by an independent approved evaluator (55%), and to a lesser extent by PHP staff (16%), or unapproved outside evaluators (13%). Treatment was exclusively abstinence oriented utilizing the 12-step approach. The majority of initial treatment was residential or day treatment (78%) and the remainder was intensive outpatient (22%). Only one participant of the 904 was placed on methadone and that participant was not practicing medicine at the time of the study, even though opioids were the primary drug of abuse for over 300 of the participating physicians, roughly half of whom used opioids intravenously. Naltrexone was used by 6% of participants and antidepressants were taken by 32%.

Outcomes were measured in several ways. *Program completion*: Sixty-four percent of participants completed 5 years of monitoring without incident. Sixteen percent were retained in the program following difficulty (usually a relapse – see below) and 19% failed to complete "this episode" of PHP care. Of this final group who failed to complete, 55% retired, 31% did not complete because their license was revoked, and 14% died (6 by suicide). *Licensure*: 72% of the 904 participants were actively practicing at the time of the follow-up study and only 4% of the total had their licenses revoked at the time of the study. The remainder were either inactive (possibly due to moving out of state), retired, or practicing while on probation. *Relapses*: 22% had some type of substance use relapse; 16% of participants had a relapse that did not involve patient care; and 6% of participants had a relapse that, in the context of practice, could have put patients at risk. Despite this, there was only one noted episode where a patient was harmed and that involved inappropriate prescribing. *Drug tests*: The 793 physicians with known outcomes and available drug test results were separated into three groups based on the number of positive tests they had during their entire period of PHP monitoring. Six hundred and twenty-three or 79% of these physicians had no positive tests for any drug or alcohol during their monitoring. One hundred and eleven or 14% had only one positive test for drugs or alcohol. The remaining 59 physicians – 7% of this group – had more than one positive test during their monitoring, with a mean of 3.3 positive tests for this group. Of the 67.652 tests given to this group, 308 were positive (0.46%) or about one in 200 tests. The average number of random drug and alcohol tests per physician participant was 85. There were no significant differences among the three groups on demographic variables or primary drug of abuse, but there was a significant difference in the outcome of their PHP care. In the large group with no positive tests, 16% failed to complete their care successfully compared to 24% of the physicians with one positive test and 45% of the physicians who had more than one positive test for alcohol or drugs. We believe that these drug test results are without equal in any clinical sample of substance abusers in terms of the intensity, comprehensiveness of the testing (many drugs plus alcohol), and results of the tests. In fact, there are few records of populations without any known drug problems who have such a low positive test rate (0.46%) with similarly comprehensive testing (cite our LTE in process).

Wider Applicability of the PHP System of Care Management

The most obvious application of the PHP model is in other workplace settings where employees have a high motivation to retain their jobs and where the employer has a high motivation to keep the employee. Unlike physicians, some employees are not valued highly. Other employees are so highly accomplished in their field that they can simply and easily move to a new job. For physicians, this is far more difficult because licensing is tracked by a National Practitioner Databank, designed to prevent physicians from "escaping" their transgressions by moving. Few physicians have the option of leaving the practice of medicine and replacing their lost income and the lost nonmonetary rewards they reap from their medical practices. Nevertheless, when there are employment situations where the motivations to retain the job and the employee are high, then the conditions are similar to that with physicians.

Contingency management studies have shown that even tiny positive and negative reinforcements linked to drug testing make a dramatic difference in outcomes. Therefore, PHP concepts, tied to tight monitoring of compliance including random drug testing, can be built upon minor positive and negative consequences that can almost always be found, if sought, with any patient.

One group of patients that deserve special mention are those in the community under the supervision of the criminal justice system, including drug courts. While this population of substance abusers could hardly be more different from physicians, a similar system of care management has evolved in some locations. A program called HOPE Probation (Hawaii's Opportunity Probation with Enforcement) in Honolulu has produced similar outstanding long-term outcomes. This program uses similar intensive random monitoring linked to swift, certain but not severe sanctions, in this case a few days in jail.

Early research results that compare 6-month follow-up data to 3-month baseline data show that HOPE participants have better outcomes than regular probationers reporting fewer arrests, probation revocations, and missed probation appointments [11]. HOPE participants in a specialized unit showed a 91% reduction in positive drug tests and an 85% reduction in missed appointments, while non-HOPE offenders in the same specialized unit showed no improvement on drug test results and a 23% increase in missed appointments. Under general probation without HOPE, 36% of offenders tested positive on drug tests compared to only 11% of HOPE participants. Rates of general arrests for HOPE participants were 34% lower than for nonparticipants. Additionally, rates of nontechnical violations for HOPE participants were 111% lower.

A similar program has emerged to deal with DWI offenders in South Dakota. In this innovative program, the 24/7 Sobriety Project, in which, instead of offenders being required to simply refrain from driving after drinking, they are required to refrain from any alcohol or drug use. This program, like HOPE Probation, relies on intensive testing linked to swift, certain, but mild consequences (brief jail time) to produce remarkable results. Unlike many programs, 24/7 utilizes specific drug tests based on geography to enhance results. Offenders may be subject to twice daily urine testing at their local sheriff's office or, if in rural areas of South Dakota, they may be subject to ankle bracelet monitoring 24 h a day.

In a pilot study of over 1,000 DUI offenders in which participants were drug tested for an average of over 100 days, two-thirds were 100% compliant and drug free. Seventeen percent failed to be compliant once and less than 10% failed twice. Only 6% of offenders failed more than two times. This pilot study initiated state-wide authorization of the 24/7 program, which has continued to demonstrate remarkable results. Of all participants given urinalysis tests, 98% were compliant, testing alcohol free. Seventy-eight percent of offenders who wear alcohol monitoring bracelets remained alcohol free and program compliant. Finally, 92% of participants who wore drug sweat patches remained clean.

These programs share obvious similarities to PHPs and deserve further consideration. Their successes support the contention that PHP-type care should be more widely utilized and that the outstanding results found in PHPs are not solely the result of special characteristics of physicians or the unusually high level of treatment the PHP physicians receive.

Barriers to Wider Application of the PHP Model of Care Management

There are significant barriers to wider application of the PHP model. These include cost, public opinion, tradition, cynicism about the possibility of long-term recovery, and anger toward addicted people. Philosophically, there are two extreme views that disagree with PHP-type care, those that want to protect addicts from consequences and those that want harsher consequences. First, there is a deeply held view among many people treating substance abusers that relapse is part of the disease and thus to be expected and tolerated even if passively discouraged. It is thought in this view known as "harm reduction" that to "punish" an addicted drug user for continued drug use is similar to punishing a diabetic for having a crisis or a heart attack patient who does not stop smoking cigarettes.

Those at the other extreme believe addicts should receive harsher punishment. They do not want PHP-type care because they believe addiction is a crime that should be punished exclusively through the legal system. In many ways, the harm reduction stance is a political or ideological reaction to this legal position. Both are barriers to expanding PHP-type care. These law and order folks who want PHPs ended also believe that addicts should receive harsher "punishment."

We see PHP care is a middle ground between these two extremes. Like diabetics who are not careful with their diets, there are natural consequences of further testing, more frequent doctor visits and possible hospitalization. There is also the ever present risk that a diabetic episode could cause more serious debility or even death. PHP care delivers similar "reality-based" consequences to its participants. Failing to attend required treatment and support groups may result in heightened testing frequency. Relapse outside the context of practice may result in 3–4 days inpatient evaluation with attendant loss of income and cost. Major relapse causing risk of harm to patients typically results in license suspension or revocation. We contend that between the two extremes of withdrawing direct consequences in the "harm reduction" model vs. excessive consequences in the "law and order" model, the PHP model is the correct balance. In the end, this is not a question of ideology or politics; it is a question of scientific evidence. The 3 decades of PHP experience have established one of the longest and best studied records of care in the substance abuse field. That record validates the PHP model and helps to shape attitudes. For example, it has demonstrated that a strict no use standard not only for the patients' primary drug of abuse but also for any alcohol or other drug use leads not to high levels of failure and termination of care but to the opposite – to remarkable compliance and long-term success. That evidence turns the usual ideological arguments on the head. Is it more compassionate to let a drug user continue to use drugs or to use serious, long-term contingencies to insist on monitored compliance with the absolute abstinence standard? The PHP gives a clear answer to that question: it is not scientifically valid, nor is it compassionate to expect and to tolerate continued alcohol and drug use among people with substance use disorders. In reality, it may not be possible to provide most patients with the quality and level of care that typical PHP patients receive. To the extent that the outstanding outcomes of the PHPs are dependent on outstanding treatment, this is a barrier to wider application of this model. The HOPE probation model offers a different view of this, as their treatment is what is available in the community, and more than half of the participants succeed for up to 6 years with monitoring and consequences alone, without treatment beyond their once-a-month visits to their probation officers.

In our view, the most appropriate way to look at the PHP outcome data is first to see that it disproves the claim that relapses are inevitable or even common in this biological brain disease. When the conditions in which the decision to use or not to use alcohol and other drugs change so does the behavior. In the case of the

PHP participants, an environment rich in support and utterly intolerant of continued alcohol and drug use results in outstanding outcomes over the course of many years.

We favor integrating the concepts and elements of PHP care management more widely within the framework of national drug and alcohol treatment policy.

Summary

Addicted physicians involved in PHPs have exceptionally high long-term recovery rates. They recover in such high numbers not necessarily because they are physicians, but at least in part because they participate in programs that differ significantly from usual substance abuse treatment in the USA. The eight components of PHPs that we consider to be the keys to quality enhancement are (1) find a motivational fulcrum, (2) provide comprehensive initial assessment and extended treatment, (3) provide care management for many years, (4) have a high expectation for abstinence-based recovery, (5) assertively link to recovery support groups, (6) sustain monitoring and support and, when necessary, reintervene, (7) reintervene at a higher level of intensity at any sign of relapse, (8) integrate these elements, where possible, within a comprehensive program.

The nation's state PHPs are rooted deeply in the recovery community. They have been the embodiment of the recovery view of addiction as a serious, potentially fatal, progressive disease that can be overcome to produce lifelong abstinence and greatly enhanced quality of life through the use of the recovery programs, especially the 12-step programs. Recognizing that relapse is a continuing threat even after abstinence is obtained for people with substance abuse disorders, the PHPs include long-term and intensive monitoring in the context of the highest level of professional treatment not only of addiction but also of comorbid disorders, which can be barriers to recovery. Not only are these programs a model on which others can build, but they are also an inspiration to improve care management and treatment for all people suffering from substance use disorders and many other behavior disorders. The PHP model of care management was not built around any ideology. It evolved over decades in separate – but communicating – state programs. This model of care was based on what worked as judged over long periods of time and intense and direct involvement with the diverse individual physician participants.

Even if the PHP model is unattainable for all patients with substance use disorders today, the data compiled by the nation's state PHPs offer a beacon to future developments in managing substance use disorders. It shows the way forward, and even more importantly, this still growing body of evidence dispels the self-defeating pessimism about substance use disorders that normalizes relapse failure to achieve long-term recovery. The PHP experience makes clear the limits of recovery from substance use disorders that do not lie in the biology of the disease but in the context in which it is managed and treated. The PHP experience clearly supports the role of intensive, long-term recovery management participation.

Key Points

1. PHPs have a high expectation for successful abstinence-based recovery and have developed their programs to help physician participants achieve this goal.
2. PHPs utilize a primary care paradigm for substance-use disorders, one where early detection is encouraged, nonconfrontational interventions are performed with dignity and care, thorough evaluation and treatment are obtained, and long-term monitoring with contingency management are carried out.
3. A motivational fulcrum or "leverage," based on maintenance of medical license, is subtly or overtly utilized through every step of PHP care.
4. Interventions are directed at encouraging evaluation rather than treatment.
5. Much emphasis is placed on good evaluations, conducted by selected providers who meet stringent criteria.
6. The conditions of the physicians' relationships with the PHP and the terms of extended monitoring are clearly detailed in simple language in an agreement between the PHP and the physician and signed by both.
7. PHP care could be thought of as a long-term high stakes example of contingency management.
8. PHP care and monitoring are a very successful example of the management of addictions as chronic illnesses.
9. Aspects of PHP care that can be used in other populations include finding and defining leverage, intervention directed at obtaining good evaluation, adequate treatment, long-term monitoring under a contingency contract, reintervention and reevaluation as needed for relapse.
10. Drug courts are similar in many ways to PHPs and have been shown to be successful.

References

1. http://www.himsprogram.com/HIMS_about.html. Accessed 28 Aug 2009.
2. McLellan AT, Skipper GE, Campbell M, DuPont RL. Five year outcomes in a cohort study of physicians treated for substance use disorders in the United States. BMJ. 2008:a2038. doi:10.1136.a2038.
3. Petry NM. A comprehensive guide to the application of contingency management procedures in clinical settings: a review. Drug Alcohol Depend. 2000;58:9–25.
4. Crawshaw R. An epidemic of suicide among physicians on probation. JAMA. 1980;243 (19):1915–17.
5. Anonymous. The sick physician. Impairment by psychiatric disorders, including alcoholism and drug dependence. JAMA. 1973;223(6):684–7
6. DuPont RL, McLellan AT, Carr G, Gendel M, Skipper GE. How are addicted physicians treated? A national survey of physician health programs. JSAT 37 2009;1–7.
7. Skipper GE. Treating the chemically dependent health professional. J Addict Dis. 1997;16 (3):67–74.

8. Dennis MI, Scott CK, Funk R. Main findings from an experimental evaluation of recovery management checkups and early re-intervention (RMC/ERI) with chronic substance users. Eval Program Plann. 2003;26:339–52.
9. Domino KB, Hornbein TF, Polissar NL, Renner G, Johnson J, Alberti S, et al. Risk factors for relapse in health care professionals with substance use disorders. JAMA. 2005;293:1453–60.
10. Hawken A, Kleiman M. (February, 2009). Research brief: evaluation of HOPE probation. http://09conferencecd.nadcp.org/Handouts/F-14%20Hope%20Eval%20Summary%20-2009.pdf. Retrieved 31 Aug 2009
11. Long L. The 24/7 Sobriety Project. The Public Lawyer. 2009;17(2):2–5.

Part IV
Future Directions in
Recovery Management

Chapter 16
Recovery Management and the Future of Addiction Treatment and Recovery in the USA

John F. Kelly and William L. White

Abstract Scientific understanding of addiction as a chronic disorder has increased substantially in the past 15 years stemming from the results of several retrospective and prospective studies. This research has revealed that among individuals with severe alcohol and other drug problems periods of relapse and poor functioning are common over many years and even decades, despite the receipt of intermittent interventions. Because these interventions typically occur only following acute substance-related crises, treatment typically takes the form of acute biopsychosocial stabilization and is delivered in discrete, self-contained, programs that typically end the service relationship shortly after discharge with little focus on providing adequate linkage to continuing care or recovery support. The predominant acute care paradigm is insufficient and mismatched to the realities of the chronic illness of substance dependence. In this chapter, we provide an overview of recovery management (RM) and recovery-oriented systems of care (ROSC) as new guiding paradigms for the future treatment of, and recovery from, severe alcohol and other drug problems. We also summarize notable examples of RM and ROSC implementation efforts at the program, system, city, and state, levels. Results from these efforts provide a foundation for confident optimism that a cost-effective system of care can be successfully established that is well suited to managing the undulating and enduring risks associated with the chronic illness of substance dependence.

Keywords Addiction recovery management · Recovery-oriented systems of care · Addiction treatment systems · Alcoholics anonymous · Narcotics anonymous

J.F. Kelly (✉)
Massachusetts General Hospital, Center for Addiction Medicine,
60 Staniford Street Suite 120, Boston, MA 02114, USA
e-mail: jkelly11@partners.org

J.F. Kelly and W.L. White (eds.), *Addiction Recovery Management: Theory, Research and Practice*, Current Clinical Psychiatry, DOI 10.1007/978-1-60327-960-4_16,
© Springer Science+Business Media, LLC 2011

Introduction

Scientific understanding of addiction as a chronic condition that requires ongoing monitoring and intermittent management to achieve and maintain recovery has increased substantially in the past 15 years [1–5]. This has come about through the long-term retrospective, and increasingly, prospective study of individuals with substance-related conditions. Results have brought forth a clear realization that among those with substance dependence, especially severe dependence, and few recovery resources, periods of relapse and poor functioning are common over many years and even decades, despite the receipt of intermittent and various interventions [2, 3, 6–9]. These interventions typically occur only following an acute substance-related crisis. Consequently, care typically takes the form of acute biopsychosocial stabilization and symptom reduction. Furthermore, treatments are often delivered in self-contained programs, which typically end the service relationship shortly following discharge, with little sensitivity or time devoted to facilitating ongoing support to cope with the enduring environmental triggers and risks in the homes and communities in which patients live. Thus, adequate linkage to continuing care or recovery support is often lacking [10–12]. It is estimated that between 50 and 70% of individuals following a treatment episode will resume alcohol/drug use in the first year, most within the first 90 days [13]. Furthermore, 25–35% of patients treated in addiction programs will be readmitted within 1 year, and nearly 50% will be readmitted within 2–5 years [14–16]. These accumulating scientific findings echo the voice of recovery advocacy groups and amplify the experience of affected individuals and their families: the existing acute care paradigm is clearly insufficient and mismatched to the realities of the chronic illness of substance dependence.

In this chapter, we outline recovery management (RM) and recovery-oriented systems of care (ROSC) as new guiding paradigms for the future treatment of, and recovery from, severe alcohol and other drug problems (AOD). We begin by discussing briefly the nature of "recovery" on which the RM and ROSC approaches are based. We then describe the broad range of substance-related concerns and where RM and ROSC fit within this broader picture and provide a rationale for the necessary implementation of RM and ROSC. We end by summarizing some notable RM and ROSC real-world exemplars and their impact.

What is Recovery? Definition and Conceptual Boundaries

The term "recovery" is the organizing concept of this book and forms the paradigmatic basis for a "recovery management" approach. But what is recovery exactly? Defining addiction "recovery" is a challenging task that evokes passionate and wide-ranging opinion [17]. However, its current "conceptual fuzziness" [17] has not prevented its use as an organizing paradigm nor its integration into major consumer, advocacy, and federal agencies (e.g., SAMHSA/CSAT, 2006) including the National Institutes of Health [18]. Its increasingly widespread use and acceptance as an organizing concept has led to attempts in producing operational definitions (e.g., [17, 19]). While broad consensus has not been reached, several definitions have been proffered.

Multiple terms are used in the field to define improvement following AOD problems [20–23]. Perhaps the most commonly used are "sobriety," "remission," and "recovery." It has been suggested that "sobriety" or "remission" might represent the elimination of problems from one's life (e.g., individuals no longer meet DSM criteria for "abuse" or "dependence"), whereas the term "recovery" might convey, in addition to remission, a broader achievement of global health [24]. Thus, the former emphasizes what has been removed, and the latter what has been added to one's life [17]. What does it mean when an individual states, "I'm in recovery"? Typically this means, "I am abstinent and I don't want to use alcohol or other drugs anymore and I'm taking steps in my life to ensure that doesn't happen." Taken separately, constituent parts of this statement include current abstinence (presumably for at least a month or longer), a desire for continued abstinence, and a realization that in order for abstinence to persist, a variety of other activities must be pursued in order to support and facilitate it. Abstinence is the principal constituent and goal because without it little progress can be made, and reinstatement of the disorder is highly likely if the individual has suffered previously from dependence [25, 26]. Also, RM approaches that have focused explicitly and intensively on abstinence have been associated with remarkable long-term recovery rates [27]. However, there is an equally powerful realization that abstinence is unlikely to be maintained without ongoing engagement in supportive and rewarding activities that can compete effectively with substance use for time and attention. Engagement in such activities comes under the broad rubric of "recovery capital" [28, 29]. Unlike acute models of addiction care that focus on deficits and pathology, the RM and ROSC approaches assess and place greater emphasis on strengths, assets, and recovery capital. White [17] describes recovery as the experience of healing from addiction while actively managing a continued vulnerability to relapse and building a healthy, productive, and meaningful life [17].

RM and ROSC Within the Broad Range of Approaches to Substance-Related Problems

Substance-related problems and conditions are viewed as the number one public health problem in the USA [30]. These problems encompass a vast range of substance-related involvement and impairment ranging from mild and intermittent to chronic and severe. Thus, characterizing addiction as a chronic illness does not mean that all substance-related problems have a prolonged course, high potential for relapse, or require ongoing monitoring and management [31, 32]. Even diagnosed "substance use disorders" (both DSM IV "abuse" and "dependence [addiction]") represent a huge range of substance involvement and impairment, and the syndrome of "dependence/addiction" itself possesses a graded intensity [26]. Substance-related conditions are marked also by their heterogeneity in cause, clinical course, physical and psychiatric comorbidities, and pathways to recovery [11, 31, 33–35]. In contradistinction to less severe or transient problems for which briefer, nonspecialty, interventions may suffice, RM and ROSC are best suited to treat that segment of the population for whom severe AOD problems tend to be chronic and who possess only limited recovery assets and resources.

The chronically relapsing course and harmful and hazardous health risks associated with severe addiction problems are analogous to other chronic medical illnesses, such as hypertension and diabetes. Thus, approaches to the management of these chronic disorders make sense and have intuitive appeal for the management of addiction [36]. Such sustained preventative and early detection/intervention approaches provide a valuable and fitting model to minimize the potentially harmful and frequently lethal consequences of addiction [3]. Such models do not wait for crises to occur, but rather attempt to avoid crisis through proactive monitoring and collaborative management of sobriety-based symptoms and relapse warning signs [37], as well as early reintervention if and when lapses do occur [3]. Recovery management (RM) and recovery-oriented systems of care (ROSC) approaches [11], based on a chronic disease conceptualization akin to the management of hypertension and diabetes, can help reduce the enormous burden of disease and prodigious social and economic costs associated with severe substance-related conditions by reducing reliance on costly, crisis driven, systems of care [27, 38–40].

As noted [31], the survival of specialty treatment for severe AOD problems as a social institution depends on the ability to move toward RM and ROSC. The current acute care treatment system has vastly oversold what can be achieved with regard to a given treatment episode (one addiction rehabilitation center even advertises its specific "cure rate" at "84.4%"). The mantra "treatment works" is as popular as it is vague, surviving through its rhetorical indistinctness. Consumers are more likely to see and experience alarmingly high rates of relapse following treatment, especially during the first 90 days post discharge [41–43]. While continuous abstinence is the exception, the reality is that treatment does produce substantial clinical improvements in continuous measures of change, such as the percent of days an individual is abstinent, increased lengths of continuous abstinence, and decreased intensity of use, in the months following a treatment episode. However, even these short-term gains often decay, especially for those most addicted and severely impaired and who have few recovery assets or resources. Yet, and as ludicrous as it may seem when exposed to the light of day, there remains an implicit expectation of a "cure" (i.e., lifelong full sustained remission) following a single episode of addiction care. Even the best addiction treatment evaluation scientists have been susceptible to the exaggerated potency of a single episode of care as measurements of addiction treatment effectiveness have typically taken place 6–12 months or longer following a single treatment episode [44]. This is an acute care model evaluation paradigm.

RM and ROSC are part of a larger shift toward a recovery paradigm reflected in the growth and diversification of recovery mutual aid groups, new recovery support institutions, and a new recovery advocacy movement that further reflects the cultural and political awakening of individuals and families in recovery. The addiction treatment industry has oversold the long-term recovery outcomes that can be achieved for people with severe AOD problems from a brief episode of professionally directed biopsychosocial stabilization. We believe the acute model of care is culturally, economically, and politically unsustainable. Flexible treatment approaches that are able to assess and build on individuals' assets and strengths, as well as attend to deficits, and readily adapt to the variety in presentation and manage undulating relapse risk *over the long term* are deemed critical in order to provide appropriate levels of care at optimal times and thus maximize addiction treatment effectiveness and cost-efficiency.

The inability of our society to cope effectively with the immense burden of disease attributable to substance-related conditions using professional efforts alone has been reflected in the growth in number and size of addiction-specific mutual help organizations during the past 75 years [44–46]. Assertive linkage to communities of recovery through mutual-help groups (MHGs) [45, 47] represents important opportunities to sustain and potentiate treatment benefits. There have been eight rigorously conducted, randomized controlled trials of assertive linkage to mutual-help groups, such as Alcoholics Anonymous (AA), which have used twelve-step facilitation (TSF) approaches. Each of these studies reveals clinically meaningful gains for TSF over standard referral practices and when compared to cognitive behavioral therapy alone [47, 48]. These studies have used different methods including TSF as an independent, stand alone, addiction therapy (Brown et al. 2004) [48–50]; TSF integrated into an existing therapy (e.g., CBT) [50, 51]; TSF as an additional, but independent, group component of a treatment package [52, 53]; and TSF as a modular appendage used to enhance effective linkages to 12-step groups at the end of a standard treatment phase [54–56]. Such linkage epitomizes the type of synergism that can amplify and extend the effects of formal care by facilitating engagement with free, peer-led, community recovery resources. However, by itself, this type of RM intervention would represent an appendage or "additive," rather than "transformative," change [38].

Models of, and Benefits from, RM and ROSC Transformation and Implementation Initiatives

The process of transforming addiction treatment from an acute care model to a model of sustained recovery management is already underway as evidenced by federal, state, and local "systems transformation" efforts and growing calls for a recovery-focused research agenda to guide and support these transformation efforts. However, diffusion of innovations is notoriously slow. Certain factors are associated with more rapid diffusion. According to Rogers (2003) [57], diffusion of innovation is likely to be enhanced when (1) the innovation is seen by adopters to have "simplicity", (2) there is an opportunity to "try it out" for a while before committing entirely ("trialability"), (3) there is an obvious "relative advantage" to the new innovation, (4) it makes an observable difference ("observability") when implemented, and (5) it is compatible with existing practice and infrastructure ("compatibility"). When one compares the types of systems changes and innovations discussed and exemplified in RM and ROSC approaches, it is clear that these types of innovations are likely to take time, may be a long time, to disseminate, be adopted, and shape the delivery of service to the ultimate benefit of primary sufferers, their loved ones, and our broader society and public health. Yet, we believe that such changes are entirely necessary if addiction treatment as a social institution is to survive. Furthermore, as described in more detail below, the efforts of the city of Philadelphia, the state of Connecticut, and many other organizations highlight the fact that these changes are wholly possible, are beneficial on a broad scale, but are likely to require concerted and persistent effort and integrated approaches from multiple stakeholder groups.

The "observability" element in diffusion of innovation noted above means that not only is the implementation of evidence-based practices important within RM and ROSC but also measurement of process and outcomes. The vastness and complexity of systems changes mean that change will take time, but in the meantime, stakeholders will need to know that these efforts are having some actual real-world impact. For example, rates of treatment access, engagement, and retention should increase, and treated persons and their families at least should experience better outcomes and less suffering. Such changes also ultimately should lead to better stewardship of available resources and enhanced cost-efficiency through a lowered need for emergency/crisis care. Most important is the measurement of implementation and system change efforts. Without such measurement, the impact on patient outcomes of these large-scale undertakings will be assumed to be better, but unknown, with accountability absent. Further, without embedded measurement of processes and outcomes innovation will be stymied, as systems and practitioners within systems will be unable to assess the impact of their own innovations and adaptations to meet the recovery needs of their own patients or particular patient subgroups more effectively.

Adoption, Implementation, and Maintenance of RM and ROSC

There are now outstanding recent exemplars of RM and ROSC implementations [3, 27, 38, 40, 58–60]. These have taken place at the treatment system [3, 27, 59, 61], city [38], and state [39, 40] levels. Achara-Abrahams et al. [38] describe different levels of system change that can occur in ROSC that produce different impacts. The first is "additive" change, in which a component of RM and ROSC is added as an appendage (e.g., peer support services or telephone support services). While a step in the right direction, this level of change is unlikely to produce lasting changes, may be difficult to sustain in an otherwise acute care-oriented system, or produce large impacts. The second level of change is "selective," in which certain programs or levels of care within a larger system undergo shifts to align themselves with a RM/ROSC orientation, while others do not. Although significant efforts are expended in the selective change approach, this type of change can result in service user and provider confusion and, ultimately, may introduce disintegrative forces. The third level is "transformative" level change in which the entire philosophical and practice basis of the system undergoes radical change. Below we summarize some of the documented benefits arising from the implementation of RM and ROSC at different levels of scale, beginning with treatment systems and followed by city and state level transformations.

Two of the most heavily evaluated examples of sustained RM approaches have been conducted through Recovery Management Checkups initiatives [3] and the Physician's Health Program (PHP) [27]. Scott and Dennis [3] describe a groundbreaking five-point protocol for managing addiction as a chronic condition. The acronym "TALER" provides a summary of the protocol. It consists of (1) tracking, (2) assessing, (3) linking, (4) engaging, and (5) retaining. In order to provide ongoing assessment and intervention the patients' whereabouts must be continually "tracked." Second, valuable and reliable assessment instruments are needed to objectively "assess" which individuals need early reintervention. Third, "linkage" assistance helps motivate and link individuals to formal treatment or other recovery support services. Fourth, assertive follow-up helps ensure that after assessment, individuals actually "engage" in recommended services. Fifth, support for "retention" is needed to prevent early dropout, which is a major risk factor for relapse. The core RM assumption of this approach is that long-term monitoring and early reintervention facilitate early detection of relapse, reduce the time to treatment, and thus improve long-term outcomes. Scott and Dennis describe an iterative improvement process using "lessons learned" from the evaluation of earlier RM implementation efforts to improve TALER approaches. For example, they were able to substantially improve treatment linkage rates from 30 to 44% by adding transportation help for patients, and improve treatment retention rates from 40 to 62% by helping clinicians avoid unnecessary and premature discharges. Relative to those individuals not receiving TALER recovery management checkups (RMCs), those receiving them were significantly more likely to enter treatment sooner, to receive more treatment, experience more abstinent days, and spend less time in the community needing treatment. These findings indicate that using the TALER protocol, RMCs are able to more adeptly address the enduring and cyclical nature of substance dependence via ongoing monitoring and linkage to treatment.

A further study of RM implementation on a national scale has been conducted with physicians suffering from a substance use disorder (SUD) [27]. This is a further example of how early detection and intervention with physicians with SUD, coupled with high-quality treatment, extensive monitoring, and assertive linkage to ongoing abstinence-focused recovery support can produce impressive

5-year abstinence rates of 79% and return-to-work rates of 96%. This RM approach as noted by Skipper and Dupont [27] is based on eight components (1) finding a motivational fulcrum, (2) providing comprehensive initial assessment and extended treatment, (3) providing care management for many years, (4) having a high expectation for abstinence-based recovery, (5) assertively linking participants to recovery support groups, (6) sustaining monitoring and support, and, when necessary, reintervening, (7) reintervening at a higher level of intensity at any sign of relapse, and (8) integrating these elements, where possible, within a comprehensive program. This eight-point PHP program might be seen as a concise practical summary of the RM approach [32]. Given the broad range of substance involvement, impairment, and range of available recovery capital for physicians within this program, the PHP experience strongly suggests that "the limits of recovery from substance use disorders do not lie in the biology of the disease but in the context in which it is managed and treated" [27]. The PHP is perhaps the best evidence to date that high-quality, sustained, RM initiatives of this type can produce outstanding long-term rates of addiction remission and recovery.

A further study of RM and ROSC implementation was conducted across an entire behavioral health care system in the state of Illinois. Boyle et al. [61] initiated transformative level RM changes that included professional recovery coaches (RC). The RC model was based on a community case management model to help individuals build on their recovery assets and strengths. There are six essential components inherent in this model: (1) RC services are voluntary – based on clients' willingness to meet. (2) Services are time-unlimited – service is delivered for as long as individuals need or want to receive them. (3) Services are community based – RC services are delivered primarily in the community, but treatment setting meetings can be conducted to help engage clients early. (4) The RC–client relationship is open-ended: Clients have the option of working with RCs after they complete, or if they withdraw early, from treatment. (5) Services are designed to reduce harm – RCs never stop working with clients because they become symptomatic and begin using substances. Rather, they attempt to link and reengage them with treatment or other peer-support services. (6) Services operate on the "Vegas Rule" – what is communicated to RCs stays with RCs and confidentiality is upheld. As of June 2009, 503 patients had enrolled in the new RC initiative. Preliminary evaluation research that examined proximal outcomes among enrolled women found that women who chose to receive ongoing support and treatment via a RC were significantly more likely both to engage in continuing care outpatient services (an explicit goal of the treatment continuum of care) and to stay engaged in treatment longer [61].

A more traditional but potent RM example has been the provision of ongoing recovery support and monitoring through residential recovery homes (e.g., Oxford Houses). These community-based, peer-led, residential resources have been shown to be highly cost-effective. Prospective research studies of the Oxford House model reveal that these resources are able to retain some of the most relapse-vulnerable individuals in a supportive living environment, minimizing relapse risk, while simultaneously building individuals' recovery capital. In one experimental study, 150 individuals with SUD were randomly assigned either to live in an Oxford House or receive community-based aftercare services (Usual Care). At a 2-year follow-up, about one-third of participants assigned to the Oxford House condition reported substance use compared to nearly two-thirds of those assigned to Usual Care. Also, just over three-quarters of Oxford House participants were employed versus just under half of those assigned to Usual Care. Illegal activity among Oxford House participants during this follow-up was half that of Usual Care. Among women, compared to those receiving Usual Care, those entering Oxford Houses were substantially more likely to be deemed stable enough to regain custody of their children. Earning capacity was also greater among Oxford House participants who earned roughly $550 more per month than the participants in the Usual Care group resulting in an annualized productivity difference of approximately $494,000. The lower rate of incarceration among Oxford House participants compared with Usual Care participants resulted in annualized savings for the Oxford House sample of roughly $119,000. Together, productivity and incarceration benefits yielded an estimated $613,000 in savings accruing to Oxford House participation.

On a broader scale, Achara-Abrahams et al. [38] provide a detailed example of the processes, challenges, and benefits that resulted from the transformative level change undertaken in the city of Philadelphia. The city undertook large-scale initiatives to transform its behavioral health care system. Preliminary results from these broad-ranging efforts indicated that populations with serious behavioral health conditions were experiencing substantially improved quality of life, were participating in the community at increased levels, and utilizing emergency care at significantly lower levels. Also, cost efficiencies were demonstrated as a result of the provision of recovery-oriented care. Provider agencies implementing integrated peer- and professionally led services experienced increased higher retention rates in the magnitude of 50% to over 75% [38].

Perhaps most ambitiously, Connecticut has conducted a transformative, state-level, initiative to redesign its entire public/private behavioral healthcare system treating approximately 100,000 individuals annually, producing some compelling results. This transformation resulted in a 62% decrease in use of acute inpatient services and a 78% increase in use of ambulatory services while simultaneously experiencing 14% lower annual costs, even after adding extensive recovery-support services, such as housing and transportation. There was also an increase in access by 40% for first time admissions, while experiencing a simultaneous 24% decrease in average annual costs per client. This decrease was even larger for high service users [39]. As a further piece of this transformational level change effort within the state of Connecticut, community-based peer recovery support services have made an impact on the receipt of continuing care for individuals leaving treatment. In 2009, for example, 268 volunteers contributed almost 15,000 h of service mostly within the walls of Connecticut's recovery community centers. Almost 37,000 outbound calls were made through telephone recovery support calls to 1,420 individual recovering persons. The peer-based continuing care initiative provided the equivalent of nearly $400,000 in service provision [40], and is likely to result in significantly improved remission and recovery rates for those individuals in receipt of these services [62, 63].

Deepening and Broadening the Transformation to RM and ROSC

As cultural shifts in treatment conceptualization and service system delivery occur at multiple levels, the reach of ROSC is beginning to broaden and deepen to address the needs of special populations (e.g., young people; dually diagnosed) and settings (e.g., rural areas) and to make use of new computer and Web-based technologies (e.g., self-assessment and recovery monitoring; online support groups).

From a life course perspective, it is adolescents and emerging adults who are at the highest risk to encounter AOD problems [64], and it is during this life stage that SUD has its onset in nearly all cases. Yet, surprisingly, this age group has received comparatively little attention and has remained drastically underserved. Given that early detection and early intervention in almost every disease or disorder increases the chances of early remission and a better prognosis for recovery, including in addiction [2], a broadening of RM and ROSC approaches to address this highest risk segment of the population is likely to yield considerable subsequent public health benefit. Because these young people are often the least intrinsically motivated to seek and remain in treatment, proactive assertive outreach and screening in work places, colleges and schools, and primary care settings are most likely to detect cases and begin the treatment process earlier, thereby preventing long-term problems [2]. There have been increasing initiatives for screening, brief intervention, and referral to treatment (SBIRT) that are designed specifically for this purpose [65, 66]. Clinical collaboration with employers and employee assistance programs and criminal justice can provide a "motivation fulcrum" [27] that can aid treatment retention, which has been shown to improve rates of SUD remission.

The use of technology has been shown to improve the quality and effectiveness of health care and reduce related costs. However, the adoption and implementation of computerized assessment and monitoring systems in health arenas lags far behind that in other business community sectors. In the management of severe AOD problems, this medium is rarely used but has the potential for broad reach in risk assessment, providing automated individualized feedback, and for providing ongoing support and monitoring of relapse risk following an index episode of stabilization. The emergence too of online addiction recovery support groups means 24/7 access to supportive communities globally either to augment or, for some, replace professional and peer-led face-to-face recovery support contact. Such Web-based programs and resources may be invaluable in rural area where access to recovery support services is limited.

Conclusions

Perceptions of the possibility of long-term recovery from the chronic illness of addiction have been pessimistic and even nihilistic. This perception has been perpetuated by a pervasive treatment mismatch between an acute care delivery system and its attempts to treat a chronic condition. These examples of, and results from, RM and ROSC implementation efforts paint a discernibly more hopeful and optimistic picture of what can be achieved when concepts and practices converge and are aligned to fit the true chronic and complex nature of addiction. Transformation efforts to RM and ROSC take time to achieve and, as work in the State of Connecticut and City of Philadelphia illustrate, will involve sustained processes of conceptual alignment, practice alignment, and contextual alignment (policy, regulation, funding mechanism, and stakeholder relationships). However, while undoubtedly challenging, we believe such efforts to be vital. The future of addiction treatment as a social institution may rest with this ability or inability to align itself with a model of sustained recovery management.

References

1. Cunningham J. Untreated remission from drug use: the predominant pathway. Addict Behav. 1999;24:267–70.
2. Dennis M, Scott C, Funk R, Foss M. The duration and correlates of addiction and treatment careers. J Subst Abuse Treat. 2005;28:s51–62.
3. Scott C, Dennis M. Recovery Management Checkups with Adult Chronic Substance Users. In: Kelly JF, White W, Editors. Addiction Recovery Management: Theory, Research and Practice. New York, NY: Springer Science and Business Media; 2011.
4. McLellan AT. Have we evaluated addiction treatment correctly? Implications from a chronic care perspective. Addiction. 2002;97(3):249–52.
5. Hser Y, Anglin D. Addiction Treatment and Recovery Careers. In: Kelly JF, White W, Editors. Addiction Recovery Management: Theory, Research and Practice. New York, NY: Springer Science and Business Media; 2011.
6. Brown SA, Ramo D, Anderson K. Long-term trajectories of adolescent recovery. In: Kelly JF, White W, Editors. Addiction Recovery Management: Theory, Research, and Practice. New York, NY: Springer Science and Business Media; 2011.
7. Hser Y, Longshore D, Anglin MD. The life course perspective on drug use: a conceptual framework for understanding drug use trajectories. Eval Rev. 2007;31:515–47.
8. Moos R, Schutte K, Brennan P, Moos B. Older adults' alcohol consumption and late-life drinking problems: a 20-year perspective. Addiction [serial online]. 2009;104(8):1293–302.
9. Vaillant G. The natural history of alcoholism revisited. Cambridge, MA: Harvard University Press; 1995.
10. McKay JR. The role of continuing care in outpatient alcohol treatment programs. In: Galanter M, editor. Recent developments in alcoholism: services research in the era of managed care. New York, NY: Plenum Publishing; 2001. p. 357–73.
11. White WL. Recovery management and recovery-oriented systems of care: scientific rationale and promising practices. Pittsburgh, PA: Northeast Addiction Technology Transfer Center, Great Lakes Addiction Technology Transfer Center, Philadelphia Department of Behavioral Health/Mental Retardation Services; 2008.
12. Godley M, Godley S, Dennis M, Funk R, Passetti L. The effect of assertive continuing care on continuing care linkage, adherence and abstinence following residential treatment for adolescents with substance use disorders. Addiction. 2007;102(1):81–93.
13. Hser Y, Grella C, Chou C, Anglin M. Relationships between drug treatment careers and outcomes: findings from the National Drug Abuse Treatment Outcome Study. Eval Rev [serial online]. 1998;22(4):496–519.

14. Simpson DD, Joe GW, Fletcher BW, Hubbard RL, Anglin MD. A national evaluation of treatment outcomes for cocaine dependence. Arch Gen Psychiatry. 1999;56:507–14.
15. Simpson DD, Joe GW, Broome KM. A national 5-year follow-up of treatment outcomes for cocaine dependence. Arch Gen Psychiatry. 2002;59:539–44.
16. Brown SA, Ramo DE. Clinical course of youth following treatment for alcohol and drug problems. In: Liddle HA, Rowe CL, editors. Adolescent substance abuse: research and clinical advances. Cambridge, NY: Cambridge University Press; 2006. p. 79–103.
17. White WL. Addiction recovery: its definition and conceptual boundaries. J Subst Abuse Treat. 2007;33(3):229–41.
18. Substance Abuse and Mental Health Services Administration. Results from the 2005 National Survey on Drug Use and Health: National findings. (NSDUH Series H-30, DHHS Publication No. SMA 06-4194). Rockville, MD: Office of Applied Studies; 2006.
19. Betty Ford Institute Consensus Panel. What is recovery? A working definition from the Betty Ford Institute. J Subst Abuse Treat. 2007;33:221–8.
20. Kelly JF. Evidence for adolescent participation in Alcoholics Anonymous and Narcotics Anonymous: further steps needed. Brown Univ Dig Addict Theory Appl. 2004;23:31.
21. Kelly JF, Westerhoff C. Does it matter how we refer to individuals with substance-related problems? A Randomized study with two commonly used terms. Int J Drug Policy. 2010;21 (3):202–7.
22. Milgram G. The need for clarity of terminology. Alcohol Treat Q [serial online]. 2004;22 (2):89–95.
23. Substance Abuse and Mental Health Services Administration. National Survey of Substance Abuse Treatment Services (N-SSATS): 2003. Data on Substance Abuse Treatment Facilities, Office of Applied Studies. DASIS Series: S-24, DHHS Publication No. (SMA) 04–3966. Rockville, MD: Office of Applied Studies; 2004.
24. CSAT. Definitions and terms relating to co-occurring disorders. COCE Overview Paper 1 (DHS Publication No. (SMA) 06-4163). Rockville, MD: Substance Abuse and Mental Health Services Administration and Center for Mental Health Services; 2006.
25. Koob GF, Le Moal M. Neurobiology of addiction. New York, NY: Elsevier; 2006.
26. Edwards G. The alcohol dependence syndrome: a concept as stimulus to enquiry. Br J Addict. 1986;81:171–83.
27. Skipper GE, DuPont RL. The Physician Health Program: A Replicable Model of Sustained Recovery Management. In: Kelly JF, White W, Editors. Addiction Recovery Management: Theory, Research and Practice. New York, NY: Springer Science and Business Media; 2011.
28. Cloud W, Granfield R. Natural recovery from substance dependency: lessons for treatment providers. J Soc Work Pract Addict [serial online]. 2001;1(1):83–104.
29. Granfield R, Cloud W. Social context and 'natural recovery': the role of social capital in the resolution of drug-associated problems. Subst Use Misuse [serial online]. 2001;36(11):1543–70.
30. Schneider Institute for Health Policy. Substance abuse: the nation's number one health problem. Princeton, NJ: Robert Wood Johnson Foundation; 2001.
31. White and Kelly, this volume.
32. White W, McLellan AT. Addiction as a chronic disease: key messages for clients, families and referral sources. Counselor. 2008;9:24–33.
33. Hesselbrock V, Hesselbrock M. Are there empirically supported and clinically useful subtypes of alcohol dependence? Addiction [serial online]. 2006;101 Suppl 1:97–103.
34. Jellinek EM. The disease concept of alcoholism. New Haven, CT: Hillhouse; 1960.
35. Moss HB, Chen CM, Yi H. Prospective follow-up of empirically derived alcohol dependence subtypes in wave 2 of the National Epidemiologic Survey on Alcohol and Related Conditions (NESARC): recovery status, alcohol use disorders and diagnostic criteria, alcohol consumption behavior, health status, and treatment seeking. Alcohol Clin Exp Res. 2010;34(6):1–11.
36. McLellan AT, Lewis DC, O'Brien CP, Kleber HD. Drug dependence, a chronic medical illness: implications for treatment, insurance, and outcomes evaluation. JAMA. 2000;284:1689–95.

37. Gorski T, Miller M. Staying sober: a guide for relapse prevention. Staying sober workbook: A serious solution for the problem of relapse. Independence. Missouri: Herald House/Independence Press; 1992.
38. Achara-Abrahams I, Evans A, King J. Recovery-Focused Behavioral Health System Transformation: A Framework for Change and Lessons Learned from Philadelphia. In: Kelly JF, White W, Editors. Addiction Recovery Management: Theory, Research and Practice. New York, NY: Springer Science and Business Media; 2011.
39. Kirk TD. Connecticut's Journey to a Statewide Recovery-Oriented Healthcare System: Strategies, Successes and Challenges. In: Kelly JF, White W, Editors. Addiction Recovery Management: Theory, Research and Practice. New York, NY: Springer Science and Business Media; 2011.
40. Valentine P. Peer-Based Recovery Support Services within a Recovery Community Organization.–The CCAR Experience. In: Kelly JF, White W, Editors. Addiction Recovery Management: Theory, Research and Practice. New York, NY: Springer Science and Business Media; 2011.
41. Hunt WA, Barnett LW, Branch LG. Relapse rates in addiction programs. J Clin Psychol. 1971;27(4):455–6.
42. Brown SA. Recovery patterns in adolescent substance abuse. In: Marlatt GA, Baer JS, editors. Addictive behaviors across the life span: prevention, treatment, and policy issues. Newbury Park, CA: Sage Publications, Inc; 1993. p. 161–83.
43. Tims FM, Dennis ML, Hamilton N, Buchan BJ, Diamond G. Characteristics and problems of 600 adolescent cannabis abusers in outpatient treatment. Addiction. 2002;97:46–57.
44. Kelly JF, Yeterian JD. Mutual-help groups. In: O'Donohue W, Cunningham JR, editors. Evidence-based adjunctive treatments. New York, NY: Elsevier; 2008. p. 61–105.
45. Humphreys K. Circles of recovery: self-help organizations for addictions. Cambridge: Cambridge University Press; 2004.
46. White W. The mobilization of community resources to support long-term addiction recovery. J Subst Abuse Treat. 2009;36:146–58.
47. Kelly JF, Yeterian JD. The role of mutual-help groups in extending the framework of treatment. *Alcohol Res Health*. in press.
48. Project MATCH Research Group. Project MATCH (Matching Alcoholism Treatment to Client Heterogeneity): rationale and methods for a multisite clinical trial matching patients to alcoholism treatment. Alcohol Clin Exp Res. 1993;17(6):1130–45.
49. Brown BS, O'Grady KE, Farrell EV, Flechner IS, Nurco DN. Factors associated with frequency of 12-Step attendance by drug abuse clients. American Journal of Drug and Alcohol Abuse, 2001;27(1):147–160.
50. Litt MD, Kadden RM, Kabela-Cormier E, Petry NM. Changing network support for drinking: network support project 2-year follow-up. J Consult Clin Psychol. 2009;77(2):229–42.
51. Walitzer KS, Derman KH, Barrick C. Facilitating involvement in Alcoholics Anonymous during out-patient treatment: a randomized clinical trial. Addiction. 2009;104:391–401.
52. Kaskutas L. Alcoholics anonymous effectiveness: faith meets science. J Addict Dis [serial online]. 2009;28(2):145–57.
53. Kaskutas L, Subbaraman M, Witbrodt J, Zemore S. Effectiveness of making Alcoholics Anonymous easier: a group format 12-step facilitation approach. J Subst Abuse Treat. 2009;37(3):228–39.
54. Timko C, DeBenedetti A, Billow R. Intensive referral to 12-step self-help groups and 6-month substance use disorder outcomes. Addiction. 2006;101(5):678–88.
55. Timko C, DeBenedetti A. A randomized controlled trial of intensive referral to 12-step self-help groups: one-year outcomes. Drug Alcohol Depend. 2007;90(2–3):270–9.
56. Kahler C, Read J, Stuart G, Ramsey S, McCrady B, Brown R, et al. Motivational enhancement for 12-step involvement among patients undergoing alcohol detoxification. J Consult Clin Psychol. 2004;72:736–41.
57. Rogers EM. Diffusion of innovations. 5th ed. New York, NY: Free Press; 2003.

58. Boyle M, Loveland D, George S. Implementing Recovery Management in a Treatment Organization. In: Kelly JF, White W, Editors. Addiction Recovery Management: Theory, Research and Practice. New York, NY: Springer Science and Business Media; 2011.

59. Jason LA, Olson BD, Mueller DG, Walt L, Aase DM. Residential recovery homes/Oxford Houses. In: Kelly JF, White W, Editors. Addiction Recovery Management: Theory, Research and Practice. New York, NY: Springer Science and Business Media; 2011.

60. Kirk TD. Connecticut's Journey to a Statewide Recovery-Oriented Healthcare System: Strategies, Successes and Challenges. In: Kelly JF, White W, Editors. Addiction Recovery Management: Theory, Research and Practice. New York, NY: Springer Science and Business Media; 2011.

61. Boyle M, Loveland D, George S. Implementing Recovery Management in a Treatment Organization. In: Kelly JF, White W, Editors. Addiction Recovery Management: Theory, Research and Practice. New York, NY: Springer Science and Business Media; 2011.

62. McKay JR. Is there a case for extended interventions for alcohol and drug use disorders? Addiction. 2005;100:1594–610.

63. McKay JR. Continuing Care and Recovery. In: Kelly JF, White W, Editors. Addiction Recovery Management: Theory, Research and Practice. New York, NY: Springer Science and Business Media; 2011.

64. Substance Abuse and Mental Health Services Administration. Results from the 2008 National Survey on Drug Use and Health: National Findings (Office of Applied Studies, NSDUH Series H-36, HHS Publication No. SMA 09-4434). Rockville, MD; 2009.

65. Substance Abuse and Mental Health Services Administration. National Registry of Substance Abuse Programs and Practices. Washington, DC: US Department of Health and Human Services; 2008.

66. Madras B, Compton W, Avula D, Stegbauer T, Stein J, Clark H. Screening, brief interventions, referral to treatment (SBIRT) for illicit drug and alcohol use at multiple healthcare sites: comparison at intake and 6 months later. Drug Alcohol Depend [serial online]. 2009;99(1–3):280–95.

Appendix

RM and ROSC Web Resources

1. Behavioral Health Recovery Management Project: http://www.bhrm.org
2. Faces & Voices of Recovery: http://www.facesandvoicesofrecovery.org
3. Philadelphia Department of Behavioral Health and Mental Retardation Service: http://www.dbhmrs.org/
4. Connecticut Department of Mental Health and Addiction Services: http://www.ct.gov/dmhas/site/default.asp
5. Great Lakes Addiction Technology Transfer Center: http://www.attcnetwork.org/regcenters/index_greatlakes.asp
6. Northeast Addiction Technology Transfer Center: http://www.attcnetwork.org/regcenters/index_northeast.asp

J.F. Kelly and W.L. White (eds.), *Addiction Recovery Management: Theory, Research and Practice*, Current Clinical Psychiatry, DOI 10.1007/978-1-60327-960-4,
© Springer Science+Business Media, LLC 2011

Index

A

AA. *See* Alcoholics anonymous
Abstinence-based recovery, 286
Abstinent living environment, 153
ACC. *See* Assertive continuing care
A-CRA. *See* Adolescent Community
    Reinforcement Approach
Acute-care (AC) model
    addiction treatment, 69
    AOD problems, 2
    attraction/access to treatment, 71
    behavioral health, 239
    contrasting assessment procedures, 72
    core characteristics, 1–2
    health treatment system, 232
Addiction as a chronic disorder
    AOD problems, 66
    characterizing addiction, 67
    conceptualize addiction and recovery
        processes, 68
Addiction as a chronic illness
    long-term care models, 21–22
    recovery-oriented system, 10
    treatment delivery system, 22
Addiction recovery
    conceptual framework, 10–11
    conceptualization and definitions, 15–16
    current treatment services, 20
    drug users, 13–14
    general population, 12
    emerging long-term care models, 21–23
    drug use and recovery trajectories, 24
    longitudinal intervention studies, 25
    ROSC movement, 24–25
    treatment programs and services, 23
    integrated systems approach, 10
    long-term follow-up studies, 16
    predictors, 16–18

substance abuse patterns, 9–10
theory-based process, 18–19
treatment outcomes and cumulative
    treatment effects, 20–21
Addiction recovery management. *See*
    Recovery management
Addiction RM and ROSC
    "additive" change, 304–305
    average annual costs, 307
    behavioral healthcare system,
        redesign, 307
    components, RM approach, 306
    Oxford House model, 306–307
    PHP program, 306
    selective and transformative level change,
        305
    deepening and broadening,
        transformation, 308
    abstinence, 301
    conceptual fuzziness, 300–301
    sobriety and remission, 301
    guiding paradigms, as, 300
    "cure rate" and "treatment works", 302
    flexible treatment approaches, 303
    SUD and dependence/addiction syndrome,
        301–302
    survival, specialty treatment, 302
    diffusion of innovation, 303–304
    "observability" element, 304
Addiction treatment
    conceptual framework, 10–11
    current treatment services, 20
    definition and conceptualization, 15–16
    drug users, 13–14
    general population, 12
    emerging long-term care models, 21–23
    drug use and recovery trajectories, 24
    longitudinal intervention studies, 25

Addiction treatment (*cont.*)
    ROSC movement, 24–25
    treatment programs and services, 23
    integrated systems approach, 10
    long-term follow-up studies, 16
    predictors, 16–18
    substance abuse patterns, 9–10
    theory-based processes, 18–19
    treatment outcomes and cumulative
        treatment effects, 20–21
Addiction treatment and mutual aid
        recovery resources
    group TSF, 37
    individual TSF, 35
    group format, 36
    intensive referral condition, 34–35
    MAAEZ, 37
    motivational interviewing, 34
    alcohol abstinence rates, 33
    psychiatric severity, 34
    relapse prevention (RP) condition, 36
    intensity and length, 33
    public payors and private insurers., 32–33
    support resources, 32
    psychiatric comorbidity, 38
    religiosity, 39
Addiction treatment systems
    acute care, 302
    RM and ROSC implementations, 304, 305
Addictive disorders
    family, 48–49
    friend and peer, 49
    behavioral economics, 45–46
    family process, 46–47
    friends and broader, 47–48
    rewarding activities, 50–51
    self-efficacy and coping skills, 49–50
    abstinence-oriented norms and models, 53
    rewarding activities, 55
    self-efficacy and coping, 53–55
    support, goal direction and
        structure, 51–52
    social control theory, 44–45
    social learning theory, 45
    stable recovery components, 56
    stress and coping theory, 45
Adolescent Community Reinforcement
        Approach (A-CRA), 108
Adolescent recovery
    composite use, 128–129
    identify factors, 130
    longitudinal patterns, 128
    substance-related outcomes, 126

    symptoms, 126–127
    long-term course, 126
    binge drinking, 134–135
    developmental patterns, 134
    self-efficacy, 135
    alcohol and marijuana consumption, 133
    diagnosis classification, 133–134
    drinking patterns, 132
    longitudinal patterns, 131
    polysubstance use, 132–133
    diagnostic thresholds., 131
    self-awareness, 130–131
Adolescents
    appointments, 113
    assertive approach, 114
    case management services, 110
    clinical outcomes, 116
    continuity of care, 103
    drug courts, 105
    follow-up interviews, 115
    juvenile justice system, 108
    outpatient treatment, 107
    residential treatment, 104
    treatment system, 102
Alcohol and other drug (AOD) problems
    addiction treatment, 76
    characterizing addiction, 67
    low-to-moderate severity, 71
    personal vulnerability, 66
    RM, 70
Alcoholics anonymous (AA)
    alcohol and drug abstinence, 33
    assertive linkage, 39
    motivational interviewing, 35
    psychiatric problems, 38
    12-step programs, 32
    steps, 37
    TSF subjects, 34
Alcoholics anonymous, PHP, 282, 286
Alcohol-use disorders (AUDs), 132
Anti-Drug Abuse Act, 142
AOD problems. *See* Alcohol and other
        drug problems
Assertive continuing care (ACC)
    A-CRA protocol, 113
    A-CRA, 108–110
    assertive community treatment
        (ACT), 107–108
    management activities, 110
    single-group follow-up studies, 107
    homework and mid-week check-ins,
        111–112
    obtain consent, 110–111

rapid initiation, 111
staff characteristics, 112
follow-up interviews, 115
initiate and retain adolescents, 114
mental health disorders, 112
motivational incentives, 114
outpatient treatment, 119–120
practice and clinical outcomes,
    115–116
rapid initiation, 116–117
follow-up interviews, 118–119
higher initiation rate, 119
performance measures, 116–117
rapid initiation, 116
WC continuity, 118
resistance required perseverance, 113
social networking recovery, 120
clinician change, 106
discharge type, 103–104
family/personal crises, 105
fatigue/demoralization, 105–106
medical model, 104–105
resource issues, 105
treatment reimbursement
    mechanisms, 106
AUDs. *See* Alcohol-use disorders

B
Behavioral economics
protective activities, 45
salient elements, 46
Behavioral health recovery management
    (BHRM)
addiction, mental health and physical
    conditions, 236–237
addressing culture, 237–238
chronic care model, 232–233
disease management approach, 232
academic settings, 235
advantages, 234
supervision-training protocol, 235
guidelines, 234
new technology development and
    utilization, 247–248
organizational and administrative
    structures, 236
outpatient buprenorphine-assisted
    program, 250
principles, 233
case management, 240
challenges and modifications,
    245–247

program, 241–243
recovery capital, 239–240
research, 243–245
reimbursement and regulatory challenges,
    238–239
restructuring residential treatment,
    248–249
true-north solutions, 250–251
Behavioral health units (BHUs), 223
BHRM. *See* Behavioral health recovery
    management

C
Care management, PHPs, 282–283
Children of alcoholics (COAs), 133
Cognitive behavior therapy (CBT), 33
Community Reinforcement Approach
    (CRA), 242
The Connecticut Community for Addiction
    Recovery (CCAR)
activities, addiction treatment, 274
cable public access TV shows, 258
community, recovery, 259
DVDs and videos, 258–259
frequent speaking engagements, 258
recovery poster series, 258
Recovery Walks, 259
website, 259
family education and support, 273
winners circle support group, 273
coaching, recovery, 269–271
"err on the side of being generous", 262
"err on the side of the recoveree", 261
"focus is on the recovery potential, not the
    pathology", 261
"there are many pathways to
    recovery", 261
"you are in recovery if you say you
    are", 260
milestones, 263
origin, 256–258
peer-led recovery social activities, 274
RCCs, 262–266
Recovery Housing Project, 271–272
ROES, 272–273
TRS, 267–269
training series, recovery, 273–274
VMS, 266–267
Continuing care and recovery
addiction treatment system, 162
and drugs, 177
use outcomes, 173

Continuing care and recovery (*cont.*)
    deficits *vs.* strengths, 167–168
    fixed *vs.* flexible, 168–169
    patients' preference, 168
    effectiveness, primary treatment, 164
    actively link patients, 176–177
    incentives for participation, 175
    leverage when available, 175–176
    reduce patient burden, 174
    self-help organizations, 169
    extended monitoring program, 170–171
    effective life skills, 164
    effective management, 163–164
    shapes and sizes, 163
    inpatient samples, 165
    intensive case management
        intervention, 172
    low-level incentives, 173–174
    consideration, 166–167
    and service providers, 172–173
    recovery-oriented approach, 178
    retention problem, 169
    chronic forms, 162
    treatments, 163
    traditional treatment models, 166
    transition problem, 170
    treatment completers, 166
Continuity of care
    barriers, 106
    drug addiction, 10
    logistic regression testing, 116
    long-term patterns, 11
    performance measure, 117
    treatment system, 103

D
Department of Mental Health and Addiction
    Services (DMHAS)
    BHUs, 223
    cornerstones, 218
    health-care service agency, 210
    phases, 207
    ROSC, 208
    skill sets, 216
    website, 217
    Yale's Program, 214
Double trouble in recovery (DTR)
    active ingredients, 54–55
    mental health recovery, 54
Drug Outcome Monitoring Study (DOMS)
    follow-up protocol, 88
    tracking model, 89

E
Evidence-based treatment
    application, 233
    community reinforcement approach, 234
    effective practices, 242
    use, 249

G
General continuing care adherence
    (GCCA), 114
Global appraisal of individual needs (GAIN), 88

H
Hawaii's Opportunity Probation with
    Enforcement (HOPE) Probation,
    290–291
Health-care system, recovery movement stages
    core values and premises, 207–208
    DMHAS, 210
    establish policy, 209
    increase depth, complexity and
        preparedness, 219–227
    strategic action plan, 210–219
Holistic services
    advance practice alignment, 196
    recovery transformation, 24

I
Intensive outpatient program (IOP)
    goals, 174
    monitoring and counseling, 172
    retention problem, 169

L
Long-term abstinence
    levels, 143
    psychiatric disorders, 155
    psychological functioning, 151
    social support, 153
Long-term patterns of use
    sequences of behavioral transition, 11
    substance, 24
    trajectories, 126

M
Motivational enhancement therapy (MET), 33
Motivational interviewing (MI), 87
Mutual-help groups (MHGs), 303

N

Narcotics anonymous (NA)
  motivational interviewing techniques, 35
  social network characteristics, 39
  support post-treatment, 33

O

Oxford houses. *See* Residential recovery
        homes

P

Participatory action research (PAR) methods, 143
Peer-based recovery support services, 255
PHP. *See* Physician's Health Programs
Physicians
  behavioral problems, 278
  cost per licensed, 281
  drug test results, 289
  harm to patients, 279
  history, 281–282
  relapses level, 286
  relationships, PHP, 280
Physician's Health Programs (PHPs)
  HOPE Probation, 290–291
  24/7 Sobriety Project, 291
  extreme views, 291–292
  outcome data, 292–293
  "reality-based" consequences, 292
  care management, 282–283
  assertively link, recovery support
        groups, 286
  care management oversight role, 286
  comprehensive assessment and treatment,
        285
  elements integration, within comprehensive
        program, 287
  high expectation, abstinence-based
        recovery, 286
  motivational fulcrum, 285
  reintervene, higher level of intensity, 287
  sustain monitoring, support and
        reintervene, 286–287
  dual objectives, 278
  medical licensing boards, 278–279
  physicians confidential support, 280
  primary care paradigm, 279
  routine random drug testing, 281
  success rate, 280
  practitioners, 281–282
  primary factors, 282
  educational programs, 283–284

long-term monitoring, 284–285
  professional intervention services, 284
  referral to formal evaluation, 284
  referral to formal treatment, 284
  phase I, 287–288
  phase II, 288–290
Principles of recovery management
  application, 251
  BHRM, 232
  Fayette Companies, 232
  modifications, 247
  residential addiction treatment, 248–249
  viable funding sources, 238

R

RCCs. *See* Recovery community centers
Readiness to change, 103
Recovery
  advocacy movement, 2
  clinical treatment setting, 271
  cycle, recoveree to recovery coach
        function, 270, 271
  peer support role, 270
  training, 270
  definition, 300–301
Recovery coaches (RC), 306
Recovery coach model
  case management, 240
  fidelity Maintainance, 246–247
  professional-driven treatment program,
        245–246
  coach program, 241–243
  recovery capital, 239–240
  research, 243–245
Recovery community centers (RCCs)
  administration, 264–265
  core elements, 262–264
  general conditions, 266
  programming, 265–266
  site, 264
  volunteers, 266
Recovery core values
  classification, 208
  DMHAS, 207
  establish policy, 209
Recovery-focused behavioral health system
        transformation
  additive approach, 187
  adopters and recovery champions, 195
  connect the vision, 192
  guiding coalitions, 191
  knowledge sharing and exploration, 194

Recovery-focused behavioral health system
    transformation (*cont.*)
  perceived loss and facilitate engagement,
      194–195
  sense of urgency, 190–191
  stakeholders, nature, 192–193
  transparent and participatory approach,
      193–194
  administrative components, 200
  indigenous recovery capital, 202–203
  long-term sustainability, 201–202
  organizational structure alignment, 201
  political agendas, 203
  attitudinal change and skill building, 198
  celebrating sucess, 200
  create short-term wins, 199–200
  empower stakeholders, 198–199
  establish priorities, 196
  identify practice changes, 196–197
  behaviors, 190
  components, 189
  contextual alignment, 189–190
  selective approach, 188
  transformative approach, 188–189
Recovery Housing Project, CCAR, 271–272
Recovery management (RM)
  AC model, 69–70
  BHRM, 232–239
  challenges and modifications, 245–247
  addiction and treatment careers, 66
  AOD problems, 67
  posttreatment monitoring, 68
  coach model, 239–245
  Fayette companies' transformation,
      247–251
  long-term, 71
  assessment and level of care placement, 72
  attraction/access to treatment, 71
  delivery locus, 74–75
  dose, scope and duration, 74
  linkage to communities, 75
  posttreatment monitoring, 76
  relationships/roles, 73
  team composition, 72–73
  time-sustained process, 69–70
Recovery management checkups (RMC)
  continuing care, 96
  control group participants, 94
  re-admission to substance treatment, 92, 94
  relative effectiveness, 93
  DOMS, 88
  implications, 96
  intervention, 172

chronicmedical conditions, 86
substance-abusing lifestyles, 86–87
protocol from experiments 1 to 2,
    89–90
substance abuse treatment, 95–96
symptoms and resolve ambivalence, 95
definition, 87
implementation, 88, 91
objectives, 89
treatment monitoring, 22
Recovery management system, 227
Recovery movement stages
  contextual components, 208
  problems and challenge, 207
  DMHAS, 210
  establish policy, 209
  align organizational structure and health-
      care, 226
  behavioral health system, 224
  data and quality analysis, 220–221
  DMHAS, 220
  evaluation and quality management
      information unit, 226
  GA-ICM component, 223
  health-care financing, 222
  intensive case management (ICM)
      intervention, 223
  opioid dependence, 223
  QIC, 225
  reinvestment, system enhancement cycle,
      222–223
  RSSs complement treatment, 221
  system clinical managers, 225
  centers of excellence (COE), 216
  consumer satisfaction survey (CSS),
      216–217
  cross-state agency collaboration, 217
  goals, 210–211
  identify and apply tools, 214–216
  intensive and extensive process, 212
  quality improvement and collaboration,
      213–214
  spread the word, 212–213
  statewide conferences, 217–219
Recovery-Oriented Employment Services
    (ROES), 272–273
Recovery-oriented systems of care (ROSC)
  additive approach, 187
  administrative component, 200
  adoption, implementation and maintenance,
      304–307
  approaches, substance-related problems,
      301–303

behavioral health system, 224
collaborative treatment planning, 216
deepening and broadening,
    transformation, 308
designing and implementation, 206
desired practice changes, 197
DMHAS, 206
goal, 218
growth of costs, 222
guiding paradigms, 300
performance and outcome measures, 225
policy and operational drivers, 210
quality improvement and collaboration, 213
recovery and guiding principles, 191
redesign and development, 22
revenue-enhancement approaches, 226
selective approach, 188
system-level outcome evaluation, 23
tools, 211
transformation and implementation
    initiatives, 303–304
transformative approach, 188–189
Recovery training series, 273–274
Recovery Walks, CCAR, 259
Relapse prevention (RP) condition, 36
Residential recovery homes
alcohol and drug abuse facilities, 147–148
growth, 148–149
loan fund and technical assistance, 149–150
multilevel treatment scheme, 147
policy, loan, 148
potential benefits, 146
12-step options, 146–147
abstinence-specific social support, 153
communication and reasoning skills, 154
resources, substance abuse, 151–152
romantic relationships, 152
social support networks, 151
abstinence-specific social support, 143
rules and policies, 142
substance abuse problems, 142
action-oriented agenda, 143–144
community coalitions, 144–145
PAR methods, 143
random assignment design, 144
recruiters training and monitoring, 145
"chicken and the egg" concept, 154
choices and adaptations, 153
personality characteristics, 154–155
psychological benefits, 155
community opposition, 151
health programs, factors, 150
RM. See Recovery management

ROES. See Recovery-Oriented Employment
    Services
ROSC. See Recovery-oriented
    systems of care

S
Self-efficacy and coping skills
stable recovery, 49
substance-specific, 50
Self-help groups (SHGs)
abstinence-oriented norms and
    models, 53
key ingredients, 51
rewarding activities, 55
motivation, 53
Project MATCH, 54
emphasis, 54–55
group beliefs, 51
12-step, 52
24/7 Sobriety Project, 291
Social control theory
key elements, 46
social bonds and surveillance, 57
strong bonds with family, 44
Social learning theory
attitudes and behaviors, 45
key elements, 46
stable recovery components, 56
Socioeconomic status (SES), 130
Step-down care
continuing care, 116
description, 102
Strategic action plan, DMHAS
centers of excellence (COE), 216
consumer satisfaction survey (CSS),
    216–217
cross-state agency collaboration, 217
goals, 210–211
identify and apply tools, 214–216
intensive and extensive process,
    212
quality improvement and collaboration,
    213–214
spread the word, 212–213
statewide conferences, 217–219
Stress and coping theory
life circumstances, 45
self confidence, 46
Substance use disorders (SUDs)
adolescents, 126
community-based treatments, 126
diagnostic criteria, 128

Substance use disorders (SUDs) (*cont.*)
   professional-based intervention, 240
   prognosis, 130
   residential treatment, 247
   RM implementation, 305
   12-step groups, 52
   symptoms, 128

T
Telephone Recovery Support (TRS)
   enrollment, recoverees, 269
   as evidence-based practice, 269
   model description, 267–268
Tracking, assessing, linking, engaging
      and retaining (TALER)
   approach, 305
   components, 88
   definition, 87
   implementation, 90
   monitoring and linkage, 95
   monitoring mechanism, 96
   objectives, 90
   recovery process, 89
Trajectories of substance use
   alcohol patterns, 128
   alcohol symptom severity, 127
   community and clinical
      samples, 135
   definition, 126
   drug-use disorders, 135–136
   gender differences, 136
   longitudinal research, 132
   marijuana and alcohol, 133
   psychiatric diagnosis and
      symptomatology, 130
Treatment as usual (TAU), 173
Treatment careers, addiction, 66

Treatment outcomes for adolescents
   composite use, 128–129
   identify factors, 130
   longitudinal patterns, 128
   substance-related outcomes, 126
   symptoms, 126–127
Treatment system
   addiction specialty care, 167
   continuing care effectiveness, 162
   substance use disorders, 162–163
TRS. *See* Telephone Recovery Support
TSF approach. *See* Twelve-step facilitation
Twelve-step facilitation (TSF)
   AA/NA steps, 33
   approach, 303
   cocaine dependence, 35, 37
   effectiveness, 35
   intervention, 38
   Kahler's study, 35
   Project MATCH, 34
   religious beliefs, 39
   treatment, 32–33

V
VMS. *See* Volunteer Management System
Volunteer Management System (VMS)
   description, 267
   growth, 267, 268

W
Washington Circle (WC) group, 116
Women in Recovery through Enhanced
      Design (WIRED), 274
World Health Organization Quality-
      of-Life instrument
      (WHOQOL), 216

9781603279598